What People A[…]
Brain Cha[…]

Brain Changers 365 *is a resource that will be welcomed by anyone seeking to improve brain health individually, within groups, classrooms, social activities, care centers, clubs, and other settings. It contains a wealth of informative material as well as easy to follow directions that will allow participants to interact, have fun, and improve brain functioning all at the same time. Whether you select specific activities or work your way through the book daily, it will help your brain become healthy.*

—Lory Nels Johnson, Iowa Dept. of Educ.
Consultant and Ad Hoc Professor

Because we're living longer, most of us are concerned about maintaining memory and healthy brain function. Brain Changers 365 *is a perfect prescription for such concerns. The only side effects are an increase in brain health and some good fun! As a life coach, I especially appreciate this book's holistic approach. Its well-rounded exercises inspire, increase mind-body connection, boost creativity, assist in problem-solving and enhance the use of logic while promoting brain health. There's an activity set for each day of the year. It's not often you can actually enjoy your "medicine," but I guarantee this will go down easily! This looks like an amazing resource for any and all of us. I really am impressed!*

—Sonia C. Solomonson, Life Coach with
www.Way2GrowCoaching.com and former managing editor
of The Lutheran magazine in Chicago

I always have thought that one of the best ways to keep fit was to exercise, not only physically but also mentally. Through fun and thought-provoking activities that can be done almost anywhere, the authors have created a way to stimulate and exercise key brain functions. The daily activities, which focus on seven brain functions and take only a few minutes, will cause both young and old to keep their minds active and think in new ways.

—Dr. Paul Bucci, President, PTB & Associates
in the Washington DC area

Thank you very much for manuscript of your new book, Brain Changers 365. *I like it! Please let us know where I will be able to buy it in Japan.*

—Dr. Michiya Murata, University Professor in Kobe, Japan

In my experience as an acupuncturist, people need easy and user-friendly ways to anchor information to create real changes. Brain Changers 365 *definitely accomplishes this goal by creating an easy to access way to incorporate cognitive tools in a simple and fun daily activity to begin to transform your life. As our neural pathways integrate new information and ground the old information in new ways, we will be able to think with more clarity and have more energy. I love this book, and would recommend it to young and old as a clever way to enhance brain function and memory retention.*

—Rose Thomas, Licensed Acupuncturist in California

As a person with Parkinson's Disease, I have lost some of my cognitive skills. I read Brain Changers 365 *and found it helpful and stimulating. It helped me identify areas of my cognitive functioning that needed improvement. The 365 days of exercises helps develop a routine that can lead to improvement and a sense of accomplishment.*

—Dr. Roger Hadley, Retired College Vice President

Bringing my "old" brain to Renie's Brain Boosters class has added sparkle to my life the last five years. The activities are groovy, we socialize, reminisce, laugh, and even stretch our muscles in each class. It is more like a social club than a class, and helps one to slow down or prevent dementia. Renie's Brain Changers 365 *will help you do the same.*

—Nancy Smith, Tai Chi Instructor in New York

Living next door to a beautiful young woman and dear friend who has severe dementia, watching my daughter-in-law's mother, also a dear friend, struggle with the beginnings of dementia, and thinking of other people in my life whom I love, I am wishing that I had had this book earlier. But it is not too late. I will hope to have opportunities to use Brain Changers 365 *with people I care about and to recommend it to people who also have loved ones who would benefit from the exercises or are in leadership roles where they can use the exercises with groups of people. It would be fun to use it in one of my classes of young people. And I hope to use it myself!!! Thank you for all the research and work that makes this a practical book to use for a growing problem.*

—Kathleen K. Beal, English as a Second/Foreign Language Teacher (multiple ages) and Author, in the U.S., Singapore and South Korea

BRAIN CHANGERS 365

BRAIN CHANGERS 365

BUILD a BETTER BRAIN with 7 ACTIVITIES EACH DAY

LORENE "RENIE" LENNING, MS • OSCAR LENNING, PhD • ALISHA SOLAN, PhD

With foreword by Pat Sievers – National Speaker with Dr. Pat Wolfe's Brainy Bunch

ISBN-10: 1548993476
ISBN-13: 978-1548993474

Library of Congress Control Number: 2017911314
CreateSpace Independent Publishing Platform, North Charleston, SC

Printed in the United States of America

Interior Design: Ghislain Viau

Contents

Foreword

We all know that our muscles need exercise to stay healthy and strong throughout life. Likewise, our brain cells can change physically and grow with that same stimulation and exercise. The old saying "use it or lose it" remains as important today as it was decades ago in the science and education community. The old science of limiting brain growth to childhood is just wrong. The brain can remain strong and fit throughout life if we take care of it.

The activities in this book consciously provide a well-balanced meal for the brain. The brain thrives on variety, so the authors created a daily "menu" of accessible, practical, and adaptable prompts and exercises that can be done in 10-15 minutes to activate fitness in seven different brain functions. Readers find a year's worth of daily mental stimulation activity sets that: 1) inspire, 2) deepen self-awareness, 3) practice recall, 4) challenge logical thinking, 5) encourage innovative and creative thinking, 6) provide new learning, and 7) invite increased mindfulness and well-being. What distinguishes *Brain Changers 365* is its focus on specific, well-rounded sets of activities for each day to provide *multiple* types of brain stimulation all in one easy place. There are unique activity sets for each day of the year with emphasis on diversity to reflect the importance of exposure to new things each day.

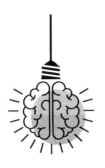

Brain Changers 365 will especially appeal to a number of audiences for personal use. Doctors often advise patients who have a known family history or early diagnosis of Parkinson's or Alzheimer's to engage in mentally stimulating activities to delay symptoms of cognitive impairment. As the U.S. population ages, many people who witness the aging and mental decline of their parents and/or grandparents may also want goals to improve their physical and cognitive health so as not to become a burden or suffer as they see their parents and grandparents doing.

In addition, teachers, activity directors and other group leaders can follow the model of Renie's "Brain Booster" class, for a beneficial, structured group activity. Teachers at all levels can adapt or directly use many of these activities to stimulate critical and creative thinking with their classes, for instance as warm-up activities at the start of the day.

I love the Brain Changers 365 book! It is long overdue for everyday people. Humor, which is a critical part of maintaining brain health, permeates the book! The activity sets that focus on seven different voluntary functions of the brain are easy for anyone to do, but so relevant for everyone! These kinds of practical activities are valuable for any person who wants to stay sharp through all phases of life, as well as seniors and those who are disabled. I definitely use these exercises myself!

Pat Sievers, MS, Education Leadership Graduate Instructor and a National Speaker with Dr. Pat Wolfe's Brainy Bunch at Mind Matters, Inc. http://patwolfe.com, Specializing in the Brain and Learning

Acknowledgements

We are grateful for the support of many people who contributed in various ways to this project.

Many thanks to Renie's former supervisor and close friend, Pat Sievers. She is a nationally-known expert on improving the brain, has taught university courses on that topic, and has made numerous presentations on improving the brain to audiences of many kinds. She was the one who more than anyone else motivated Renie to focus on the brain in working with her elementary and college students, and with retired citizens in her "Brain Boosters" class. In addition, we appreciate more than we can say Pat's willingness to review our book manuscript, suggest changes, and provide a foreword for the book.

Special thanks to Ghislain Viau of Creative Publishing Book Design for a wonderful job of reformatting and designing the interior of our book, and to Heidi Kotzian for support, encouragement, and marketing ideas. Many thanks also to Mary Johnson for her superb reviewing and editing, to Dr. Roger Hadley for reviewing the manuscript and providing helpful feedback, to Janice Steinberg for her encouragement and insights on the publishing process, to Rose Thomas who suggested acupuncture TABs, and to occupational therapist Shuan Goose who tested some of these activities with her patients.

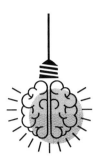

We sincerely thank many residents from Tucson Estates who have attended Renie's *Brain Boosters* class for serving as a "test class" for trying out many of the exercises included in the book, and for encouraging Renie to write a book that would include such activities. Thanks also to all of Renie's students and co-workers from her 40 years of teaching.

Special thanks to Carol Warneke, who led tai chi exercises in each Brain Boosters class period for three years. Thanks also to Nancy Smith (a long-time outstanding PE teacher) who took over the role of movement leader. Both did a wonderful job and offered helpful ideas and suggestion for inclusion in the MMM section, for which we are immensely grateful.

Special thanks are also due to Kirti Khalsa and Valerie Powers of the Alzheimer's Prevention and Research Foundation for their encouragement to write the book and the commitment of the Foundation to promote the book. We honor the important work this foundation is doing.

Finally, much gratitude goes to our friends and family. Deepest appreciation goes to Jade Solan for her patient love, support and advice. Additional thanks to Oscar and Renie's other two children (Denise and Chris), their spouses (Jeremy and Jennifer), and Oscar and Renie's five grandchildren and Alisha's nephews and nieces (Aspen, Johnny, Bradyn, Jackson and Hannah) for all of their love and support. It is appreciated more than we can express in words.

Renie and Oscar Lenning,
Alisha Solan

Introduction and How to Use This Book

If you are hungry and desire a fine meal prepared by a professional, do you want a food scientist or do you want a chef? So then, if your brain is hungry for mental stimulation to stay fit and healthy, do you want a book by a neurologist who can tell you the latest research on brain health? Or do you want a teacher who can take that brain research and craft it into a flavorful feast of ready-made activities you can directly bite into? *Brain Changers 365* is practical brain-training, written by and rooted in the experience, research and intuition of long-time educators with over 100 years combined professional experience.

Brain Changers 365 offers delicious, well-balanced and practical brain-training. The exercises are grounded in scientific brain research findings and have been informally tested over the years with students of various ages to be challenging, motivating, and fun. In particular, Renie has developed and taught a weekly "Brain Boosters" class for people in her Arizona retirement community for the last seven years. When members of the class strongly encouraged her to write a book to make these materials more available to them and others, she turned to Oscar and Alisha for help. This book is the result.

What distinguishes *Brain Changers 365* from other brain fitness and self-help books is its focus on specific, well-rounded sets of brief activities for each day.

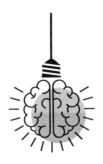

The brain functions as a marvelous and complex system, with all parts intertwined rather than functioning in isolation. Just as your body would not be happy and healthy if you ate only one thing day after day, your brain is not happy doing only one type of thinking to keep fit, such as the classical, "go-to" brain puzzle games like crosswords or Sudoku. Instead, our brains thrive on variety. So, this book is designed to provide a daily "menu" of seven different prompts and exercises to activate fitness in seven different voluntary brain functions.

Seven Ways to Stimulate the Brain

If your heart is beating, congratulations! Not only are you still alive, but you are using your brain. Much of the brain's activity functions involuntarily below the level of our consciousness. And that is a good thing; we don't want to have to stay up at night reminding our heart to beat and our stomach to digest dinner. However, many of us go through much of our lives with the rest of our brain also on some level of auto-pilot, just responding to routine stimuli in our daily lives. But, autopilot does not stimulate and increase brain function.

The healthy brain is alert, playful, curious, and open to new experiences. New scientific research demonstrates that some parts of the brain can actually create new brain cells throughout an entire lifespan. In addition, learning contributes to increasing the number and strength of connections between brain cells. To maintain brain health, you must actively engage in new experiences and stimulate your mind in a variety of thought processes to activate new growth and a variety of connections.

The activities in this book are intended to keep the brain active and healthy by stimulating multiple brain areas daily. Each page of the book contains a "daily dose" of activities that invite conscious brain activation in seven overlapping mental functions: 1) inspirational thinking, 2) personal memory and self-awareness, 3) objective memory recall, 4) problem solving, 5) creative thinking, 6) processing new information, and 7) mind-body connection. Each day you will find seven different categories of activities designed to target or emphasize each of these functions. Each category has a fun title and identifying acronym. The following sections detail the particular benefits and guidelines for approaching each category of activities. At the end of the introduction, you will find a quick-reference table summarizing them.

1. **Words of Wisdom (*WOW*)** – *WOW* activities target *inspirational thinking*; includes ability to engage in positive inspiration and motivation. *WOW* activities consist of inspirational quotes from writers, philosophers, leaders, and other intellectual or well-known individuals. As you read the quotes, consider the meaning and how they might inspire or motivate you.
2. **Reminiscing, Recollecting and Reflecting (*3Rs*)** – *3Rs* activities target *personal memory and self-awareness*. Personal memory functions include the ability to remember past experiences and to reflect on one's life. Self-awareness includes exploration of identity, preferences, values, and goals to gain insight into one's self now. Recalling personal memories stimulates the limbic area of the brain connected to emotions, learning and memory. In addition, neurological research demonstrates that by consciously visualizing events in detail, the areas of the brain related to those thoughts and memories are also stimulated. So if you recall the scent of a rose, the area of the brain associated with smell lights up. If you visualize riding a bike, the areas of the brain that manage the muscles used to ride a bike are also stimulated. Thinking on self-awareness can be a renewing experience. It helps bring meaning, boosts confidence and mental clarity, maintains a sense of self-continuity, improves self-esteem, and promotes overall life satisfaction.

   3Rs activities consist of prompts that invite you to remember some past events or experiences and/or to reflect on yourself now in a way that creates a useful mental image that can positively affect the future. Its value is not so much in re-living past events, but in seeing things anew and possibly framing memories differently. As you spend a few moments reflecting on the prompts for each day, visualize specific situations in detail. Where were you? With whom? What were your feelings then? What are your feelings now? To stimulate more of the brain, apply all five senses as you visualize and relive those memories. Then, think about the relevant meaning these thoughts can have for you today and for your future.
3. **Knowledge in School Subjects (*KISS*)** – *KISS* activities target *objective memory recall*, which is sometimes referred to as semantic memory. Objective memory recall includes the ability to access past learning and to

recall objective knowledge or factual information. With objective memory recall, there are right and wrong answers. Regardless of whether or not you successfully recall specific information accurately, the act of searching for it has benefit in increased brain activity, process and concentration. KISS activities consist of factual questions that recall information often taught in school or learned through reading or other media. To trigger activity in more areas of the brain, each *KISS* in the "daily dose" is made up of questions from several different subject areas such as fine arts and language, science and health, and history and geography. Depending on factors such as when and where you went to school, you may or may not have actually learned certain *KISS* items in your schooling and you may or may not have encountered the information in other ways. Even if you have never learned the information, make your best educated guess based on the knowledge you do have and then check the answers to learn something new.

4. **Searching Out Solutions (*SOS*)** – *SOS* activities target *problem solving* which includes the ability to use abstract thinking, apply reason and logic, solve problems, make inferences, and have insights. These activities are somewhat more open-ended than objective memory recall, but "correct" solutions are still limited by logic and the given information. For example, suppose we are challenged to determine who stole the cookies. If we know that William was out of town when the cookies were stolen, then it is unlikely that William is the correct answer. Logical reasoning stimulates the brain to make connections and seek out "Aha!" moments of insight that are both pleasurable and beneficial for brain health. Each *SOS* activity is a "mini brain workout." *SOS* focuses on discovering solutions that stimulate us to analyze, deduce, and determine solutions based on known ideas. The approach to solve or try to solve a problem is often not immediately obvious and may involve traditional step-by-step logic as well as making creative connections that may go beyond the obvious.
5. **Imagination, Creativity & Elaboration (*ICE*)** – *ICE* activities target *creative thinking*, which is the ability to think in a variety of ways and to make connections. Creative thinking includes the ability to generate multiple ideas, to think flexibly, to use the imagination, and to extend or

elaborate on concepts. Research suggests that flexible and creative thinking generally correlates with increased activity across more areas of the brain. To improve your skill in creative thinking, you should work to:

- **Develop a large number of responses (Fluency)** – Think of as many ideas as you can. Include obvious responses as well as unique, outrageous, or downright silly responses. Push yourself to keep thinking of other options or elaborate on possibilities without censoring what comes to mind. Use the "hot pen" technique; write down whatever comes to your mind. Don't judge or edit your ideas!
- **Generate a variety of responses (Flexibility)** – Notice if your responses fall into distinct categories or not. For example, if you were asked to list foods, were all your responses fruits or do you have items from many food categories? Consider what other categories might apply like meats, dairy, snacks, deserts, junk food, etc.
- **Create novel and original responses (Originality)** – Consider different angles. Think beyond the ordinary. Maybe go a little crazy. For example, some cultures eat seaweed or insects. And if the prompt did not specify foods eaten by people, consider other types of food such as dog food or food for thought.
- **Elaborate on ideas (Elaboration)** – Add to previous ideas by adding details or building on a theme. Once you have thought of cake, you can add details such as lemon cake with seven layers of whipped cream, lemon curd, and butter cream icing with rainbow sprinkles on top. Or you can build on the cake theme to add angel food cake, cheese cake, birthday cake, pancake, something "caked on", etc.

Notice that creative thinking by its nature generally moves beyond right and wrong solutions and may have any number of "correct responses." For the ICE activities, we have provided some *possible* solutions just to inspire your thinking and to encourage you to consider a variety of solutions. These are far from the only possibilities, and **it is best to generate a number of your own solutions before checking**. Then you can use the provided solutions to stimulate some additional possibilities.

6. **Tidbits about the Brain (*TAB*)** – *TAB* activities target *new information processing*, which includes the ability to learn, apply, and adapt to new information. Much research has been done on how brain health improves when we expose ourselves to new information such as studying a new language or learning to play an instrument or learning a new game. For the purposes of this book, new information processing will be related to the brain. The brain is an amazing organ, and a number of the *TAB*s reveal fascinating information about brain functioning that show just how spectacular a system the brain is. Other *TAB*s provide useful information for maintaining the health of your brain in terms of what will hinder and what will help maximize its functionality and effectiveness.

   As you read the informational tidbits for each day, let your brain wander and make connections. Focus for a moment on whatever you sense will positively impact your ongoing actions and habits. Where the findings are based on a number of studies, the individual studies will not be identified. The studies will be identified if the findings are based on only one or two research studies. Much new brain research will continue to be conducted that will extend or shift our current understandings.

7. **Mindfulness, Movement and Meditation (*Mmm*)** – *Mmm* activities target *mind-body connection.* They promote concentration, visualization and relaxation. Mind-body connection includes the ability to use the body consciously, to be aware of sensations and emotions, to calm and relax body and mind, and to keep the brain alert and in tune with the present moment and environment (the body is always in present time and in a particular place). Strong mind-body connection can help maintain sensory awareness, calm emotions, create a sense of well-being, and reduce tension and stress.

   There is a great deal of recent research into how mindfulness, meditation, and physical exercise benefit memory and brain health. A 2001 five-year pre-post comparison study of 4,615 individuals, all of them free from cognitive impairment, demonstrated that high levels of physical activity were associated with a 42% reduction in the risk of cognitive impairment in the future for those individuals, a 50% reduction in Alzheimer's disease risk, and a 37% reduced risk of dementia from any other cause[1] Researchers recommend 150 minutes a week of moderate-intensity aerobic exercise and strength training two or more times a week.[2]

Furthermore, in 2016 a carefully-done Finnish study of rats suggests that some forms of physical exercise may be much more effective than others in helping improve brain health.[3] In particular, exercise that involves intentional mind-body connection is generally even better for the brain. For example, recent research indicates that yoga (a form of physical exercise which has a direct mind-body dimension) demonstrates greater benefit to brain health than stretching alone (a similar exercise without any conscious mind-body component); and a 2014 study at Harvard indicates that "meditation literally rebuilds the brains grey matter in just eight weeks"[4]

Brain benefits demonstrated in the research include: improved working memory capacity, increased accuracy and speed in information recall, greater concentration, reduced anxiety, and greater mental flexibility. In particular, researchers suggest that attention to somatic or sensory awareness, conscious breathing, meditation, and relaxation may have contributed to the observed benefits. Therefore, many of the physical activities in the Mmm section are based on exercises from mind-body practices such as yoga, Nia, and martial arts such as tai chi and qi gung.

Mmm activities involve very brief exercises in controlled breathing, sensory awareness, mindfulness, movement, visualization, and mind-in-body techniques. They emphasize such activities as breaking patterns, breathing, playfulness, crossing the midline of the body, activating the spine as an extension of the brain, and various forms of meditation and conscious visualization. In general, unless specified, do 3-10 repetitions of simpler activities. If you are a beginner, do meditations for several minutes or for about ten breath cycles. If you are an experienced meditator, you may choose to set a longer time

---

1 http://brainblogger/2014/10/24/exercise-reduces-the-risk-of-alzheimers-disease/

2 http://sharpbrains.com/blog/2012/05/01/aerobic-exercise-or-weight-training-to-boost-brain-function/

3 http://www.bch.org/Blog/2017/March/Which-Form-of-Exercise-Does-Your-Brain-Like-Best.aspx

4 http://www.collective-evolution.com/2014/12/11/harvard-study-unveils-what-meditation-literally-does-to-the-brain/

With many of the Mmm activities, it would be beneficial to repeat activities for better mastery and/or greater depth of experience. However, since one of the goals of the book is to help you to create new experiences for the brain, we have provided a variety of types of movement, meditation, and mindfulness activities, and similar activities are generally scattered across the sets. In some cases, similar activities may build on one another or create better contrast by experiencing them closer together in time. Some of these have been placed closer together in the sets for that purpose. When similar activities are closer together in the sets, you can deepen your mindfulness experience by taking the opportunity to notice subtle differences and dialogue between the different experiences of the activities.

We recommend that you read through the whole activity before attempting it. If doing any activity will cause a physical problem for your current situation—such as not having needed space, potential pain or discomfort, or seems like it might cause harm or aggravate any health condition—modify the activity for comfort or skip it as needed. For example, when sitting on the floor, you may want to sit with your hips elevated on a cushion or a folded towel or blanket. Also although not ideal, some standing or lying down activities can be done seated if standing or lying down is difficult or uncomfortable. Unless specified otherwise, most activities on the floor can be done on a bed. (However, be aware that one of the best ways to maintain good physical mobility is to get up and down from the ground on a regular basis.) Another option if an activity does not seem appropriate is to go back and do a related Mmm from another day. For example, if the activity of crawling is too strenuous, you could repeat one of the "pre-crawling" activities from a previous day.

Again, since novelty is one of our goals for brain health, if the discomfort you feel is more about awkwardness or unfamiliarity and not health-related, give it a chance. In fact, some activities, such as using the non-dominant hand, are specifically intended to stimulate the brain by bringing the novelty of a new sensation or awareness that may seem awkward at first. Many times a new activity may take a few tries to find comfort and success in it.

Please note that Mmm activities are not intended to be a fitness program. We suggest that you supplement these activities with 30 to 60 minutes of a mind-body class and/or other pertinent physical activity at least three times per week. And as always, consult your healthcare provider as appropriate before engaging in any physical activity.

Tips for Using This Book

This book is designed to present a variety of noncompetitive questions and activities to stimulate the different parts and functions of the brain. Each page has a set of seven activities that can be completed in as little as five minutes. Feel free to think about and dwell on them longer. These can be done once a day or more often. Before beginning the section for the day, glance over it quickly to get a feel for the content and variety of the entire set of activities. This will help prepare you to move through it effectively and efficiently. Generally, the only additional tools you might want or need are a pencil and paper to record thoughts and responses from the day's activities. Some additional tips for how to use the book:

- Keep this book in a handy place, such as where you like to relax, next to your bed, in your bathroom, in the car, in the office with your appointment book, or next to your bath tub. It can also be helpful to choose a relatively consistent time to set aside for your brain health practice —morning, noon, or night. Make brain care a good habit that leaves you feeling that you missed something enjoyable whenever unexpected occurrences cause you to miss a session. If you do miss a day or two, just start where you left off.
- Another way to use the material is to make a regular date with friends to practice brain fitness together. Just remember to keep it non-competitive, and do not put anyone "on the spot." To illustrate the importance of this suggestion, the members of the "Brain Boosters" class—who served as a primary inspiration to write this book—have often commented that Renie's ongoing strong emphasis on non-competition and not asking the class members to announce their solutions has been a key to the popularity and success of the class.
- There is a wide range of difficulty in the items and activities. Some may seem familiar and quite accessible, others may seem more challenging. But watch your language! In the Brain Boosters class, "Easy" and "hard" are

four-letter words! Saying things are "easy" may diminish your felt need to do the activity and could put yourself or someone else down. Saying things are "hard" is discouraging to you and others. Instead say, "This is a challenge, and I'm going after it!" Even if you cannot come up with a response that makes sense to you, you have still succeeded because your brain has been engaged and thinking. And that is what it's all about: thinking!

- Give every item quality time, even if it feels too easy or too difficult for you. You are the one who will benefit. So do your best and keep on thinking. Keep in mind that sometimes there is no "right" solution or that there may be a number of appropriate solutions. When you get "stuck," try a new direction. Sometimes moving on and coming back to an item works when the solution is on the "tip" of your tongue. There is no hurry; you are not being graded. No one else knows what your solutions are, and no awards or prizes are given. All of your solutions are acceptable! Just let your brain percolate!
- **Possible solutions are given at the end of the book beginning on page 275 for items in the KISS, SOS, and ICE sections for all 365 sets of exercises in the book.** We try here and there to introduce some humor in the possible solutions we provide because humor has been proven to be beneficial for the brain. **But don't look, unless you must, until you are done.** It is not a matter of whether a solution is right or wrong. Just thinking is enough! Even if no solution comes to mind, you still benefit from the attempt. It is like trying to lift weights to develop your muscles. Looking at the weight and saying it is too heavy will not have any positive effect. However, even if you are unsuccessful, attempting to lift a heavy weight still engages the muscles. And, as you try, continued effort over time does develop strength.

In addition to the activities provided in this book, we strongly encourage you to practice ongoing good brain health in other ways as well. Try out new activities and new skills, meet new people and socialize, laugh regularly, spend time with friends and loved ones, get enough quality sleep each night, avoid excessive alcohol consumption (yes, it does kill brain cells), eat healthy food, learn how to manage stress, and do a variety of physical exercise 3-5 times a week—especially mind-body practices.

Think and have fun! Have a happy brain!

Table: How to Use This Book

Category	What You'll See	What It Does	What To Do
WOW = **W**ords **O**f **W**isdom	Inspirational quotes	Inspirational Thinking	Read quote and consider: • How is this meaningful? • How does it apply to you and your life?
3Rs = **R**eminiscing, **R**ecollecting, **R**eflecting	Prompts to remember past events or experiences and/ or to reflect on yourself	Personal Memory, Self-Awareness, & Visualization	Reflect on the questions and what the answers say about you; visualize specific situations in detail, using all five senses. Consider: • Where were you? • With whom? • How did you feel then? • How do you feel now? • How is this relevant today and in the future?
KISS = **K**nowledge **I**n **S**chool **S**ubjects	Factual questions from three subject areas: • fine arts & language • science & health • history &geography	Objective Memory Recall	Answer the question to the best of your ability. If you do not know, make an educated guess before you check the possible solutions provided.
SOS = **S**earching **O**ut **S**olutions	Brain teasers, traditional and nontraditional logic problems, and puzzles	Problem Solving	Use your knowledge and logic to analyze, deduce, and problem solve. Use both traditional step-by-step logic as well creative connections.

ICE = **I**magination, **C**reativity, **E**laboration	Prompts to find new ideas, generate novel solutions, elaborate/adapt familiar things in new ways	Creative Thinking	• Think of as many responses as you can. • Include responses from a variety of categories. • Don't judge or edit ideas! Include the obvious, unique, outrageous, and silly. • Elaborate on earlier ideas by adding detail or building on a theme.
TAB = **T**idbits **A**bout the **B**rain	Facts about the brain	New Information Processing	Read the information and let your brain make connections. Focus on how you can apply the information in a positive way.
Mmm = **M**indfulness, **M**ovement, **M**editation	Guided meditations, Movement exercises, Breathing exercises, Sensory stimulation, Mindfulness techniques	Mind-Body Connection	Read through the activity first. Relax and do your best. Stay in touch with your breathing, body sensations and emotions. Based on current health and conditions, modify or replace with earlier activities as needed.

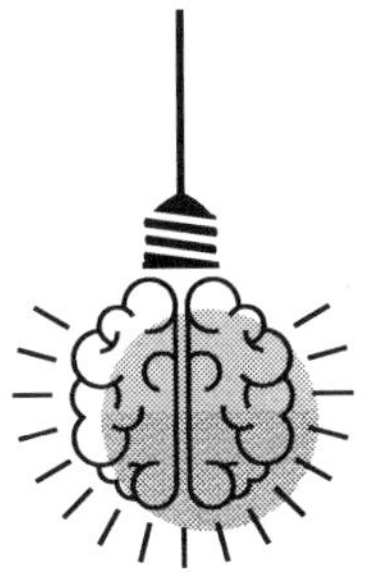

The Activity Sets

(NOTE: Solutions for KISS, SOS, and ICE are provided starting on page 275)

— SET 1 —

WOW All of the flowers of tomorrow are in the seeds of today. – Margaret Lindsey

3Rs What was your favorite and least favorite food as a child? Have your "food tastes" changed over the years? What are your favorite foods right now? What would be the hardest food for you to give up?

KISS 1. Name three adjectives that describe the person you are.

2. What American scientist discovered more than 300 uses for peanuts?

3. Which former U.S. presidents are on the penny, nickel, dime, and quarter?

SOS Dave and Bev are twins. One of them always tells the truth, and one of them always lies. What statement would you never hear Dave or Bev make?

ICE How many common words and phrases can you list using the word "hand"?

TAB According to Swanson (2001)[1]: "You'll never have to worry about running out of room to store memories. If you stashed away 1000 new bits of info every second of your life, you'd still be using only part of your total storage space" (p. 5)

Mmm Observing the Rhythm and Flow of Breath – Lie down in a position of comfort. Place your hands on your belly. Close your eyes and bring your attention to your breath. Do not alter the pattern of your breathing, just observe it. Notice the rhythm and flow of your natural breath. Do some parts of the breath seem stronger or weaker, faster or slower, tenser or

1 Swanson, D. (2001). Hmm? The most interesting book you'll ever read about memory. New York: Scholastic.

easier? Are there times when the breath seems ragged or wheezy? How are the inhalation and exhalation similar and different? What about the pauses between breathing in and breathing out? Observe the breath in this way (without judgment) for several minutes.

— SET 2 —

WOW You have brains in your head and feet in your shoes, so you can steer yourself any direction you choose. – Dr. Seuss

3Rs What advice would you give to your fifteen-year-old self? Would that younger self take your advice?

KISS 1. Name as many characters from *Little Women* as you can.
2. Name some astronauts.
3. List the original 13 colonies.

SOS Decipher the following: doc doc; oturnedut (Example: irighti = right between the eyes)

ICE Add something to sunglasses to make them unique.

TAB Through stimulating the production of alpha and theta waves in the brain, music stimulates creativity.

Mmm Music March – Put on some music (or make your own) and march to it.

— SET 3 —

WOW Happiness is as a butterfly which when pursued is always beyond our grasp, but which if you will sit down quietly may alight upon you. – Nathaniel Hawthorne

3Rs At what age did you first vote in a Presidential election? Who did you vote for? Who or what influenced your vote? Did your candidate win?

KISS 1. At the age of 5, what popular childhood song did Mozart compose?
2. What diseases have been reduced because of vaccinations?
3. Which of the 50 states comes first and last alphabetically?

SOS Using homophones (e.g. to and too), which pair is a vegetable and a weight?

ICE What might George Washington and Abraham Lincoln have to say to each other?

TAB The brains of older people are not slower because of cognitive decline, they are slower because they are filled with so much information to sift and organize; actually, a 2014 research study at the University of Tübingen in Germany found that the elderly know more and use that information better than those who are younger.[2]

Mmm Seated Meditation: Rooting & Grounding – Sit in a position of comfort with your back upright. If you sit on a chair, sit with your legs uncrossed on the front edge of the seat (about two-thirds away from the chair-back). Close your eyes. On an in-breath visualize the breath extending down though the pelvis and sit bones and sending roots down into the earth. With each in-breath continue to extend roots down deep. This is a visualization meditation: you do not need to make any conscious physical effort to change the body, nor do you need to resist any of the body's own subtle adjustments.

— SET 4 —

WOW The really happy person is the one who can enjoy the scenery while on a detour. – Sir James Jeans, English physicist, astronomer & mathematician

3Rs Based on your experiences and observations of people you know, has TV made the world a better place to live? How or why not?

KISS 1. Think of three sentences using the word "fan," as a noun, verb and adjective.

2. What are some fruits that do not grow on trees?

3. In ancient Greece, tossing what to a girl was a traditional proposal of marriage, and catching it meant that she accepted?

SOS What comes next? Worm, chicken, bear, fly, _______.

ICE What are some things that are hollow?

TAB The brain thrives on novelty, challenge and unpredictability. Moving beyond the routine is important for maintaining cognitive fitness. Therefore, periodically take different routes to familiar places and park in different locations. Or, try something new: new friends, new stores, new hobbies, etc.

Mmm Change of Scenery – When you go out today, take a new route to get wherever you are going and home again.

— SET 5 —

WOW Snowflakes are one of nature's most fragile things, but just look what they can do when they stick together. – Vesta M. Kelly

3Rs At what other time in history would you rather have lived? Why?

2 https://www.sciencedaily.com/releases/2014/01/140120090415.htm

KISS 1. Who was the author of *Winnie the Pooh*?

2. Which is warmer, 100°Fahrenheit or 100° Celsius?

3. Name some African countries.

SOS The answers to all of the following clues contain the letters "bat": (1) Burrowing Australian marsupial = _______; (2) A mixture used in baking = _______; and (3) Warfare = _______.

ICE You are in a restaurant and want to get the server's attention. List five crazy ways you might do this.

TAB A multitude of both environmental and genetic factors are reflected in a person's brain, so just like a snowflake or a thumb print every human brain is unique. Not only are the five senses different for each of us, we all have very personal interpretations of what information those senses send the brain.

Mmm Tense to Relax – Starting with the shoulders, you will tighten and release the muscles of the body one-by-one. This can be a good way to relax chronically tight muscles.

— SET 6 —

WOW All our knowledge has its origins in our perceptions. – Leonardo da Vinci

3Rs If you could pass down one physical item from your life to someone in the future, what would you give and to whom? What story or stories would you want that person to know about that item?

KISS 1. What is America's largest piece of art?

2. What three numbers come next in this series of prime numbers? 1, 2, 3, 5, _____.

3. What presidents are on Mount Rushmore in S. Dakota?

SOS What is it that belongs to you but is used by others more than you?

ICE How would you feel and what would happen if one day you just started floating three feet above the ground?

TAB The brain is primarily concerned with survival rather than learning for learning's sake. Therefore, your brain will only concentrate on learning after primary survival needs (food, safety, etc.) have been satisfied and if the learning is perceived to be meaningful or useful in some way.

Mmm Tie Me Up / Tie Me Down – See how many ways you can "tie yourself up in knots" by crossing or twisting limbs and body parts. Do this without hurting yourself, of course; muscle strains and broken bones definitely do not count. ☺

— SET 7 —

WOW Always be a first-rate version of yourself and not a second-rate version of someone else. – Judy Garland

3Rs What experiences have you had with farming or growing plants? Did you ever have a garden or grow your own food? House plants? What did you grow? Do you have a green thumb?

KISS 1. List words that begin with a silent letter.
2. What are the four basic blood types?
3. Name some early explorers of our country.

SOS Leo has six sons and they were all born on the first day of the month. Only the twins were born in a month that has the letter "r." The rest of the sons were all born in different months. Leo remembers that he was preparing to file his taxes when Harold was born. Junior is the oldest son, but his birthday comes last in the year. The youngest son's birthday comes first each year. Walter is older than Mike, but younger than Kevin. Mike and Arnold were both born in months that begin with the same letter as their names. Kevin was born between May 21 and June 21. The older twin's name comes before the younger twin's name in the alphabet. What is the birth order of Leo's sons and what are their respective birthdays?

ICE The following are common sayings with the ending listed in parentheses. Replace the words in parenthesis to create new alternative endings: A friend in need (is a friend in deed); It's no use crying (over spilt milk); Every dog (has its day); haste makes (waste).

TAB The neocortex is the gray matter that forms the surface of the brain. It is involved in higher functions such as conscious thought, generation of motor commands, language, spatial reasoning, and sensory perception.

Mmm Thread the Needle – Get down on your hands and knees. Make sure that your knees are hip-width apart and your hands are directly under your shoulders. Lift one hand off the floor. With the palm of your hand facing up, slide the hand and arm along the ground underneath your torso. Your arm and hand are the "thread" going through the "eye of the needle" formed by space between your torso and the floor. Allow the elbow of the supporting hand to bend as you extend "through the needle." Gently rest into the stretch on that side for a few breaths. Then "unthread," and repeat for the other side.

— SET 8 —

WOW A candle loses nothing by lighting another candle. – James Keller

3Rs Did you ever try to run away? If so, what were the results? If not, what made you change your mind?

KISS 1. Musical instruments can be classified as percussion, woodwind, brass, stringed, or electronic. Which type of musical instrument is a xylophone?
2. Which of these trees are conifers: Dogwood, maple; redwood; spruce?
3. How many senators serve in the U.S. Senate?

SOS Which timepiece or device created by humans to track time has the smallest number of parts? Which timepiece has the largest number of parts?

ICE Make a long and sensible sentence using only words beginning with the letter "S."

TAB Our brains release dopamine in anticipation of a desired effect as part of rewarding our ability to predict outcomes accurately, so anticipation *is* half the fun of good things.

Mmm Writing "Wrong" – Using your dominant hand, write your full name in cursive backwards. Next write your full name upside down. Finally, write your full name with your non-dominant hand.

— SET 9 —

WOW Ability is a wonderful thing, but its value is greatly enhanced by dependability. – Robert Heinlein

3Rs Tell of a time when you were upset with someone else. Who was involved and what was it about? Was your being upset justified? Why or why not? How was your concern resolved? If not, why not? How is your being upset with someone else different from another person being upset with you?

KISS 1. Name four woodwind instruments.
2. At what temperature does water freeze?
3. Name at least three of Thomas Edison's inventions.

SOS If a doctor gives you three pills and says to take one every half hour, how long would you be taking a pill?

ICE A man has a terrified look on his face. List at least five reasons for his fright.

TAB Recent studies clearly indicate that regular exercise helps reduce physical shrinkage of the brain and improves cognitive adaptability.[3]

---

3 Gretchen Reynolds *New York Times Magazine*, How Exercise Could Lead to a Better Brain, April 18, 2012

Mmm Jumping – Be mindful to protect your knees and joints for this one. Jump up and down ten times. Hop on your left foot five times. Hop on your right foot five times. Then hop around in a circle first clockwise and then counter-clockwise. Repeat 2-3 times.

Nov 2, 2018

—— SET 10 ——

WOW Contentment is not the fulfillment of what you want, but the realization of how much you already have. – Anonymous *spread medicine*

3Rs Describe a time you really wanted something and then regretted getting it later? What were your underlying motives for wanting it? What did it cost you to get it? Why did you later regret it? What happened to the "item"? *everyone had one / gained wt. / gave away*

KISS 1. When spelling the 50 states in the U.S., what one letter is **not** used?
2. What do we call the latitude line that is zero degrees? *equator*
3. In what country would you find the Black Forest? *germany + cold*

SOS Read the clues to figure out what this is: It's skinny. It comes in many different colors. Sometimes you see it and sometimes you don't. It begins up open and ends up closed. All people can use it. If it breaks, it's hard to fix. It often gets stuck. It's filled with teeth. It holds things together. *ZIPPER*

ICE Imagine you are only 12 inches tall. What is your story?

TAB The typical adult human brain is about the size of your two fists placed together. It is wrinkled like a walnut with a surface that feels somewhat like a ripened avocado, and it is soft enough that it could be cut with a butter knife.

Mmm Gratitude Meditation: Relax the Body – Lie down in a comfortable position and close your eyes. Bring your awareness to the sensation of the breath for a few breaths. Then bring your awareness down to your feet. Think of all the steps they have walked for you. Thank them and let them rest. Next bring your awareness to your lower legs. Thank them for helping you to stand and then let them rest. Continue moving up the body in this way—knees, thighs, pelvis, belly, ribs, shoulders, arms, hands, and head. Sense the body part, recognize how it serves you, thank the body part, and then invite it to rest. At the end, acknowledge your body as a whole.

—— SET 11 ——

WOW The same sun which melts wax hardens clay. – Charles Spurgeon

3Rs As a child, did you have time limits on watching TV or specific program restrictions? What reasons did your parents give for limiting TV watching or forbidding certain programs? What do you feel was the effect of such limits/lack of such restrictions?

KISS 1. In American folklore, what is the name of the giant lumberman with a blue ox named Babe?

2. Where in your body would you find the hammer, anvil, and stirrup?

3. Who were the first six presidents of the United States?

SOS What common item is seen every day and rarely seen without its mate. It has a tongue you can see, but no voice. It moves often but does the same job. It may squeak and sometimes is known to pinch.

ICE What would you say to a giant who sneezes on your home?

TAB The brainstem is located just above the spine. It performs involuntary functions like heartbeat, digestion, and breathing.

Mmm Spinal Roll – Stand in a comfortable hip width stance with the spine upright and the chin parallel to the floor. Breathe in deeply. As you exhale, let your chin drop softly and slowly down towards your chest. Keep the ribcage lifted and do not curve the shoulders. Hold this position as you breathe in again. Then, as you exhale, begin to slowly release the spine, allowing the body to roll forward. Relax and take your time. Imagine that you can feel each vertebrae of the spine releasing one-by-one until you are dangling over from your hips. (There are a total of 33 vertebrae in the human body, but seven are in the neck and the five in the sacrum are fused.) Relax and breathe for a moment. Then, on an inhale, reverse the process, stacking each vertebrae back up on top of one another "one-by-one" until you resume your original stance.

— SET 12 —

WOW The grass may be greener on the other side, but it still has to be mowed. – Anonymous

3Rs Visualize a time when someone told you a secret, but did **not** swear you to secrecy. Did you keep it a secret or tell someone else? Why? Who was the person with the secret? What was the secret? Who did you tell if you told?

KISS 1. Who painted the ceiling of the Sistine Chapel?

2. Name as many reptiles as you can.

3. New York City was originally a colony of which European country?

SOS If an electric train is rolling down the track going northwest at 100 miles per hour and the wind is blowing 100 miles per hour in exactly the opposite direction (southeast), which direction does the smoke blow?

ICE Which is stronger, "tick" or "tock"? Justify your answer in a creative way.

TAB A number of recent long-term studies concluded that drinking coffee improves memory and other important cognitive functions of the brain. Drinking coffee can positively affect memory within 24 hours of consumption. Drinking 3-5 cups of coffee daily throughout one's lifetime definitively lowers the risk of developing both Alzheimer's disease and Parkinson's disease. One study estimated that the mid-life risk of contracting such disease was cut by up to 65%.[4]

Mmm Seated Meditation: Breathing – Sit in a position of comfort with your back upright. Close your eyes. Bring your awareness to your breath. Whenever, you find your mind wandering, return your focus back to your breathing. Let your breath be natural. Do not alter your breath; simply observe it with your mind.

— SET 13 —

WOW It is the mark of an educated mind to be able to entertain a thought without accepting it.

– Aristotle

3Rs Describe a time when you (or someone you know) had car trouble. Where were you? What happened?

KISS 1. Using each letter of the alphabet, list an adjective for each letter.

2. What element does the symbol *Fe* stand for?

3. What are the three largest cities/metropolitan areas in the U.S. in terms of population?

SOS **What is the activity described below?**

It is actually quite simple. First, you arrange things into different groups depending on their makeup. Of course, one pile may be enough depending on how much there is to do. If you don't have your own equipment, you may want to go somewhere else to do it. It is important not to overdo any particular part of the job. That is, it is better to do too few things at once than too many. In the short run, this may not seem important, but trouble from doing too many can easily arise. A mistake can be expensive as well.

4 http://www.webmd.com/alzheimers/news/20090116/coffee-strong-enough-to-ward-off-dementia#1.

Working the equipment should be self-explanatory. At first, the whole procedure will seem complicated. Soon, however, it will become just another facet of life. It is difficult to see an end to the necessity for this task in the immediate future, but then one can never tell. Just be careful things do not get too soapy. What activity do you think is being described?

ICE Name things that light up.

TAB In a recent study, participants who practiced mindfulness ("the intentional, accepting and non-judgmental focus of one's attention on the emotions, thoughts and sensations occurring in the present moment") for 20 minutes per day performed better and faster on a cognitive test after only four days.[5]

Mmm Body Scan – Sit or lie down in a comfortable position. Close your eyes and become aware of your body. Just observe your sensations without judging them or attempting to change them. Notice how each part of the body feels. Start at the toes and move up the body, one body part at a time until you get to the top of the head. Notice each body part's relation to gravity, its temperature, and the sensation of anything that touches it—such as clothing, furniture, the floor, or the air. Notice any comfort and/or discomfort, tension and/or relaxation, pain and/or pleasure.

— SET 14 —

WOW Blessed are they who can laugh at themselves, for they shall never cease to be amused. – Anonymous

3Rs Relate about a time when you were scared. Was there a legitimate reason to be scared? How did the situation turn out? Are you still frightened in this type of situation?

KISS 1. Who was the author of *Poor Richard's Almanac*?

2. I have 12 inches of string. How many cuts would I need to make if I want 1-inch strips?

3. The oldest colonial settlement in the U.S. is in which state?

SOS Take away the jumbled letters of something sweet to find (in correct order) something sour: DLEACMNOYN.

ICE What is the quietest thing in the world? Be creative.

5 http://www.ncbi.nlm.nih.gov/pmc/articles/PMC3277272#B23

TAB The heaviest human brain ever recorded weighed 5 lb. 1.1 oz. Compare that with the average elephant's brain at 10.5 lbs. and the average sperm whale's brain at 17.5 lbs.

Mmm Do the Hokey Pokey – Yes, we mean it. Singing aloud is optional.

— SET 15 —

WOW Truly great friends are hard to find, difficult to leave, and impossible to forget. – G. Randolf

3Rs Think of a time you created something. What was it? What happened to it? What did you learn from the experience of making it?

KISS 1. Who painted the Mona Lisa?
2. Name some organs of the body.
3. Which two states in the U.S. are shaped like a rectangle?

SOS What do these foods have in common? Beans, Bread, Cabbage, Dough, Lettuce.

ICE Compare an umbrella to a porcupine.

TAB The brain benefits from activities that contribute to emotional fitness, such as having solid, caring, ongoing social support networks, participating in enjoyable and fun group activities regularly, supporting others emotionally, and participating in volunteer work.

Mmm In the Swim: The Crawl – Do the swimmer's crawl around the room.

— SET 16 —

WOW Don't mind criticism. If it's untrue, disregard it; if it's unfair, keep from irritation; if it's ignorant, smile; if it's justified, learn from it. – Anonymous

3Rs Visualize what your bedroom looked like when you were a child. How was it decorated? Where was it located in your home, and how far was it from your parents' bedroom? Who did you share it with, if anyone?

KISS 1. What are the plurals forms of deer, moose, Mrs. goose, octopus, ox, and tooth?
2. True or false: Some bees sting only once.
3. Name some vice presidents of the United States.

SOS What three different English words can be made by rearranging the following letters: GYRLEAL?

ICE How would it affect your daily life if all numbers disappeared? List as many ways as you can.

TAB Brain diseases and disorders include: addiction, Alzheimer's disease, bipolar disorder, depression, epilepsy, expressive aphasia, head trauma, Huntington's disease, multiple sclerosis, Parkinson's disease, rabies, stroke, and Wilson's disease.

Mmm Pre-Crawl: Doggy – Get down on your hands and knees. Gently rock your body over your hands and knees—forward-and-back, side-to-side. Wag your pelvis like the tail of a dog. Turn and look over your shoulder to see if you have grown a tail. Look for it over the other shoulder, too.

— SET 17 —

WOW As the blossom cannot tell what becomes of its fragrance, so no one can tell what becomes of his [or her] influence. – Henry Ward Beecher

3Rs Describe a time you misjudged a person or situation. What happened? How did you find out you were wrong? How did you feel after you realized you had been wrong?

KISS 1. Who wrote the novels *The Color Purple* and *For Whom the Bell Tolls*?
2. Which insect tends, herds, shelters, and milks plant lice like a dairy farmer?
3. Name some Native American nations.

SOS Lenora, Melissa, David, and William went out for dinner. Melissa is a vegan, and she is lactose intolerant. The one who ate steak had New York cheesecake for dessert. William did not have the chocolate cake or the vanilla ice cream. Lenora wanted to order the same dessert as the person who ate chicken, but she is allergic to chocolate. David did not have apple pie for dessert, but the person who ate salad did. What entrée and dessert did each person have?

ICE You are creating a new welcome mat for your house. It says "Welcome to the ______." What would your mat say and what does it look like?

TAB A University of Cincinnati study suggests that people's concentration and performance improves after smelling either peppermint or muguet, "a scent similar to lily of the valley."[6]

Mmm Seated Meditation: Flower Fresh – Close your eyes. Bring awareness to your breath. On your next inhale begin to visualize yourself as a flower; fresh, sweet-smelling. Imagine the type of flower you would be; whatever appeals

---

6 *Washington* Post, The Power of Peppermint Is Put to the Test, by Lori Aratani, March 20, 2007.

to you is fine. Imagine the sensation of the stem of the flower growing up your spine and your face is the blossom of the flower. Then as you exhale, visualize the freshness of the flower within you. As you inhale, say in your mind, "Breathing in, I see myself as a flower." Then, as you exhale, say, "Breathing out, I feel fresh." Continue for at least 10 breath cycles.[7]

—— SET 18 ——

WOW A friend is a person who goes around saying nice things about you behind your back. –Thomas Fuller (paraphrased)

3Rs Bring to mind a time you needed to be emotionally strong. What was the situation?

KISS 1. Name five or more classical composers.
2. Name the instrument doctors use to listen to your heart and lungs.
3. All Interstate highways that run east to west end in what kind of number? What about those running north to south?

SOS Put a different woman's name in each of the blanks and make a word: rea_ _ _e and tis_ _ _.

ICE Create a sensible sentence by replacing the underlined words:
"When the <u>opur</u> hits the <u>wingle bisser</u>, check the <u>liposcooter</u> for signs of <u>whipdoodle</u>." What does this "wild" sentence mean?

TAB A clear, colorless liquid called cerebral spinal fluid surrounds the brain and spinal column. This fluid serves as a cushioning buffer, clears away wastes, carries hormones between areas of the nervous system, and keeps the brain buoyant to reduce the weight of the brain at the base of the neck.

Mmm Pre-Crawl: Snaky Spine – Get down on your hands and knees. Keeping your hands on the floor, imagine that your neck and spine have turned into a snake and allow your snaky spine to slither and writhe. Alternately open and close your elbow joints to allow more movement in the shoulder joints and to move the spine closer to and away from the ground.

—— SET 19 ——

WOW I prefer to call a nap a "horizontal life pause." – Anonymous

3Rs What was your first day of school like? How did you feel? Scared? Excited? Were you the oldest child from your family to go to school? What did you like most/least about your school?

---

7 Nhat Hanh, Thich. (2009). The Blooming of a Lotus. (Revised). Boston: Beacon Press.

KISS 1. List words using "qu", but not at the beginning of the word.
2. Name at least three simple machines.
3. What did the 19th amendment do?

SOS The alphabet has been divided into two groups as follows: AEFIKLMNTVWXYZ and BCGJOPQRSU. In which group would you place the letters D H and Q?

ICE How could you share a birthday cake if you had no type of knife or utensil? Think of at least three ideas.

TAB Napping isn't just for kids! Recent studies show that adults who indulged in midday naps performed 20 percent better on memory exercises than those who did not nap.

Mmm Gratitude Meditation: Internal Organs – Lie down in a comfortable position, and close your eyes. Use a combination of sensory awareness and visualization in this meditation to acknowledge and thank your internal organs. First bring your awareness to the sensation of the breath as it fills your lungs. Acknowledge and thank your lungs for the way they sustain your life. Bring your awareness to the beating of your heart. Acknowledge and thank your heart for the way it sustains your life. Repeat for each internal organ. You may want to place your hands over the appropriate area of the body to help with awareness—stomach and pancreas (beneath the heart on the left side of the body); liver (below ribs on the right side); kidneys (bottom of ribs on the backside); intestines (belly below the ribs). And, of course, don't forget your brain inside your skull!

— SET 20 —

WOW A minute of thought is greater than an hour of talk.—John C. Maxwell

3Rs Remember a time you spilled or broke something. What happened? Where were you and what thoughts entered your mind when it happened? Was the damage able to be repaired?

KISS 1. Name as many Shakespeare plays as you can.
2. Which is more likely to win in a battle between a cobra and a mongoose?
3. Which country has the most English speakers, China or the U.S.?

SOS Add three letters to each of the following to make words: l_ _ _g; d_ _ _d; p_ _ _p; and t_ _ _l. See how many words you can make for each one.

ICE What things are round and have a hole in the middle? Be creative.

TAB David Farrow is a two-time Guinness Record Holder for The World's Greatest Memory. In 2007, he broke the record a second time by memorizing and correctly recalling the exact order of 59 decks of cards (3068 cards), exceeding his previous record of 52 decks (2704 cards).[8]

Mmm Finger Crawl – Sit at an open desk or table. Place your fingertips on the table. Imagine your hands are little animals and your fingers are their legs. Let your hands crawl all around the table. Walk them together and separately, forward and backward, to the left and to the right. For an extra challenge, add music and let your hands do a dance number.

— SET 21 —

WOW The mind is a wild white horse and when you make a corral for it make sure it's not too small – Laurie Anderson

3Rs What were some of your favorite vacations? What made them memorable?

KISS 1. Shakespeare's tragedies end with at least one death. How do his comedies end?

2. Describe the three main parts of the water cycle.

3. Why does it take longer to hoist a flag to half-mast than to full-mast?

SOS The letters "ph" almost always are pronounced "f", e.g., phone. What are some words where this is not true?

ICE The following are common sayings with the ending listed in parentheses. Replace the part in parenthesis to create new alternative endings: "Don't bite off more (than you can chew)." "He who laughs last (laughs best)." "A bird in the hand (is worth two in the bushes)." "The more things change (the more they stay the same)."

TAB Several studies suggest that practicing the martial art of Tai Chi may contribute to improved cognitive function and reduced risk of dementia.[9]

Mmm Pulling Chi – In Eastern martial arts and acupuncture, chi refers to life force energy. This exercise uses visualization and movement to cultivate awareness of chi. Find a stable stance with knees slightly bent. Bring your hands in front of your belly button; place the palms facing each other close together, but not touching. Now imagine that a strong rubber

8 http://www.worldsgreatestmemory.com/

9 Zhu, W., Guan, S., & Yang, Y. (2010). Clinical implications of Tai Chi interventions: A Review. *American Journal of Lifestyle Medicine*, 4, 418-432: http://harvardmagazine.com/2010/01/researchers-study-tai-chi-benefits

band is attached to the center of each palm and connects them. Keep your mind focused on the imaginary band between the two palms throughout the exercise. Pull the hands apart and stretch the rubber band open wide. Then let the rubber band contract back, drawing the palms back towards one another. Don't let the palms touch. Continue to stretch and contract the rubber band in many directions. When you are done, close your eyes and hold the palms about 8-12 inches from each other. What sensations do you notice in and around your hands?

— SET 22 —

WOW Among my most prized possessions are words I have never spoken. – Orson Rega Card

3Rs Did you ever witness someone doing something wrong? What did you do?

KISS 1. There are three root words in the English language that begin with "dw". What are they?

2. Name the planets that circle the sun in order from closest to the sun to the furthest away.

3. Which of the Ancient Seven Wonders of the World is still standing?

SOS In the following, take away the scrambled letters of a big thing to find a little thing with the remaining letters in the correct order: ALEMHOPTUSENE.

ICE What if you fell asleep today and slept 20 years; what would your new world be like?

TAB The cerebrum is the largest part of the brain. It does all the higher-level thinking functions. When someone says, "Use your brain," they probably mean "use your cerebrum."

Mmm Standing Meditation: Three Point Balance – Stand with your feet in a narrow to hip-width stance. Close your eyes. Sense the feet on the ground and the vertical line of your body. Sense the heel of each foot. Press into the center point of the heel of both feet. Then sense a point on the ball of each foot below and between the big toe and the second toe, and press into that point. Finally, sense a point on the ball of each foot below and between the fourth toe and the little toe, press into that point. Allow your body to rock back-and-forth slightly between these three points on the feet until you experience a sense of balance. Then gently press through all three points at once to create a stable, solid stance. Notice if your posture has changed. Hold in this balanced place for several breaths.

— SET 23 —

WOW Achieving starts with believing. – Anonymous

3Rs Who would you most appreciate having as your next-door-neighbor? Why?

KISS 1. What red month is in the title of a bestselling Tom Clancy novel?
2. What main function does the liver, your second largest organ, perform in your body?
3. Name some Asian countries.

SOS Use the same three letters to fill in the blanks to create legitimate words from the following: be___ble, gu___ntee, c___van.

ICE List reasons you can't close the front door.

TAB Your brain's cerebrum is divided into two hemispheres. The right hemisphere deals especially with attention, rhymes, poetry, tunes, music, awe, inspiration, emotions, creativity, etc. The left hemisphere deals more often with sounds, words, meanings, logic, analysis, synthesis, active reflection, application, etc.

Mmm Supine Twist – Lie on your back in a comfortable position with your knees bent and your feet on the floor. Spread the arms out at the shoulders like at "T." Exhale and pull your knees in towards your belly. Keep both arms and shoulders firmly on the ground, and on the next exhale, allow the knees to fall to one side. This will gently twist the lower spine. For more of a stretch, turn your head in the opposite direction of the knees. Relax and breathe in the pose for a while. Then on an in-breath, bring the knees back to the center. Repeat for the other side. When you are done, use your hands and arms to hug your knee in close to your body for a few seconds before getting up.

— SET 24 —

WOW Blessed are those who can give without remembering and take without forgetting. – Princess Elizabeth Bibesco

3Rs What did you like about your "hometown" community? What would you change about it if you could? What parts would you not change at all?

KISS 1. What movement in art is Picasso associated with?
2. What are Tasmanian devils and where are they found?
3. Which one state in the continental U.S. does not follow Daylight Savings Time?

SOS Put down four 9's so that they will equal 100.

ICE The following are common sayings with the ending listed in parentheses. Replace the part in parenthesis to create alternative endings: The early bird (gets the worm); A penny saved (is a penny earned); The grass is always (greener on the other side); It's always darkest (before the dawn).

TAB Recent studies suggest that cinnamon can promote brain activity and may be able to serve a primary role in preventing age-related brain diseases such as Alzheimer's and Parkinson's. Cinnamon can be included in food or as a supplement. But be careful, too much cinnamon can cause toxicity; the typical recommended dosage is 2-4g cinnamon powder a day.[10]

Mmm Spinning – Be sure you have a clear floor space of about six feet around you. Stand with your arms out and palms down. Focus your eyes on one hand to reduce the likelihood of getting dizzy. At your own speed, turn in a full circle to the right. Then turn in a full circle to the left. Repeat several times. Or for more of a challenge, see how many turns you can comfortably turn in one direction before switching directions. If you get dizzy stop and pat your lower belly to help you get grounded again.

— SET 25 —

WOW An inch of gold will not buy an inch of time. – Chinese Proverb

3Rs As you were growing up, did you ever play "car games" to pass the time when traveling? If so, what games did you play? If not, how did you pass the time when traveling?

KISS 1. How many basic parts of speech are there? Name them.
2. Name some insects that live in colonies.
3. Name some European countries.

SOS Three men are walking in the rain with no umbrellas or hats. Two get their hair wet and one doesn't. Why doesn't the third man get his hair wet?

ICE Make up song titles that could be on next week's Top 10 chart.

TAB Research indicates that the brain is hard-wired to fear first and reflect second. However, the amygdala in the brain provides tools one can use to overcome a tendency toward fear and achieve a full and contented feeling of freedom. Techniques such as the *"Focus, Expose, Approach, Rehearse"*

---

10 http://www.benefitsfromcinnamon.com/benefits/benefits-of-cinnamon-for-the-brain

system proposed by Dr. Pamela Garcy at the Texas School of Professional Psychology at the University of Texas-Dallas can be used.[11]

Mmm Breathing Meditation: Torso – Sit or lie down in a comfortable position. Close your eyes. After a few breaths, consciously let the in-breath grow deeper, and the out-breath grow longer and stronger. With each in-breath consciously begin to visualize the air coming into the lungs, and then filling your whole torso with vitality. With each out-breath, visualize the used air carrying away toxins and tension from your body.

— SET 26 —

WOW A goal is not always meant to be reached, it often serves simply as something to aim for. – Bruce Lee

3Rs Do you enjoy sports or physical activity of any kind? If not, why not? Did you play any sports in school? If so, which ones? Were you a sports fan in school? What physical activity/activities do you do now? Are you now a sports fan? What sport and sports team do you like best at this point in your life?

KISS 1. Who wrote: *Roots*? *Leaves of Grass*? *A Raisin in the Sun*?
2. What's the greatest number you can get when you add two three-digit numbers?
3. Who was the first woman prime minister of Britain?

SOS What do these seven words have in common? Assess, Banana, Dresser, Grammar, Potato, Revive, and Uneven. Hint: Has nothing to do with the meaning of the words.

ICE What if everyone looked the same?

TAB Research indicates that ongoing creative challenges are good for the brain and can prevent or delay the onset of dementia because creative activities stimulate the brain to form new synapses/pathways for new thoughts and ideas.

Mmm Prize Fighter – Imagine you are in a boxing match. Throw some good punches and dodge/weave. Upper cut. Lower cut. Left hook/right hook. Sock it to 'em!

---

11 http://www.psychologytoday.com/blog/fearless-you/201311/fear-busting-formula-you-can-remember.)

— SET 27 —

WOW Deep roots are not reached by frost. – J. R. R. Tolkien

3Rs What talent would you especially have liked to have had as you were growing up? Why? If you could have been the best in the world in one talent, what talent would that have been? Why?

KISS 1. What does not fit in this list: Beethoven, Picasso, Rembrandt, Renoir?
2. Which part of our body is always the same size from birth?
3. What is the first sentence of the Gettysburg Address?

SOS Start with the word "Boy" and change one letter at a time to get to the word "Man", making real words at each step. Boy _____ _____ Man.

ICE Prince Charming has bad breath. How will you tell him?

TAB There are about 100 billion neurons in the brain, and each neuron makes 1,000 or more connections to other neurons, adding up to some 100 trillion in total.[12]

Mmm Standing Meditation: Tree Roots – Stand with your feet in a narrow to hip-width stance. Close your eyes. Sense the feet on the ground and the vertical line of your body. With each in-breath visualize the breath extending down though the legs and feet and sending roots down into the earth. With each out-breath, visualize yourself growing taller from these roots like a tree. This is a visualization meditation: you do not need to make any conscious physical effort to change the body, nor do you need to resist any of the body's own subtle adjustments based on the visualization. Simply visualize yourself extending beyond the limits of your physical body, up toward the sun and down into the earth.

— SET 28 —

WOW It is when we forget ourselves that we do things that are most likely to be remembered. – Anonymous

3Rs During this past year, what are things you saw, heard, felt, visited, thought about, or imagined for the first time?

KISS 1. Make a list of words that are spelled the same forward as backwards (Palindromes); e.g., "toot."
2. Cats can see in the dark. True or false?

---

12 https://www.scientificamerican.com/article/new-estimate-boosts-the-human-brain-s-memory-capacity-10-fold/

3. What lake does the U.S. and Canada share that is the largest fresh water lake in the world?

SOS The answers to these questions end in the sound "sea". What sea is a southern state? What sea can talk clearly? What sea can read and write? What sea doesn't change much? What sea is an omen?

ICE List at least five creative ways to wake someone up.

TAB Apples may offer a healthier alternative to keep people awake (and the brain alert) in the morning as effectively as caffeine.[13]

Mmm Eating Meditation: Sensory Awareness – Get a small apple or other fruit that you like to eat. You are going to eat the fruit with as much mindful awareness as you can. Start by noticing the smell, shape, color, texture, temperature, and weight of the fruit in your hand. Take your first bite and set the fruit down. Close your eyes and bring full awareness to the sensations of the fruit in your mouth. Notice the taste and texture of the fruit. Continue to bring full awareness to the sensation of the fruit in your mouth as you chew. Notice the movement and sensation of jaw, teeth, tongue, lips cheeks and soft palate. Count how many times you chew each bite, and notice how the textures and taste of the fruit change as you chew. This meditation can also be done as part of a silent meal or anytime you are eating something.

— SET 29 —

WOW There is no key to happiness. The door is always open. – Mother Teresa

3Rs Everyone has had unique experiences. What situations or experiences have you had that few other people have had? Describe the experience and how it affected you.

KISS 1. Name some writers associated with the Harlem Renaissance.

2. What two gases primarily make up the Earth's atmosphere?

3. What famous American is supposed to have said "Give me liberty or give me death"?

SOS What is the relationship that your father's sister's sister-in-law could be to you if this person is actually related to you?

ICE You're a pilot and your plane is late. Think of at least three unique excuses why it is late.

13 http://haveanamasteblog.com/2011/08/apples-vs-caffeine-how-apples-can-help-keep-you-awake/

TAB Memories can sometimes be altered or modified by stimuli the person is exposed to after the event. This is why eyewitnesses to crimes are sometimes found to be unreliable.

Mmm Army Crawl: Leg Positions – Lie face down, resting your head comfortably on your bent arms. On an inhale, bend the left leg and rotate the leg out at the hip to place the inner-thigh-side down on the ground. (The legs now create the shape of the numeral four.) Keep the torso in contact with the ground throughout. Rest in this position for a few breaths. Then on an exhale, straighten the bent leg along the ground and rotate the other leg out at the hip to place the inner-thigh-side down on the ground to switch sides. Repeat.

— SET 30 —

WOW All things are difficult before they are easy. – Thomas Fuller

3Rs Describe your family's favorite activity while you were growing up.

KISS 1. Name some characters in *Winnie the Pooh*?

2. If you were on the moon, what would you hear?

3. What is the only U.S. state that formed as a result of a popular vote to separate from another state?

SOS What nationality goes with each of these pairs: Bath and Delight; Steak and Cheese; Ice and Bread; and Beetle and Lantern.

ICE What are some unusual things you "own" that you could never throw out?

TAB The amygdala, an almond-shape set of neurons located near the center of the brain, is the part of the brain that especially deals with emotion and motivation. In response to perceived danger, it stimulates the release stress hormones (glucocortoids) that immediately result in a "fight or flight" adrenaline rush. Experts think that autism, depression, phobias, post-traumatic stress disorder, and excessive anxiety are linked to damage, developmental problems, or neurotransmitter imbalances related to abnormal functioning of the amygdala.

Mmm Clearing Interference Meditation – Sit in a position of comfort with your back upright. Close your eyes. Bring your awareness to your breath for a while. Then ask yourself if there is anything that clouds your mind or interferes with your being in the present moment. Whatever comes to mind, imagine it draining out of your body and sinking down into the earth to be transformed. Notice how you feel. Is there anything else? If so, let that drain away, too. When you feel clear and solid, thank yourself for letting go and return to the breath for a few seconds before opening your eyes.

— SET 31 —

WOW And the trouble is, if you don't risk anything, you risk even more. – Erica Jong

3Rs Have you ever been a patient in a hospital? If so, how long were you a patient there and what were the circumstances for your being there? If you've never been a hospital patient yourself, what experiences have you had visiting others in the hospital?

KISS 1. What are some words you could use instead of the word "said"?
2. Stare at your finger and slowly bring it close to your nose. Your finger should appear to split. Why?
3. What country has more lakes than the rest of the world combined?

SOS The answers to the following clues all contain the letters "sit" in them: 1) An easy target (two words); 2) A person who provides childcare; 3) A stringed instrument from India; 4) Chief who fought at the battle of Little Bighorn; 5) Form of protest.

ICE The people you are supposed to accompany on a prepaid vacation have begun to annoy you. What are some creative reasons you can give them for not going?

TAB The average human brain weighs about 2.7 pounds, approximately 2% of one's total weight. Furthermore, in 2010, a study at the Salk Institute in La Jolla, CA found that the human brain's memory-storage capacity is ten times greater than previously thought, to around one quadrillion bytes.[14]

Mmm Army Crawl: Head and Arm Positions – Lie face down. Stretch one arm out along the floor above your head with the palm down. Bend the other arm up next to your body and press the hand and forearm into the ground to gently lift your head and shoulders off the ground slightly. Keep the torso in contact with the ground. Leading with the eyes, look around and above you for several breaths. Then on an exhale, reverse arms and repeat.

— SET 32 —

WOW As a single footstep will not make a path on the earth, so a single thought will not make a pathway in the mind. To make a deep physical path, we

14 https://www.scientificamerican.com/article/new-estimate-boosts-the-human-brain-s-memory-capacity-10-fold/

walk again and again. To make a deep mental path, we must think over and over the kind of thoughts we wish to dominate our lives. – Henry David Thoreau

3Rs Describe some of your memories about puddles, rivers, lakes, the ocean, etc. What do you most enjoy about water?

KISS 1. What artist is most commonly associated with Pop Art? (Think tomato soup.)

2. What is the main difference between viper and constrictor snakes?

3. Name some states that seceded from the Union at the start of the U.S. Civil War?

SOS Steve, Victoria, Roxanne, and Ali all have shops that sell different things on the four corners of an intersection. The person who sells shoes is on the north corner. The appliance shop is diagonal from the fruit stand. No one carries their purchases home from Steve's shop. Roxanne goes east to eat lunch at Ali's, but her dentist has told her to stop shopping at the candy store afterward. Who sells what, and on what corner is each person's shop?

ICE Think of a proper name and add other letters to make a new word; for example, TOMato.

TAB A study at the University of Pittsburgh of more than 100 men and women aged 60 to 80 found that taking a short walk three times a week increased the size of brain regions linked to planning and memory over the course of a year by more than enough to overcome the steady shrinkage doctors expected to see over the same period. Half of the participants, who all confessed to doing little if any daily exercise in their daily lives, were randomly assigned to walk for 30 to 45 minutes three days a week. The rest spent a similar amount of time doing stretching exercises. The walking reduced "the age clock by about one to two years" and led to better performance on cognitive tests.[15]

Mmm Walking Meditation: Sense Your Steps – Take yourself for a mindful walk. Bring your mind and your full awareness to the sensation of walking. Feel your feet touch the ground with each step. Sense your leg lifting and your body moving through space. If you find your mind wandering, it can be helpful to walk at a slower pace and return your focus back to your steps on the earth and the sensations of walking. This walk can be done indoors, outdoors, or even walking to and from your car in a parking lot.

---

15 https://www.theguardian.com/society/2014/feb/17/brain-walk-delaying-dementia-memory .

— SET 33 —

WOW Correction does much, but encouragement does more. Encouragement after censure is as the sun after a shower. – Johann Wolfgang von Goethe

3Rs Did your mom and/or dad make you do something or wear something that you did not like? Did you end up doing it? What happened? Were you embarrassed?

KISS 1. What song in the English speaking world is sung most often?
2. What is the largest living bird?
3. Which national park in the northeastern U.S. is the second most visited of all the national parks?

SOS Can you pass this candy "Bar Exam": Which candy bar has three pronouns in its name? Which candy bar is a do-it-yourself misspelled pet? Which candy bar is an infant and a book of the Old Testament? Which candy bar is where pitchers stand?

ICE What could you do if your parachute was full of holes?

TAB Be careful in making judgments about one's potential cognitive abilities. For example, Albert Einstein was unable to speak until four years of age, and unable to read until he was seven, which led his parents and teachers to think he was mentally retarded.

Mmm Army Crawl: Full Body Positions – Lie face down. Take the Army Crawl Head and Arm position so that right arm is stretched out in front, left arm is bent, head and shoulders are lifted, and torso is on the ground. Bend the left leg (opposite from long arm) and rotate the leg out at the hip to place the inner-thigh-side down on the ground. (The legs now create the shape of the numeral four.) Leading with the eyes, look around and above you for several breaths. Then on and exhale, reverse which arm and leg is bent or straight. Alternate positions for a total of ten on each side. For more challenge, "army-crawl" along the ground—pulling your body weight forward by pressing down into the straight arm as you bend it and pushing against the floor with the bent leg as you straighten it. Keep the torso in contact with the ground throughout.

— SET 34 —

WOW Be calm when things go wrong, persevere when things are difficult, be helpful to those in need, and be sympathetic to those whose hearts are heavy. – Anonymous

3Rs Have you ever experienced road rage or been in the car when someone else did? What happened?

KISS 1. "The quick brown fox jumped over the lazy dogs" is a sentence that includes all 26 letters of the alphabet. Which words in that sentence are adjectives?

2. What is the process by which the cortex is severed and keratin-containing cells are removed?

3. What did the Emancipation Proclamation do?

SOS Find a one-word answer to the following so that the last two letters of each answer are also the first two letters of the next answer. Where you see your reflection: An instrument played in a cathedral: Happening every year: A harsh type of soap: A bright color.

ICE Every day on the way to work you end up spilling your coffee. What are some novel ways to solve this problem?

TAB Neurons, or nerve cells, within the brain and throughout the body, carry messages through electrochemical processes. Charged sodium, potassium and chloride ions move in and out of these cells to create an electrical current.

Mmm Breathing Meditation: Whole Body – Sit or lie down in a comfortable position. Close your eyes. After a few breaths, consciously let the in-breath grow deeper and the out-breath grow longer and stronger. With each in-breath, consciously begin to visualize the air coming into the lungs and then extending deeper and deeper into the rest of the body right down to the toes and fingers. Then right up to the brain! Imagine and sense each in-breath, bringing aliveness and vitality to each part of the body. Imagine and sense each out-breath, clearing toxins and tension away from that part of the body. If, at any point, the breathing becomes overwhelming or if you get dizzy, return to a normal breath.

— SET 35 —

WOW Be humble, do not brag; let others "brag" about you. – Bernard Baruch

3Rs Have you ever had any serious injuries such as stitches or broken bones? If not, what accounted for your good fortune? If so, what is the story of your injury? What was your experience as the injury was treated, and what were the results of the treatment? Did you learn a lesson?

KISS 1. Why is Noah Webster famous?
2. What sports are commonly referred to as individual sports rather than team sports, even though the individuals can be members of a team in that sport?
3. In what western state are the ten highest mountains in the U.S.?

SOS What is the missing letter in this logical series: D, R, M, F, _, L, T, D? Hint: Music.

ICE Think of things that bend.

TAB Exposure to learned material a second time within 15-30 minutes can double your ability to remember it, and repeated exposure thereafter increases your memory of it significantly more.[16]

Mmm In the Swim: Backstroke – Do a swimmer's backstroke around the room.

— SET 36 —

WOW As long as one keeps searching, the answers come. – Joan Baez

3Rs What was one of the silliest things you did as a child? How about after you became an adult?

KISS 1. Name three or more female poets?
2. What three things are necessary for a fire to burn?
3. In what country would you find the Leaning Tower of Pisa?

SOS Find a word for each letter of the alphabet that both starts and ends with that letter.

ICE Name things you will never see.

TAB Imagine a line traveling down the center of your nose and dividing the body in half top to bottom. Any movement that involves one part of the body crossing over that imaginary midline to the opposite side is considered a cross lateral movement. For example, putting your right hand on your left shoulder. According to Eric Jensen, practicing cross lateral movement seems to enhance brain coordination and is linked to improvements in academic performance.[17]

Mmm Cross Body: Ears – Take your left hand and pinch your right earlobe. At the same time pinch your right earlobe with your left hand. Your forearms will form an "X" across your body. Massage your earlobes with the fingers of the opposite hand.

---

16 http://www.indiana.edu/~pcl/rgoldsto/courses/dunloskyimprovinglearning.pdf

17 Jenson, Erik. (2007) *Brain Based Learning*. Cheltenham, Australia: Hawker Brownlow Education.

— SET 37 —

WOW Be sure to form good habits because they are as hard to break as bad habits. – Anonymous

3Rs Have you ever hitchhiked or "begged" a ride? Why or why not? What was the situation?

KISS 1. There are 17 punctuation marks. Name as many as you can.
2. What silvery liquid was formerly used in thermometers?
3. Name some states that were bought in the Louisiana Purchase?

SOS I have three U.S. coins totaling 55 cents. At least one of them is not a nickel. What are the coins?

ICE Name things that have a middle. Be creative.

TAB People with autism and Alzheimer's disease have high levels of the "beta amyloid" protein plaques. Scientists believe these plaques block cell-to-cell signaling. They are working on vaccines to prevent or remove the plaques.

Mmm Hand Reflexology – According to reflexology, the brain corresponds to an area on the top, inner half of each thumb. Use one thumb to "dance" all over the fingerprint area of the opposite thumb. Then switch.

— SET 38 —

WOW When you own your breath, no one can steal your peace. – Anonymous

3Rs Have you ever pretended to be sick to get out of doing something? What was the "illness"? Why did you choose it and how did you fake it? Did your pretending work? Why? Would you ever do it again? If you have never pretended to be sick to get out of doing something, what sort of situation might you be tempted to fake sickness?

KISS 1. Why is Sequoia famous?
2. What is the formula associated with Einstein's Theory of Relativity?
3. What is the smallest country (in area) in the world?

SOS Read the clues to figure out what this is: You can hold it in your hand. Sometimes it has flowers on it. It starts up fat and ends up slim. Usually it has more than 100 parts. If you are not careful, it can roll away. It's kept in a spherical place. Anyone can use it. You can see through the middle of it. It is easy to tear.

ICE What would be unusual things to think about while descending in a parachute?

TAB Deep breathing is a scientifically proven way to reduce stress. Stress reduction positively affects the brain, heart, digestion and immune system.[18]

Mmm Breathing Meditation: Deep Belly Breathing – When we breathe with our belly, we get more oxygen. Lie on your back in a comfortable position. Close your eyes and place your hands on your belly. Focus on the sensation of your belly rising and falling with each inhale and exhale. Do this for at least ten breath cycles.

— SET 39 —

WOW Do all the good you can, by all the means you can, in all the places you can, at all the times you can, to all the people you can, as long as ever you can. – John Wesley

3Rs Did you (or someone you heard about) ever have a fire or other emergency in your home? What happened? How extensive was the damage and what was determined to be the cause? Was anyone hurt?

KISS 1. Which German composer had five sons who became musicians and had a grandfather whose sons were all musicians?

2. What part of the human body has twelve bones, but none to spare?

3. What people were forced from their homeland in the Trail of Tears?

SOS A farmer had 17 sheep and all but nine died. How many does he have left?

ICE Choose an object in the room where you are now. How could you change it?

TAB A long-term study found that people who eat seafood at least once a week have a 30 percent lower risk of developing dementia than their fish-free counterparts.

Mmm Tails – Imagine that you have grown a tail. Feel the tail growing out of your tailbone at the back of your pelvis. Wag your tail. Swing your tail. How does your tail move when you are happy? When you are angry? When you are afraid? When you are excited? What type of tail do you have? Play with having different types of tails: a bunny tail, a fishy tail, a doggy tail, a tiger tail, a stumpy tail, a long tail, a bushy squirrel tail, etc.

— SET 40 —

WOW The brain is wider than the sky. – Emily Dickinson

---

18 Cuda, Gretchen. (Dec. 6, 2010). Just breathe: Body has a built-in stress reliever. *NPR.*

3Rs Have you ever ridden a horse or other animal? What are your memories of that experience? If you have not had that experience, what do you imagine it would be like?

KISS 1. In what language does "sayonara" mean "goodbye"?
2. Is the orca a mammal or a fish?
3. What was Paul Revere carrying when he said: "One if by land; two if by sea"?

SOS Can you read this code? 100204180.

ICE Where are unusual places in your home where you might hide an expensive diamond ring? Be creative; there might be someone wanting your ring.

TAB In Traditional Chinese Medicine (TCM), what Western medicine considers to be "diseases of the brain" are viewed and treated as systemic problems? That is, rather than reducing such diseases to one organ (i.e. the brain), TCM focuses on overall function within a larger system. As such, Kaoru Sakatani of the Department of Neurological Surgery at Nihon University School of Medicine in Japan suggests TCM's "dynamic models may provide new paradigms for preventive medicine."[19]

Mmm Seated Meditation: Cloud Meditation – Sit in a position of comfort with back upright. Close your eyes. Let your breath be natural. In your mind, visualize a clear blue, cloudless sky. Whenever you find your mind wandering to thoughts or worries, see the thoughts become clouds in the sky and visualize a gentle breeze blowing the clouds far, far away past the horizon. If you want, you can incorporate the breath, such that each exhalation becomes the wind blowing the clouds further and further away from you.

—— SET 41 ——

WOW Don't lose your head to gain a minute; you need your head, your brains are in it. – Burma Shave

3Rs Have you gone to any carnivals, circuses, amusement parks, or fairs? (If not, what have you heard about them?) Where did you go and in what activities did you participate? What are your most special memories of the event?

19 http://www.fractal.org/Life-Science-Technology/Chinese-fractal.pdf

KISS 1. What kind of cat did Alice meet in Wonderland?
2. A spelunker likes to explore what?
3. Who was President of the U.S. during the Civil War?

SOS If you went to bed at 8 in the evening, wound the clock and set it for 9 in the morning, how much sleep would you get before the alarm went off?

ICE What original things could you do with a blank sheet of paper? List a number of creative ideas.

TAB Bartholomew Parker Bidder is in the *Guinness Book of World Records* for his incredible memory. In 1838, he was working for the Royal Exchange Assurance Company when the firm's records were incinerated in a building fire. In a period of six months, Bidder reconstructed all the files from memory.[20]

Mmm Embrace the Moon – Sit comfortably on the front edge of a chair with spine upright. Throughout this exercise keep the tummy in, the spine long, shoulders pulled back, and head level as if gazing at the horizon. Imagine the moon is floating just in front of your torso almost in your lap. Bring one hand and arm across the body just in front of your belly button as if circling underneath the moon. Bring the other hand and arm across the body about shoulder height as if circling above the moon. On an inhale, you will begin to switch the placement of the arms by lifting the top arm up and drawing the lower arm to the side. Following the breath, slowly continue unfurling and stretching the arms out to the side of the body in big arcs. As you exhale, complete the arcs and bring the hands and arms "back around the moon" with the opposite arms on the top and bottom. Keep the motion fluid and in tune with the breath. Repeat.

— SET 42 —

WOW Every problem contains the seeds of its own solution. – Stanley Arnold

3Rs When your parents asked you specifically not to do something and you did it anyway, what happened? What were your motivations for doing it? Did you get caught? Were you punished?

KISS 1. What do you call the dance where the dancers "go as low as they can"?
2. What is the unknown in algebra, the symbol for multiplication, and the Roman numeral for 10?
3. What is the largest library in the world?

---

20 http://www.guinnessworldrecords.com/records-1/memorizing-business-records/

SOS What do airline passengers and football players both want?

ICE You intentionally miss the bus for which you have bought a ticket. Why?

TAB If an EEG (a test that detects electrical activity in your brain) is hooked up to gelatin, it registers movements very similar to the brain waves of a healthy adult.

Mmm Feather-Duster Head – Imagine that you have feather duster growing out of the top of your head. Gently lift the head up to allow the feathers to touch the ceiling or sky. Lightly tickle the spot just above your head with the feather duster. Then if your neck feels fine gently expand the movement, making bigger swipes and circles, and maybe even dusting the corners of the room.

— SET 43 —

WOW The groundwork of all happiness is health. – Leigh Hunt

3Rs Have you kept any memorabilia from your childhood or family? If not, why not? If so, what is the "history" of the items? How special are they to you? What are your memories of "things" you no longer have?

KISS 1. Spell the word that means to spell incorrectly.

2. Which blood cells produce antibodies that fight disease, red or white?

3. Which of the following countries is not in Africa? Ghana, Guatemala, Kenya and Libya.

SOS You are on a horse, galloping at a constant speed. On the right side is a sharp drop-off, and on your left side is an elephant traveling at the same speed as you. Directly in front of you is a galloping kangaroo and your horse is unable to overtake it. Behind you is a lion running at the same speed as you and the kangaroo. What must you do to safely get out of this highly dangerous situation?

ICE A crowd has assembled; what are all the people looking at? Be creative!

TAB For our brain to be effectively attentive, it must be able to: (1) Quickly identify and focus on the most important item in a complex environment; (2) Sustain attention on its focus while monitoring related information and ignoring other stimuli; (3) Access memories that are not currently active, but that could be relevant to the current focus; and (4) Shift attention quickly when important new information arrives.

Mmm Cross Body: Hand to Foot – Sit in a comfortable position where your hands can reach your feet. Crossing your legs can help. Touch the palm of your right hand to the sole of your left foot, and the palm of your left hand to sole of your right foot. Stay with the sensation of your hands on the bottoms of your feet for a while. If it is too difficult to touch both feet at the same time, you can alternate sides, but the goal is to have the opposite hand and foot connected.

—— SET 44 ——

WOW Life is like a garden. Leave the flowers and pull the weeds. – Kelly Clarkson

3Rs How do you think others see you in terms of such things as the way you look, your personality, how you interact with them, etc.? What do you think they most like about you? Why?

KISS 1. What Pulitzer Prize winning novel is about the Joad family's migration to California?

2. What bird has the longest wingspan?

3. Name these famous pairs: Lewis and ___, Mark Anthony and ____, Juan Peron and ___.

SOS The answer to all of these questions will end with the sound "tee": What "tee" saves money? What "tee" has an inquiring mind? What "tee" is changeable and the spice of life?

ICE What would you make as a symbolic sculpture to represent you/your family?

TAB One way to help you remember what someone said is to link the information to an expression or feature on the other person's face.

Mmm Flower Gazing Meditation – Find a beautiful flower or plant that you like. Place the flower or plant about a foot or two away in a place where you will be able to look at it easily while maintaining a comfortable upright position. Breathe gently and focus your attention on the flower or plant by simply staring at it. Let your mind be filled with the image of the flower or plant; if your mind wanders, gently return your attention to it.

—— SET 45 ——

WOW A loving heart is the beginning of all knowledge. – Thomas Carlyle

3Rs Did you ever stay home alone as a child? How old were you? Describe your experience.

KISS 1. Whose famous "Overture" often accompanies fireworks on the 4th of July?

2. Name the colors of the rainbow from top to bottom.

3. The U.S. is divided into "States." Canada is divided into what?

SOS What is at the end of time?

ICE If you won a large sum of money, how would you creatively use the money?

TAB Thanking people for what they shared helps you remember what they said.

Mmm Appreciating Relationship Meditation – In this meditation you will visualize various relationships in your life—past and present—that have contributed beneficially to who you are now. You can make a list beforehand or just see who comes to mind in the meditation. Close your eyes and place your hands on your heart. . After a few breaths, identify at least one beneficial relationship that you appreciate from your life. Take the time to visualize that person as if that person were sitting in front of you right now. Look the person in the eye and smile. Tell the person how you appreciate him or her. Do this for as many relationships as you would like.

— SET 46 —

WOW Begin today! No matter how feeble the light, let it shine as best it may. The world may need just that quality of light which you have. – Henry C. Blinn

3Rs How do you wake up in the morning? Do you rely on an alarm clock, do you have someone else to wake you, do you wake up naturally, or something else? What time do you usually wake up? Is it the same each day or different? Does it take a while for you to wake up or do you wake up easily?

KISS 1. What are some words that end with the letter "i"?

2. In what galaxy is the earth?

3. What is the largest clothing manufacturer located in San Francisco? (Think denim.)

SOS What has two legs and talks behind your back?

ICE A woman comes into the kitchen with towels she just took from the bathroom. Think of possible reasons for her actions. Be creative.

TAB In a dialogue between Eastern Buddhist philosophers and Western neuroscientists, Matthieu Ricard traced the origins of the English word "emotion" to its Latin roots. He defines the Latin *emovere*, as "something that sets the mind in motion."[21]

---

21 Goldman, Daniel. (2003). *Destructive Emotions, How Can We Overcome them? A Scientific Dialogue with the Dalai Lama*. Narrated by New York: Bantam Books, p. 75.

Mmm Balancing a Book on the Head – Walk around the room with a book balanced on your head. How long can you go without dropping the book? How fast can you go?

— SET 47 —

WOW Every small positive change we make in ourselves repays us in confidence in the future. – Alice Walker

3Rs How healthy have you been as an adult? What have been your biggest health concerns?

KISS 1. What Shakespeare play begins with, "Two households, both alike in dignity, In fair Verona, where we lay our scene, From ancient grudge break to new mutiny"?

2. In which part of the body do you find the tibia?

3. What country gave the U.S. the Statue of Liberty?

SOS I took two apples from six apples. How many apples do I have?

ICE You have small children and there is chain linked fence all around the yard except for three feet in the front left corner; so you need to hook onto the neighbor's fence. You ask the neighbor if you can hook on and he says "Yes for $100." List at least three options you have, and pick the best option.

TAB The temporal lobe is on either side of the brain by your ears. It is primarily responsible for language, object recognition, and long term memory.

Mmm Temporal Lobe Meditation – Sit in a position of comfort with your back upright. Place your hands over your ears with the fingers pointing behind you. Close your eyes. After a few breaths, begin to focus on and visualize the temporal lobes of your brain. Imagine that you can actually see and sense these two areas of your brain beneath your skull where your hands are resting. What color do you visualize them as? What do they feel like? How do you imagine the sensations of the right side and left side as different, or do you? Which side seems stronger to you? Once your image is clear, play with altering the image in ways that might strengthen or nourish your temporal lobes. For example, since this area is associated with sound and language, you could imagine them as increasingly beautiful music, playing with different instruments. Thank your temporal lobes "with a thousand words" for the ways they help you to learn and function well.

— SET 48 —

WOW Disagree in an agreeable way. – Deane Beman

3Rs Remember your first "sleep over" away from home with relatives or friends? What was the occasion? How did you feel? How much did you miss your family? How much actual sleep occurred?

KISS 1. What is strung with horse hair and used to play many string instruments?
2. What insect is named for its prayerful attitude as it waits for its prey?
3. In what country can you KISS the Blarney Stone?

SOS You are driving a city bus. At the first stop you pick up eight people. At the second stop, you pick up nine and three get off. At the third stop, 13 get on and eight get off. What color are the bus driver's eyes?

ICE List things that shrink. Be creative!

TAB Different types of memories—for example, "what" and "how" memories—are stored and processed in different parts of the brain; and yet, because the brain is so well organized in its functioning, it can combine them into a "grand memory" in "the blink of an eye."

Mmm Cat-Cow – Get down on your hands and knees. Start with your back parallel to the floor and your head facing gently forward. Bring your awareness to your breath. On an exhale, pull the belly in tight, draw your chin down towards your chest, press your pelvis forward, and arch your back high (like an angry cat). Pause and hold breath out for a second. Then as you breath in, soften and round the belly, turn your eyes to look towards the ceiling, gently bring the head up, and draw the pelvis back and up to create a strong sway in the small of the back (like a cow) Pause and hold a second. Repeat for several breath cycles: Inhale – Cat; Exhale – Cow.

— SET 49 —

WOW Excellence is to do a common thing in an uncommon way. – Booker T. Washington

3Rs How would you describe one of your favorite dreams or daydreams you have experienced? Why is it a favorite?

KISS 1. List some contractions.
2. Name different types of clouds.
3. Name U.S. states that were once part of Mexico.

SOS What has cities but no buildings, and rivers but no water?

ICE You are in the airport waiting for an international flight. You have an expensive cello that you want to check at the gate but do not want to have to carry around while you wait. What creative ideas can you think of to keep the cello safe without lugging it around?

TAB A current randomized, double-blind study at UCLA focuses on curcumin for the prevention for Alzheimer's disease. Curcumin is found in turmeric and is responsible for the yellow color of curry and mustard. Curcumin is believed to protect the brain.[22]

Mmm Chair Neck and Upper Back Stretch – Sit on the front edge of a low-backed chair or stool with your with your legs uncrossed. Let your hands dangle at your sides. On a slow in-breath, gently raise your eyes up toward the ceiling allowing the neck to lengthen and curve back. Do not let the back of the neck scrunch or wrinkle. Keep your shoulders down and hands hanging heavily. Gently drop the scapula or shoulder blades as if they are reaching toward the seat of the chair. Resist the temptation to lift the shoulders. Hold briefly and release. Repeat once or twice more.

—— SET 50 ——

WOW Be who you are and say what you feel because those who matter won't mind and those who mind don't matter.—Bernard Baruch

3Rs How would you describe your personality? What part of your personality is most important to you? Why? In what ways do you see yourself as different from how others may perceive you?

KISS 1. How many syllables are in a haiku poem? (Hint: Three lines in a haiku)
2. What is "Pi" in math terms?
3. In what country is the world's largest gold mine?

SOS A professional person slaps someone until he cries. It's the right thing to do! Why?

ICE Using the letters S, T, O and P as the first letters of words, make up a complete sentence.

TAB Carotenoids and flavonoids are essential nutrients for good brain functioning. They are provided by a proper combination of apples, citrus fruits, carrots, dark leafy greens, fresh herbs, fresh beans and peas, garlic, grapes, leeks, mangos, olives, onions, red and purple berries, red bell peppers,

22 *Mind Health Report*, (2017) 8(9), 5.

spices, squashes, sweet potatoes, and tomatoes. Nutrutionists recommend one-to-two portions per day.

Mmm Eating Meditation: Gratitude – Get a small apple or other fruit or simple food that you like to eat. You are going to eat it with mindful awareness. Notice the smell, shape, color, texture, temperature, and weight of the fruit. Start to imagine where the fruit came from. Consider all the people and resources that brought it into being and into your hand. For example, it was a seed, planted by a farmer, nourished by the sun, rain and earth; it grew on a tree, was picked by workers . . . Take a bite. With each bite thank the various sources that brought the fruit to you to nourish your body and brain. Imagine you can "taste" the contribution of each of these sources in the fruit, and thank them for their contributions.

— SET 51 —

WOW Better to do something imperfectly than to do nothing flawlessly. – Robert Schuller

3Rs If you could be in any family portrayed on TV or in the movies, what family would you choose? Why?

KISS 1. Who uses a baton? A conductor, a football coach or a movie director?
2. What do you call the section of the spine that can "slip"?
3. What were the last three states to obtain statehood in the U.S.?

SOS Using people's first names, fill-in the blanks to create the given meanings. (1) Make a proposal: _____ _____ me? (2) Ask the students if they understand: _______ any questions? (3) See if anyone is in: _____ body home?

ICE Make as long and sensible sentence as you can using only words beginning with the letter "V."

TAB Researcher Brian J. Balin of the Center for Chronic Disorders of Aging at the Philadelphia College of Osteopathic Medicine theorizes that infections are a contributing factor in Alzheimer's. Evidence used to support the theory include the fact that patients with Alzheimer's given antibiotics for 3 months showed reduced rates of cognitive decline, and various studies that show increased rates (some as much as 85 higher) of certain viruses and bacteria in Alzheimer's brains compared to healthy brains. A 2016 study at Harvard University provides an explanation and lends further support to this theory.[23]

---

23 https://www.newscientist.com/article/2090925-vaccines-might-be-able-to-stop-alzheimers-plaques-from-forming/

Mmm Upper Back Arch – Kneel on the floor with the thighs and torso erect. Place the palms on the back of the thighs. Exhale and gently roll your head forward and tuck your chin in towards the chest. Hold for a few breaths. Then on an in-breath, lift the chin as you look toward the ceiling. At the same time brace your hands against the thighs and allow the back to arch gently as far as comfortable. Hold for a few breaths; then exhale as you return to an erect position. Repeat.

— SET 52 —

WOW Honesty is the first chapter of the book of wisdom. – Thomas Jefferson

3Rs Were you afraid of thunder and lightning as a child? What did you imagine was happening? How did your parents console you?

KISS 1. Name some helping verbs.
2. What big cat kills its prey by biting its skull?
3. Who are teddy bears named after?

SOS My friend and I were swimming when we saw a shark. I screamed, but my friend said, "Don't worry; we will wait until it sleeps and then sneak away." Was this sound advice? Why or why not?

ICE What ways could you keep from "tracking" dirt in the house? Be creative.

TAB There is approximately 125-150 ml of cerebral spinal fluid in your brain and spine. That's a little over a half cup.

Mmm Small Bridge – Lie on your back on the floor with the knees bent. Place the feet flat on the floor so that the heels are in line with the sit bones and the knees line up directly above the heels. Keep your arms along your sides with the palms down. Tighten the belly. Press down into the ground with your feet, shoulders, arms and hands. Inhale and push the pelvis a few inches off the floor. Hold for a few seconds. Then gently lower the pelvis back down to the original position as you exhale. Repeat once or twice.

— SET 53 —

WOW A people without the knowledge of their past history, origin and culture is like a tree without roots. – Marcus Garvey

3Rs If you could go back and relive any time in your life, when and where would it be? Why is that time in your life especially important to you?

KISS 1. What is a couplet?
2. Brass is usually an alloy of copper and which other metal?
3. Name some South American countries.

SOS What has four legs and two arms? Hint: In the house.

ICE You are a new superhero. What are your powers?

TAB A steady pace of digestion gives a more reliable flow of energy to the brain. Different foods digest at different rates.

Mmm Breathing Meditation: In Nose, Out Mouth – Sit or lie down in a comfortable position. Close your eyes. Notice whether you are breathing through your nose or through your mouth. For the next in-breath, close your mouth and breathe in through the nose. Then open your mouth and breathe out through the mouth. Repeat for at least ten breath cycles—in through the nose, out through the mouth.

— SET 54 —

WOW Give every [one] thine ear, but few thy voice. – William Shakespeare

3Rs Do you know people who have been named after people in history? What are those names? Who in history do you think it would be nicest to be named after? Why? Were you named after a person?

KISS 1. Who painted "The Night Watch"?
2. Who discovered gravity?
3. What is the most spoken language in the world today?

SOS What does no one want, but no one wants to lose?

ICE A family has a pair of identical twins. List as many ways as you can to tell them apart accurately.

TAB Research suggests that chewing gum has positive effects on the brain. It stimulates the production of serotonin and makes one much more alert.[24]

Mmm Rub Belly/Pat Head – Rub your belly and pat your head at the same time for a minute or so. Repeat switching which hand is on the belly and which is on the head. And for the true test: Can you chew gum at the same time?

— SET 55 —

WOW I wish my name was Brian because maybe sometimes people would misspell my name and call me Brain. That's like a free compliment. – Mitch Hedberg

3Rs Let's say you could invite any five famous people to a dinner party and they would all come, who would you invite? What kind of dinner would

24 Wenk, G. (Aug. 10, 2012). Gum chewing is good for the brain at https://www.psychologytoday.com/blog/yo1

you serve? How would you arrange the seating? What topic would you bring up? If you could meet any person in the world, who would it be? Why would you want to meet that person?

KISS 1. What do you sometimes add to an adjective to make an adverb?
2. What is the name of the skull bone which serves as the brain's "helmet"?
3. What mountains separate Europe from Asia?

SOS One hundred feet up in the air, it lies with its back on the ground. What would this be? (Hint: Tricky)

ICE What would you like to find in your mail? Why?

TAB Classroom tests and similar assessments of student knowledge and learning cannot verify if what the learner recalls actually came from long-term storage within the brain or short-term memory; reviewing material just before taking the test allows learners to enter the material into working memory for immediate use.

Mmm Getting Up and Down – Staying aware of your body throughout, mindfully get down on the floor. Notice how you chose to go down. As you feel ready, get back up to a standing position, still maintaining mindful awareness. Now go back down to the floor and get back up in a new way—different from the first time. Repeat, finding several different ways to get up and down. (For example, you can change speed, technique, attitude, style, etc.)

— SET 56 —

WOW A goal that is casually and lightly taken—will be freely abandoned at the first obstacle. – Zig Ziglar

3Rs When was the most memorable time you can remember when the electricity went out? Where were you? Who were you with and what were you doing? How many hours was it out? Why was it so memorable?

KISS 1. Name some musicians associated with Bebop.
2. What is the common name for *NaCl*?
3. What directions do latitude and longitude lines run?

SOS Put the same word before or after each of the words in the following sets to make common words or phrases: (1) down, in, out, walk; (2) language, neon, off, stop; (3) work, race, radish, power.

ICE What did the meatball say to the hotdog?

TAB Your brain can be conditioned to improve at any age, and dancing is one way of doing that. Researchers at the Albert Einstein College of Medicine published a study of senior citizens over a 21-year period that suggests regular dancing (3-4 times per week) improves cognitive skills at any age.[25]

Mmm Waltz Rhythm – The basic waltz rhythm consists of three beats with a strong one-count. To accomplish a waltz rhythm, step firmly on your left foot, and take two lighter steps—right then left—on the balls of the feet. Repeat, and alternate which foot does the strong first step. The rhythm is: RIGHT-two-three; LEFT-two-three. Feel free to add music and move around the room with a real or imaginary dance partner.

— SET 57 —

WOW An investment in knowledge always pays the best interest. – Benjamin Franklin

3Rs If you had only one picture left to take in your life, what picture would you take? Why?

KISS 1. What four types of instruments are in an orchestra?
2. What is No. 2 on the Elements Chart? (Hint: It's used to fill toy balloons.)
3. Which Scottish town is known as the home of golf?

SOS What month is next? April, August, December, February, January, ______.

ICE Which would you prefer? To run a mile on a deep bed of potatoes or to swim an eighth of a mile through table syrup? Why?

TAB A University of Pennsylvania Medical School study by Andrew Newberg and Dharma Singh Khalsa showed that eight weeks of daily practice of the Kirtan Kriya yoga meditation (see below) improved blood flow to the brain significantly.

Mmm Kirtan Kriya Meditation – Sit in a position of comfort with an upright spine and the back of the hands resting on the legs. One at a time, press the tip of each thumb to the tip of each finger and say the corresponding syllable as follows, starting with the index finger. As you touch your index finger, say "SA" (rhymes with "raw"). At middle finger, say "TA." At the ring finger, say "NA." At the pinkie finger, say "MA." Repeat. Do this for two minutes aloud and visualize the sound extending up and out the top of your head and forward out from between your eyebrows. Repeat whispering the syllables and again saying them silently in your head. Then go back to whispering and out loud. The Alzheimer's Research &

---

25 Verghese, J., et al. (2003). Leisure activities and the risk of dementia in the elderly. *The New England Journal of Medicine* 348:2508-2516.

Prevention Foundation (ARPF) recommends practicing the full Kirtan Kriya meditation daily for 12 minutes a day.[26]

— SET 58 —

WOW Luck favors the mind that is prepared. – Louis Pasteur

3Rs Did you like telling riddles or jokes as a child? Why? What was your favorite riddle or joke when growing up?

KISS 1. What parts of speech are these: he, her, I, me, etc.?
2. How many sides does a decagon have?
3. What country has the most volcanoes?

SOS A man is accused of a serious crime. It was legal to do it once but not twice on the same day. What did he do?

ICE You are asked to wear a tie to a performance, but you do not want to do so. What are some creative excuses you might use?

TAB Unlike any of the other senses, the sense of smell is directly connected to the limbic system, which is the part of the brain that processes emotions and stores memories.

Mmm Scent Journey – Take a nice inhale through the nose. What do you smell? Now take a walk outside or journey through the space you are in and notice what different smells you can find. For example, if you are outside, smell the plants around you.

— SET 59 —

WOW Live as if you were to die tomorrow. Learn as if you were to live forever. – Mahatma Gandhi

3Rs What brand and model was your first car? What was its color, cost and how long did you have it? Was it a good car for you at the time? What are some of your most special memories pertaining to that car? If you never owned a car, describe your experience of managing transportation.

KISS 1. H. A. Rey wrote a children's picture book with a mischievous monkey. What was the monkey's name?
2. How many permanent teeth does a typical adult have?
3. Where was the Mughal Empire?

SOS Start with the word "Mom" and change one letter at a time to get to the word "Dad", making real words at each step. Mom ____ ____ Dad.

---

26 http://www.alzheimersprevention.org/research/12-minute-memory-exercise.

ICE Make a list of things you cannot touch.

TAB Early brain surgeons and scientists used electric probes to touch different parts of the brain. They discovered that different types of memories are linked to different parts of the brain and that some parts of the brain are important to memory while others are not.

Mmm Kirtan Kriya Meditation: Reverse Order – Do the Kirtan Kriya Meditation in reverse order for two minutes. One at a time, press the tip of each thumb to the tip of each finger and think the corresponding syllable as follows, starting with the pinkie finger this time. As you touch your pinkie finger, say "MA." At the ring finger, say "NA." At middle finger, say "TA." At the index finger, say "SA." Repeat whispering; and then say them silently in your head.

— SET 60 —

WOW Always the beautiful answer who asks a more beautiful question. – e. e. Cummings

3Rs Suppose you were asked to write an article or book, what would be the topic? Why? Who would be the target audience for your book? Why?

KISS 1. Name some percussion instruments. (Hint: Ones you strike.)
2. What insect can help tell the temperature in the summer in Fahrenheit?
3. In what country is the Great Barrier Reef?

SOS Take a word for what you plant on Arbor Day, and add a letter of the alphabet (on the front or back) to get something that sounds like an agreement between nations. Example: A rubber wheel (tire) plus the letter N = All (N-Tire = Entire).

ICE Name unusual uses for an old fashioned egg beater.

TAB People's temperament is more strongly associated with the ratio of activity in the amygdala, and left and right prefrontal cortexes than with life circumstances. This explains why a 1978 study comparing paraplegics, ordinary people, and lottery winners found that within a year of a major event, people's moods shift back to the same "normal range" as before the event.[27]

Mmm Hugging the Big Tree – Sit comfortably on the front edge of a chair with spine upright. Throughout this exercise keep the tummy in, the spine long,

27 http://www.ncbi.nlm.nih.gov/pubmed/690806

shoulders pulled back, and head level as if gazing at the horizon. Start by bringing the arms out in front of just below shoulder level. The fingertips meet so that the arms form a large circle as if you were hugging a big tree. On an inhale, pull the arms apart to open up the circle. At the peak of the inhale, hold the arms still and gently close the hands. As you exhale, open the hands and following the flow of the exhale, bring the hands back to close the circle. At the peak of the exhale, you should be back in the starting position. Gently close the hands, and open them again as you inhale and start the motion again. Keep the motion fluid and in tune with the breath. Repeat.

— SET 61 —

WOW I have never seen a monument erected to a pessimist. – Paul Harvey

3Rs In which store would you choose to be "trapped" overnight, if you had a choice? Have you ever been "trapped" anyplace?

KISS 1. List times you should use a comma.
2. Give the wrong answer! Which runs faster, a grizzly bear or a squirrel?
3. The 18th amendment was the only amendment to the U.S. Constitution that was ever repealed. What did it deal with? Hint: Think of the Roaring Twenties.

SOS What do you call a fly with no wings?

ICE If you were a dentist, what fun things might you say to someone while drilling, knowing the person cannot reply?

TAB According to Wallace J. Nichols, being in, near and around water has a positive "blue mind" effect on our brains and overall wellbeing. He claims that "blue mind" contrasts with and heals stressed out, overactive "red mind" and dull, lethargic, "gray mind."[28]

Mmm Water Gazing Meditation –Many of us naturally slip into meditative states when we are near bodies of water. If you have body of water accessible, feel free to do this meditation there. If not, water gazing can be practiced with a small bowl of water. Find a beautiful clear bowl or glass, fill it with clean water, and place it where you can gaze at the water in it comfortably. Breathe gently and focus your attention on the water by simply staring at

---

28 Nichols, Wallace J. (2014). *Blue Mind. : The Surprising Science That Shows How Being Near, In, On, or Under Water Can Make You Happier, Healthier, More Connected, and Better at What You Do. New York: Little Brown.*

it. If your mind wanders gently return your attention back to your breath and the water.

— SET 62 —

WOW Birds sing after a storm; why shouldn't we. – Rose Kennedy

3Rs What favorite recipe would you share with others? Why? Have you shared it with your family and friends already?

KISS 1. Name some of the works of Jane Austen.

2. Which is longer, a day on Earth or a day on Mars?

3. Who in 27 B.C. became the 1st emperor of Rome?

SOS Starting with the word "SIDE", change one letter at a time to make "WALK" without changing the order of the letters.

ICE How many ways can you think of to keep a license plate clean?

TAB Learning takes place on both sides of the brain for nearly every human activity, although it is true that the left hemisphere of the brain processes "parts" sequentially while the right hemisphere processes wholes.

Mmm Cross-Body: Head, Shoulders, Knees and Toes – Place your Right hand on the Left side of your face. Then place your Left hand on the Right side of your face. Your forearms will form an "X" across your body. Move on down the body touching each hand to the opposite side's shoulder, knee, ankle, and toes. Then climb back up the body touching the same points across the body. Repeat several times.

— SET 63 —

WOW Both tears and sweat are salty, but they will render different result. Tears will get you sympathy; sweat will get you change. – Rev. Jesse Jackson

3Rs Did you attend a place of worship when growing up? If so, how did it affect the activities in which you participated and the values you came to appreciate? If not, how were your values/activities different from others who did participate in organized religious gatherings?

KISS 1. Five commonly recognized eras of classical music occurred from 1400AD to 2000AD. Name one or more.

2. What part of the body usually has the thickest skin?

3. What country is home to the highest city in the world?

SOS How many seconds are there in a year? Hint: Don't work too hard.

ICE A snake and a mouse are talking. What are they saying?

TAB Intentionally putting on a facial expression changes your emotion. The expression activates activity in the brain and body to shift in the direction of that emotion. So if you fake a smile or frown, you will start to feel more happy or sad as a result.[29]

Mmm Funny Face – Make faces at yourself in the mirror. Imagine you are in a contest to see who can come up with the funniest face.

—— SET 64 ——

WOW We are now in the mountains and they are in us, kindling enthusiasm, making every nerve quiver, filling every pore and cell of us. – John Muir

3Rs If you could ask anyone in the world a question, which person would it be, and what would you ask?

KISS 1. List as many synonyms for "cried" and for "grumpy" as you can; then write ten synonyms for "great".

2. What does deciduous mean?

3. What war began with an attack on Fort Sumter?

SOS Brown, Green and Black were having lunch. Green said, "Although our ties have colors matching our names, none of us has a tie matching our own name." "You are right," said Brown. "And the color of my tie doesn't even start with the same letter as my name," said the third man. What color was each man wearing?

ICE Your cell phone battery is low and you need a tow truck for your broken down car. You dial the wrong number. How can you convince the person who answers to call a tow truck for you?

TAB Animal studies have found that diets rich in blueberries significantly improved both the learning capacity and motor skills of aging rats, making them mentally equivalent to much younger rats. The blueberries help protect the brain from "oxidative stress. Some experts suggest that avocados, apples, broccoli, cranberries, kiwi, lemons, oranges, purple grapes, and spinach may have a similar positive affect.

Mmm Seated Meditation: Mountain Solid — Sit in a position of comfort with your back upright. Close your eyes. On your next inhale begin to visualize yourself as a mountain, large and stable. Imagine the sensation of your seated buttocks as the wide solid base of the mountain and your head as

29 http://ncbi.nlm.nih.gov/pmc/articles/PMC37

surrounded by cool alpine air. Then as you exhale, visualize the sensation of the stability of the mountain within you. As you inhale say in your mind, "Breathing in, I see myself as a mountain." Then as you exhale say, "Breathing out, I feel solid." Continue for at least 10 breath cycles.[30]

— SET 65 —

WOW Be wiser than other people if you can, but do not tell them so. – Earl of Chesterfield

3Rs In what ways do you relax? How might you relax more? What makes you feel most relaxed?

KISS 1. What play was Abraham Lincoln watching when he was assassinated?
2. Name the three basic kinds of rocks.
3. Which two rivers vie for the title of longest river in the world?

SOS List twelve-letter words.

ICE List as many compound or known phrases using the word "work" as possible.

TAB Every second of your life, several billion bits of information pass through your neurons and are evaluated by your brain.

Mmm Grapevine Step – The basic grapevine step consists of a sideways movement with one foot alternately crossing in front of and behind the other. Start by crossing the left foot in front of the right, and then sidestep the right foot back out to its normal position. Repeat 2-4 times moving to the right. Then shift to the left by crossing the right foot in front of the left, and sidestepping the left foot back out to its normal position 2-4 times. Put on some music or make your own. Grapevine around the room, making up your own arm movements.

— SET 66 —

WOW I learned that courage was not the absence of fear, but the triumph over it. The brave [person] is not [one] who does not feel afraid, but [one] who conquers that fear. – Nelson Mandela

3Rs If you were writing a book about your life, what chapters would you include? What were some of the best parts of your life? What were some of the hardest parts?

KISS 1. How many are singing in a duet, a solo and a trio?

30 Nhat Hanh, Thich. (2009). The Blooming of a Lotus. (Revised). Boston: Beacon Press.

2. If you were buying carpet for a 12'x12' room, how many square yards would you need to order? (Hint: A = L x W)
3. The first ten U.S. constitutional amendments are considered the Bill of Rights. Name as many of those rights as you can.

SOS Read the clues to figure out what this is: It's very complicated. It opens and closes. Sometimes it's very strong. It can hold a book. It's divided into a small part on one end and is bigger on the other. Parts of it may be painted. Everyone has it. It has five main sections. It can be lent, but not given away.

ICE You have a three-inch hole in your roof and no tarp. Rain and sleet are predicted. You can get no help, and roofing supplies are unavailable. What might be some quick fixes?

TAB Three creatures are known to be able to remember the way they look in a mirror—the orangutan, the pigeon, and the human. Of the three, humans have the shortest visual memory; they are the only ones of the three who can turn around and instantly forget what their own faces look like.[31]

Mmm Mirror Gazing Meditation – This meditation can be done seated with a small hand mirror or standing in front of a larger hanging mirror. Breathe gently and focus your attention on your reflection by simply staring at it. If your mind wanders gently return your attention back to your image in the mirror. Does your image change?

— SET 67 —

WOW I'd rather be hated for who I am than loved for who I am not. – Kurt Cobain

3Rs Did you go to any dances? What were some of the kinds of dances kids did when you were young? How did you learn to dance? Did someone teach you to dance or did you have to learn on your own? What was that like? What was the first dance you attended, and how was it? If you didn't dance, why not?

KISS 1. When do you use a colon?
2. Which bone is "no laughing matter" when you hit it?
3. What feuding Scottish clan might also make you think of soup?

SOS Sarah wrote the letters A, B, C, and D in a special order. She wrote C before B and after D. She wrote A after D and before C. What was the order of the letters?

---

31 http://www.sciencedaily.com/terms/mirror_test.htm

ICE Congress has declared a new national holiday, "Encouragement Day." You are in charge of organizing the local Encouragement Day festivities in your local community. What are your plans?

TAB The brain is 85% water and water ions are an excellent conductor of electricity. Water contributes to nerve development, more efficient storage and retrieval of information, and faster processing of higher level thinking. Drinking less than 80 ounces of water a day can adversely affect your brain function.[32]

Mmm Drinking Meditation: Body Hydration – During this meditation, you will bring awareness to water as it becomes part of your body. Get a clear glass of water to drink. Start by gazing at the water in the glass. Notice its liquid form—flowing, swishing, taking the shape of its container, etc. As you drink, visualize the water as it enters, integrates with and passes through your body. With each sip imagine that you can sense the water not just in your mouth and throat, but also in your belly, combining with your digestive fluid, becoming part of your bloodstream, nourishing your cells, lubricating your joints, purifying and eliminating toxins, and carrying messages for your brain cells!

— SET 68 —

WOW By approaching my problems with "what might make things a little better?" rather than "What is the solution?" I avoid setting myself up for certain frustration. My experience has shown me that I'm not going to be able to solve anything in one stroke. At best, I'm only going to chip away at it. – Hugh Prather

3Rs How have you shown your appreciation to loved ones and friends? How did they respond? How could you express your appreciation even more?

KISS 1. What anti-Semitic book with a title meaning "my struggles" was written in German and contributed to the Holocaust?

2. From what tree do Koala bears eat the leaves?

3. What is the lowest, driest and hottest point of land in North America?

SOS Find the favorite food of Aspen, Bradyn, Hannah, and Jack, using the following clues: (1) Jack likes catsup and mustard; (2) Hannah is allergic to cheese; (3) Bradyn eats his favorite on a bun; (4) Sometimes Jack makes

---

32 http://www.waterbenefitshealth.com/water-and-brain.html

his favorite into corn dogs; (5) The foods are chicken, hot dogs, pizza and cheeseburgers.

ICE While walking in the library, Aspen spies a large purple book. What is a good title for this book?

TAB It will help you to remember who attended a class or meeting if you can create a picture of them sitting there in your mind and then associate the names with each individual in that mind picture.

Mmm Raising and Lowering the Limbs – Lie on your back in a comfortable position. On an inhale, allow your arms and legs to rise up in the air. Then with your exhale, gently let them fall back down to the ground. Repeat for at least ten breath cycles.

—— SET 69 ——

WOW It takes both the sun and the rain to make a beautiful rainbow. – John Ruskin

3Rs Based on your experience, do you think your country is the best place to live? What would you change about your country? Why would you make those changes? What would you want to never give up about your country? Why? If you could change anything in the world beyond your country, what would it be? Why?

KISS 1. Name some of Michelangelo's sculptures?
2. True or false: Radioactivity is man-made.
3. During the late 19th and early 20th centuries, many immigrants to the U.S. passed through what New York City landmark?

SOS Put the same word before or after each of the words in the following sets to make common words or phrases: (1) wares, keeper, full, guest; (2) high, board, book, grade; (3) store, lace, horn, tennis.

ICE Denise puts spoons in the freezer. Explain. What are some possibilities?

TAB Ideal movement practices for promoting brain health involve breaking patterns, controlled breathing, and visualization. When done with intentional, relaxed awareness of emotions, sensations and thoughts, such movement can helpfully stimulate the lateral prefrontal cortex and the amygdale, which manages anxiety, emotion, and fear.[33]

Mmm Painting a Rainbow – Start with an upright spine, and hold both arms out to your sides at shoulder level like the letter "T". Turn the palms up. Keeping

33 http://www.care2.com/greenliving/6-surprising-things-that-affect-your-brain.html

one arm in place, inhale and arc the other arm up over your head, and bring it to rest on the opposite hand. Imagine that the colors of the rainbow trail behind your fingers. Paint a rainbow with the other arm. Repeat on alternating sides for a total of 12 repetitions.

— SET 70 —

WOW Anytime you see a turtle up on top of a fence post, you know it had some help. – Alex Haley

3Rs In what ways is the world a "better" place now than it was when you were growing up? Why? In what ways is the world "worse" now than when you were growing up? Why?

KISS 1. What is the most commonly used word in the English language?
2. What does the "e" in e-mail stand for?
3. In what country is the Suez Canal located?

SOS How many words can you make by adding three letters within the sets of letters that follow: c_ _ _t, f_ _ _n, g_ _ _t, h_ _ _r?

ICE Think of things that come in threes.

TAB The EEGs of a highly-trained and experienced meditation practitioner doing meditations on compassion shows a "remarkable" shift in brain activity in the area associated with happiness and joy. The degree of shift was scientifically unlikely to have occurred by chance alone.[34]

Mmm Compassion Meditation: Close your eyes, and place your hands on your heart. On the next breath, invite a memory of yourself as a very young child. See your younger self in front of you as you were then—happy or sad, active or passive, troubled or happy-go-lucky. Smile to your younger self. In your mind give that child a hug. Send the child you were gentle, loving compassion.

— SET 71 —

WOW Kind words can be short and easy to speak, but their echoes are truly endless. – Mother Teresa

3Rs In your mind, retell a story or novel you have read. What was your opinion of the story or novel? What person would especially enjoy this story or book? Why?

---

34 http://www.scmp.com/news/asia/article/1072585/buddhist-monk-matthieu-ricard-happiest-man-known-science

KISS 1. What fairy tale originally had a young woman losing a fur slipper that in later translations became a glass slipper?
2. What caused the "Black Death" that killed one-third of the population of Europe?
3. To what does Black Tuesday refer? What year did it happen?

SOS Explain: 4 cows + 2 birds + 1 spider = 28.

ICE List as many words as you can that have "ring" in them.

TAB Dr. Dean Shibata of the University of Rochester's School of Medicine, conducted MRI research that locates the part of the brain that recognizes a joke. It is in the right frontal lobe "just above the right eye."[35]

Mmm Eye Dancing – Put on some music or make your own music. Using just your eyes, "dance" to the music. You can play with changing eye directions, opening and closing lids, winking, blinking, fluttering, squinting, etc.

—— SET 72 ——

WOW Happy is the [one] who has broken the chains which hurt the mind, and has given up worrying once and for all. – Ovid

3Rs In your opinion, when and where would it have been the most interesting to live? Why?

KISS 1. In reading music, how many counts are there for a whole note in 4/4 time?
2. What is a terrarium for?
3. How long was the "100 Year War"?

SOS What word can go before "in" or "out", but follows "eye"?

ICE How many new uses can you think of for a sock with a hole in it?

TAB Unnecessary worry is a serious waste of brain power. Worry and stress negatively affect the brain's ability to apply logic and reasoning, make meaning and understanding, relate effectively to others, remember, solve problems, synthesize and think abstractly.

Mmm Breathing Meditation: Counting Breaths – As you breathe, count each breath. In-breath is one; out-breath is 2. Do not consciously alter the rhythm of the breath to ease the counting. If you lose count or your mind starts to wander return your attention to the breath and start the count again at one. How high can you count without distraction?

---

35 http://abcnews.go.com/Technology/story?id=98399

— SET 73 —

WOW Do not use a hatchet to remove a fly from your friend's forehead. – Chinese Proverb

3Rs How did you celebrate New Year's Eve growing up? Did you ever make any New Year's resolutions? What were they? How long did you successfully keep those resolutions?

KISS 1. How do you spell the word that starts with "s" and is paper used to write and send a letter in the mail?

2. What do you call vapor changing to a liquid?

3. What two Asian countries have almost half the world's population?

SOS What number can you take away half of it and leave zero?

ICE What could you do to keep the Wicked Witch of the West from melting?

TAB It has been estimated that there are 100 trillion, or more, neural connections in your brain and that messages travel through those connections at up to 250 or 300 miles an hour.[36]

Mmm Hand Shaking – Stand in a comfortable hip-width stance. Begin to gently shake your hands as if shaking water off of them. Gradually let the shaking get more vigorous so that the forearms and elbow shake, too. Eventually bring the shaking all the way up to the shoulders. Shake fast and slow. Giant shakes and mini-shakes. One side and then the other.

— SET 74 —

WOW Act as if each day were given to you as a gift. – Anonymous

3Rs What is the greatest piece of music that has ever been composed? Why?

KISS 1. Name two other characters in the tales of Robin Hood.

2. If you are going to build a fence around a yard that is 100' long and 75' wide, how many feet of fence would you need to have? Hint: $P = 2(L + W)$.

3. From what country did we get the following foods: hamburger, pretzel, pumpernickel, sauerkraut?

SOS For each of the following, fill in the blanks so that all your answers rhyme with "brain": (1) A headache is a brain ______; (2) The central genius is a _____ brain; (3) A tiresome mind puzzle is a brain _____.

ICE How many things can you think of that have numbers on them?

36 http://www.scientificamerican.com/article/100-trillion-connections/

TAB Things learned just before going to bed are usually remembered better than things learned early in the morning.

Mmm Breathing Meditation: Count Down – Close your eyes and observe your breath. Starting at 10, count backwards for each breath.) Do not consciously alter the rhythm of the breath to ease the counting. If you lose count or your mind starts to wander, return your attention to the breath and start the count again at 10. Repeat for 5 rounds of 10.

— SET 75 —

WOW A person who angers us controls us. – Elizabeth Kenny

3Rs In your opinion, what was the best television show ever produced? Why?

KISS 1. What are the four main vocal parts of a choir?

2. Hinges, pivot, and ball-and-joint socket are three types of what skeletal structure?

3. Name the four oceans of the world. Which ocean is the largest?

SOS If a daddy bull eats three bales of hay a day and a baby bull eats one bale of hay a day, how many does a mommy bull eat?

ICE You have been contacted by a large car company to improve on the standard car. What would you change?

TAB Anger and frustration manifest in the brain differently depending on how the emotion is directed or expressed. Most anger and frustration activates the amygdale and right (negative side) prefrontal cortex. However, "approach behavior" such as when frustrated by solving a very hard math problem, activates the left (positive side) prefrontal cortex.

Mmm Tango – Imagine you are in Argentina and do "your" version of a tango dance. Be dramatic. A rose between the teeth is optional!

— SET 76 —

WOW If at first you do succeed, try something harder. – Ann Landers

3Rs How did you get to school when you were young? What time did you have to be there? Were you ever late? Why or why not?

KISS 1. Make a list of homophones. For example, deer and dear.

2. How do most worms get inside apples?

3. What is located at 1600 Pennsylvania Avenue in Washington, DC?

SOS Put the same word before or after each of the words in the following sets to make common words or phrases: (1) pot, coffee, green; (2) bull, car, French; (3) chip, sweet, couch.

ICE List some squishy things.

TAB People with the rare disorder "agnosia" (damage to areas of the occipital or parietal brain lobes) can't recognize and identify objects, and they may not know whether a person's face is familiar to them.

Mmm Open and Close the Face – Open your face as wide as you can—raise your eyebrows, pop your eyes, drop your jaw fully, and open your mouth into a big "O." Stretch as wide as you can. Then close your face as tight as you can—furrow your brows, squeeze your eyes shut, scrunch up your nose, clench your jaw, and pucker your lips into a sour-lemon-mouth. Move back and forth several times.

— SET 77 —

WOW Happiness is found along the way, not at the end of the journey. – Robert R. Updegraff

3Rs Is there a particular place or type of place you like to go when you want to be alone? Where? Why do you like to go there? Do you ever bring others to that place? Why or why not?

KISS 1. What do these three men have in common: James Joyce, Homer, and John Milton? Hint: Handicap and profession.

2. What is the chemical formula for water?

3. The Maori are the native people of what island?

SOS What U.S. state is round at the beginning and end and high in the center? Tricky!

ICE Name things with the word "end" in them.

TAB Rosemary was traditionally used for concentration and mental clarity. In medieval times it was known as the herb of remembrance, and some people believed that it could restore your youth. A 2013 Study in England, seems to confirm this brain boost.[37]

Mmm Walking Meditation: Steps and Breath – Practice the mindful walking meditation again. This time while maintaining awareness of the sensations of your steps, bring awareness to your natural breathing as well. Notice how many steps you take for each in-breath and for each out-breath. Notice that it is likely that the out-breath may be longer than the in-breath or the other way round. In your mind say "IN" for each step on an in-breath and "OUT" for each out-breath—"In-in-in . . . Out-out-out-out . . ."

---

37 http://www.sciencedaily.com/releases/2012/02/120224194313.htm

— SET 78 —

WOW In the end, we will remember not the words of our enemies but the silence of our friends. – Martin Luther King, Jr.

3Rs How did you lose your first baby teeth? Did someone help you pull them out? Did a "tooth fairy" come? If so, what did the tooth fairy leave you? Did you have lots of fillings in your teeth?

KISS 1. What Greek city was the center of ancient theater?

2. Which stars are the hottest: black, blue, brown, orange, yellow, red, or white?

3. What's the name of the world's highest mountain range?

SOS In what month do Americans eat the least amount of pizza?

ICE The answer is "ridiculous." What is the question?

TAB It's no accident that telephone and license plate numbers in the United States are seven digits long. A human's short-term memory can process about seven numbers at a time and store them just long enough to get to the phone and dial.

Mmm In the Swim: Flutter Kick Front – Lie on your belly on a bed so that the legs extend off the bed. Stretch the legs out straight and point the toes. Do a flutter kick by alternately raising and lowering the legs without bending the knees. See how fast you can go and for how long. Try for at least one minute.

— SET 79 —

WOW In the spring, at the end of the day, you should smell like dirt. – Margaret Atwood

3Rs Make a list of all the things you do to take care of your body. Upon reflection, what changes are needed?

KISS 1. List ten prefixes.

2. Is the main function of the red blood cells to fight disease in the body, carry oxygen to all parts of the body, or help the blood to clot?

3. What is the name of the man who led the Chinese communist revolution and governed China until his death in 1976?

SOS Jackson's mother had three children. The first child was named April and the second child was named May. What was the third child's name?

ICE The answer is "pigeons." What is the question?

TAB When you are awake, your brain generates 25 watts of power. That's enough to light up an incandescent light bulb.[38]

Mmm Visualization Meditation: Spring – Metaphorically, spring is a time of newness: seeds sprout and eggs hatch. This meditation can be used to reflect on the season or to invite freshness and new ventures in some phase or aspect of your life. Close your eyes, and visualize yourself or some area of your life as a seed in the earth. Sense the sunlight above warming the soil and inviting you to stir and transform yourself. Send out tiny tendrils into the soil, grounding you as you reach upward toward the sunlight breaking through the surface of the earth and sprouting. Feel your fresh greenness as you stretch up toward the light.

— SET 80 —

WOW Solve the problem or learn to live with it. – Renie Lenning

3Rs List your favorite musical hits. Do you remember the words? What do they portray? Did you ever go to a concert or watch any music TV shows? What was that like for you? Has your taste in music changed?

KISS 1. According to the literature, what supposedly started the superstition that the number "13" is unlucky?

2. What kinds of mammals are involved in fox hunting?

3. What desert did Marco Polo cross to reach China? It is also the world's coldest desert.

SOS How can you build puppy pens so you can put nine puppies in four pens so that each pen has an odd number of puppies?

ICE Why did the chicken cross the road? Be creative.

TAB Several studies using MRI, found that acupuncture has a positive effect on the cerebrum, an area of the brain associated with memory and cognition.[39]

Mmm Ear "Workout" – Try to wiggle your ears. Can you do it?

— SET 81 —

WOW We are now in the mountains and they are in us, kindling enthusiasm, making every nerve quiver, filling every pore and cell of us. – John Muir

38 Banyard, P., Dillon, G., Loman, C., & Winder, B. (Eds.). (2015). *Essential Psychology*, 2nd ed. Thousand Oaks, CA: Sage.

39 http://www.healthcmi.com/Acupuncture-Continuing-Education-News/1281-acupuncture-mri-scan-shows-alzheimer-s-disease-benefit

3Rs Think of your favorite things. Why is each of them among your favorites?

KISS 1. How many keys are on a piano?
2. When lava cools, does it become igneous or sedimentary rock?
3. Since 1700, what happens every ten years to count the U.S. population?

SOS Bryan is looking at a photo. His friend asks who it is. Bryan says, "Brothers and sisters have I none; but that man is my father's son." Who is in the photo?

ICE Name things that stick to each other?

TAB The brain needs periods of high-level attention (concentration/thinking/reflection) interspersed by periods of low-level attention (downtime). Various studies indicate that down time in the form of naps, meditation, and time in nature actually increases productivity and refresh attention.40

Mmm Nature Time – Spend some quiet time moving around in nature today, whether gardening in your yard, hiking in the woods, soaking up sun, going for a walk in a park, etc.

— SET 82 —

WOW A goal properly set is halfway reached. – Zig Ziglar

3Rs How did your family discipline you? Did that need to happen a lot? What did you need to be disciplined for?

KISS 1. Make a list of compound words.
2. What makes a whip "crack"?
3. Who was emperor of Japan during WWII?

SOS Draw a circle and divide it with four straight lines. What is the maximum number of areas within the circle one can attain through this process?

ICE Why would someone listen to 24 hours of "The Flight of the Bumblebee" on the radio or watch "snow" on the television?

TAB In 1977, master chess player James Flesch played 52 chess games simultaneously while blindfolded. To do this, he had to picture each chess board in his mind, keep track of every move, and plan countermoves in each game.[41]

Mmm Leg Shaking – Lift your left foot off the ground and begin to gently shake it as if you had something stuck to the bottom of your foot that you want to get off. Really let that ankle joint move. Gradually let the shaking get

---

40 Jabr, Ferris. (October 15, 2013) *Scientific American*, Why Your Brain Needs More Downtime. http://www.scientificamerican.com/article/mental-downtime/

41 https://booksgoogle.com/books?isbn=1616080248

bigger and more vigorous until the whole leg is involved. Then put that foot down and do the other side. Once you have done both legs, you can move back-and-forth between the two legs.

— SET 83 —

WOW Make the most of the best and the least of the worst. – Robert Louis Stevenson

3Rs Of all the books and stories you have read, which character would you most like to emulate? Why?

KISS 1. What do the following have in common: Allegory, alliteration, hyperbole, Onomatopoeia, simile?

2. Round 329 to the nearest hundred.

3. Name the country where you would find the Alps, the Danube River, Innsbruck, and Vienna?

SOS The more Chris took away, the larger it grew. His parents were happy even though he got dirty and made a big mess. In the end, he helped start a new life. What was he doing?

ICE List as many "things that are equal" as you can. Be creative.

TAB Research indicates that one's mind can consciously focus on only one train of thought at a time. For the brain to be maximally effective in problem-solving, and to keep related stress to a minimum, focus on one problem at a time.[42]

Mmm Breathing Meditation: In-Breath – Observe the breath. Now focus your mind on the in-breaths only. For each in–breath, count one. Then wait for the next in-breath, and count two. And so on up to ten. If you lose count start again at one. Do two or three sets.

— SET 84 —

WOW The difference between ordinary and extraordinary is that little extra. – Jimmy Johnson

3Rs Who would you most like to trade houses with? Why? How is their house different?

KISS 1. What does *allegro* mean in music?

2. Who was the founder of the Red Cross?

3. Who won Indian independence through non-violence?

---

42 http://www.npr.org/templates/story/story.php

SOS What is the missing letter in this logical sequence: D, D, P, V, C, __, D, B. Hint: Think of Santa.

ICE You have just won 2 free tickets to any event in the world that you want, but you can buy no more. What event would you go to see?

TAB Oxford University researchers have suggested that after a trauma there's a 6-hour window when memory formation can be disrupted.

Mmm Matador – Imagine you are a famous bullfighter. Strike a pose. Wave your cape. Sidestep and turn as the bull charges by you. Continue through a full bullfight.

—— SET 85 ——

WOW Nothing is IMPOSSIBLE; the word itself says I'M POSSIBLE! – Audrey Hepburn

3Rs In your view, what are the most important characteristics for the leader of our country? Which one is the most important of all? Which presidents have had that characteristic, and which have not?

KISS 1. How many syllables are in the word "astronomical"?
2. What cat is the fastest running animal?
3. Name the country where you would find, Moscow, St. Petersburg, Siberia, and the Ural Mountains.

SOS The job required good eyesight. A blind man arrived and went right to work on it. The Hills were very pleased with his work and did not help him with it at all. Explain.

ICE Come up with words that make sense for the "made-up" words in the following nonsense sentence: "When did you creb the komyst, or did it bursk the limmer by asdumy?"

TAB *American Journal of Lifestyle Medicine* indicates that over time, regular moderate resistance training significantly helps to reduce anxiety, enhances memory, and improves overall analytical brain functioning for men and women of all ages.[43]

Mmm Downward-Facing Dog – This is a weight-bearing exercise. In the final pose, your body will form an upside-down V-shape, supporting your own bodyweight with your arms and legs. Start on your hands and knees. Spread your fingers and press your hands strongly into the floor. Turn your toes under. Lift the buttocks up and back as you start to straighten the knees. Keep

43 http://www.unm.edu/~lkravitz/Article%20folder/RTandMentalHealth.html

the back straight. Shift the weight of the body back more on the heels than on the hands. If your calves or back are tight you may want to keep the knees somewhat bent. Do not sacrifice the line of the back to straighten them.

— SET 86 —

WOW Friends are those rare people who ask how we are and then wait to hear the answer. – Ed Cunningham

3Rs Recreate in your mind the smell of an orange; the smell of lavender; the smell of peanut butter.

KISS 1. What type of literary device is the following: Sweet Sally sang several solos in September.

2. List science words that begin with C, G, M, S, T.

3. Nine presidents of the U.S. did not go to college; name four of them.

SOS A mother and her kids slept outside on a cold winter night. The neighbors knew about this and did not call the police or invite them in. Explain.

ICE Create wacky, overly literal definitions for the following terms: cupcake, log jam, spring cleaning, and turkey dressing. For example, a butterfly is "a pound of butter on the wing."

TAB The occipital lobe is located at the back of the brain, and it is primarily responsible for visual processing.

Mmm Occipital Lobe Meditation – Place your hands on the back of your skull behind your ears. Begin to focus on and visualize your occipital lobes. Imagine that you can actually see and sense this area of your brain inside your skull where your hands are resting. What color do you visualize the occipital lobes as? What do they feel like? How do you imagine the sensations of the right side and left side as different, or are they? Which side seems stronger to you? Once the image is clear for you, play with altering the image in ways that might strengthen or nourish your temporal lobes. For example, since this area is associated with vision, you could imagine it with brighter and clearer colors or as an increasingly beautiful mosaic. Thank your occipital lobe for the ways they help you to "see things clearly" and function well.

— SET 87 —

WOW Keep your head cool, your feet warm, and your mind busy! – Anonymous

3Rs Remember a time when the outdoor temperatures seemed really cold. Where were you? How bad was it? How did you manage the cold?

KISS 1. What instruments usually make up a string quartet?
2. What does URL stand for in electricity and web addresses?
3. What was the Santa Maria?

SOS Mr. Bragg said "Three of our players hit home runs and two were hit with the bases loaded. We won 9 to 0 and not a single man crossed home plate. Explain.

ICE The answer is "ole" What is the question?

TAB Once information is mastered, it behaves as a "chunk" of information. The amount of information a person can deal with at one time correlates to the ability to add more items to the chunks already in working memory. Chunking is a learned skill that is not genetically linked.[44]

Mmm Seated Meditation: Reaching to the Sky – Sit in a position of comfort with your back upright. On an out-breath, visualize yourself growing taller like a plant reaching toward the sunlight. Then imagine the crown of the head reaching up beyond the limits of your physical body.

—— SET 88 ——

WOW I cannot teach anybody anything; I can only make them think. – Socrates

3Rs How healthy were you as a child? What was your experience of going to the doctor or other healthcare provider? Did you like it or were you afraid? How about shots and other medicine? What lasting effects did your childhood health experiences have on the rest of your life?

KISS 1. Which word is not of Native American origin? kayak, kindergarten, potato?
2. Name sports that do not use a ball.
3. Name the country where you would find Mount Vesuvius, Naples, Rome and Sicily.

SOS Al, Sue, Bob, and Pam play different sports in their high schools. One plays soccer. The basketball player's school mascot is the Tiger. Only one of the young men plays a sport with a ball. Appropriately, the student who is in Track has a Road Runner for a mascot, and the swimmer's mascot is a water creature. Al does not have to run for his sport. Pam scored the winning points in the final seconds of her last game, and the same night

44 http://www.thepeakperformancenter.com/education-learning/thinking/chunking/chunking-as-a-learning-strategey/

the Shark's won on a penalty kick. Bob is not Dolphin. What sports do they each play, and what are their respective mascots?

ICE What would be the best "qualifications" to have to be the bus driver for a rock band?

TAB Choline—provided by beef, cabbage, eggs, peas, peanuts, sardines, soybeans, wheat germ, and whole grains—is an essential nutrient for good brain functioning. Nutritionists recommend one-to-two portions of cholines per day.

Mmm The Great Shake-Out – With this exercise, you will move through the major joints of the body, shaking them out. Start with the head shaking it gently like a bobblehead. Then shake your shoulders, elbows, wrists and hands, hips and buttocks, each knee and leg, each ankle and foot. Imagine you are a wet dog shaking off water after an unwanted bath.

— SET 89 —

WOW Character consists of what you do on the third and fourth tries. – James Michner

3Rs Reminisce about a particular day during your life. Where are you? Who are you with? What happened?

KISS 1. In the line "A host, of golden daffodils" from the poem "Daffodils," what literary device is represented by the repeated long-o sound, assonance or consonance? For a bonus: name the poet who wrote it.

2. What very unusual things do all crocodiles eat?

3. Two women had been on one-dollar coins prior to 2005. One was an advocate of women's suffrage and one was the Shoshone guide for the Lewis and Clark expedition. What were their names?

SOS Joy was reading a book when the power went out. She continued reading even though it was totally dark. Explain.

ICE List things that wiggle.

TAB Left-handed people are ten percent of the population. According to research, they are often more spontaneous and quicker thinkers than right-handed people, and they are better at math, remembering things, and designing in 3-D.[45]

Mmm Opposite Hand Eating – Eat with your non-dominant hand sometime today.

---

45 http://www.Seattletimes.com/nation-world/whats-so-special-about -left-handers/

— SET 90 —

WOW Give to every other human being every right that you claim for yourself.
– Robert G. Ingersoll

3Rs Some people will only buy brand names. How important is it for you to buy a brand name? What particular brands do you especially like? Is it cost or brand name that most determines what you will purchase?

KISS 1. Which composer is considered to be Father of the Symphony?
2. What is a hexagon?
3. What state has four time zones?

SOS Use the same letters in the same order to make this sentence make sense: A _o_a_l_ surgeon had _o_a_ _ _ and therefore was _o_ a_l_ to operate.

ICE We can logically connect one word to a sequence of words. For instance, the word "fudge" leads to "chocolate," leads to "candy store," etc. Think of a sequence of five or more words starting with the word "snap."

TAB From a very early age, people's brains show differences in emotional reactions to situations. The research suggests that people who can recover a calm state more quickly after being provoked, have less activation in the amygdale and more activation in the left (positive side) of the prefrontal cortex.[46]

Mmm Walk as if : Emotions – To practice emotional resilience, take a few minutes to walk as if you were a person in the following emotional states. Walk as if you were: 1) Angry; 2) Sad; 3) Afraid; 4) Excited; 5) Worried; 6) Happy.

— SET 91 —

WOW We often take for granted the very things that most deserve our gratitude.
– Cynthia Ozick

3Rs How strict were your parents? Were they too strict, not strict enough, or were they "just right"? Describe some examples of rules your parents had.

KISS 1. Name three adverbs that describe how you work.
2. Which sports use each of these terms: spare, par, love and field goal?
3. What does the acronym POW stand for?

SOS Start with the word "Wild" and change one letter at a time to get to the word "Tame", making real words at each step. Wild ____ ____ ____ Tame.

---

46 Goldman, Daniel. (2003). *Destructive Emotions, How Can We Overcome them? A Scientific Dialogue with the Dalai Lama.* Narrated by New York: Bantam Books, p. 75

ICE By mistake you have been hired to do a job that you know nothing about. What will you do the first day?

TAB Reflection is different from ranting or venting emotions. Reflection reshapes the brain's plasticity. It promotes greater problem solving tools to create positive change in the situation, whereas ranting and venting do not encourage change in the brain.

Mmm Flip It – Write a list of things you are dissatisfied with in your life. Stand up and read your list aloud one at a time. After your read each item think of a way that you can "flip it" by thinking of something that is positive about that thing. For example, if on your list you put that you hate cleaning the house, you could flip it by saying, "I am grateful that I have a home to live in and keep clean." Say each new statement out loud and strong.

— SET 92 —

WOW Remember when life's path is steep to keep your mind even. – Horace

3Rs Suppose you could have been a successful actor. Of all the movies that have been ever produced, what movie and role would you have chosen? Why?

KISS 1. Who was the Harvard Square bookstore owner whose memory was so good he made a book of quotations?

2. What is the average life span of a dog?

3. What was the sequence of the following events: 1st cultivation of land; the Pyramids; the wheel?

SOS Find a one word answer to the following so that the last two letters of each answer are also the first two letters of the next answer. Bedtime attire: Fever buster: A bluish color: A digging rodent: Wipe the board: Harsh: Go to bed.

ICE You are on the governing council for an ant colony. Create some rules for the colony.

TAB "Micro-expressions" are brief facial expressions that pass in less than a fraction of a second. Extensive research at the University of California at San Francisco Medical School indicates that people whose brain can accurately interpret emotional micro-expressions are more empathic, conscientious, reliable, efficient, curious, and open to new experiences.[47]

---

47 Ekman, Paul. (2009). *Telling Lies*. New York: Norton.

Mmm Cross Body: Arm Swing Full Circle – Stand with your feet hip-width apart. Let your arms hang loose at your sides. Twist at the waist first to the right and then to the left. Allow your arms to swing with the momentum of the movement. Gently "pump" with the legs to build momentum until the arms slap the opposite shoulder as you go.

— SET 93 —

WOW Nothing is a waste of time if you use the experience wisely. – Auguste Rodin

3Rs If you had been awarded a scholarship to develop a specific talent in one of the fine arts, which of the arts would you choose and what role would you develop within that art form? Why?

KISS 1. What does *forte* mean in music?
2. Which one of the following is an example of a chemical reaction: nail rusting, sugar dissolving, or water boiling?
3. Which U.S. ocean coast is the longest, the Atlantic or the Pacific?

SOS Bev lived in the mountains and Lea lived by the coast, and they both were boiling eggs. Who gets her eggs boiled in less time?

ICE A thought is like what?

TAB Numerous studies show that the mental clarity and judgment of someone who is sleep deprived can be as severe as someone who is legally drunk. In addition, a lack of sleep can intensify the negative effects of alcohol on reasoning and brain functioning.

Mmm Breathing Meditation: Out-Breath – Sit or lie down in a comfortable position. Observe the breath. Now focus your mind on the out-breaths only. For each out–breath, count one. Then wait. For the next out-breath, count two. And so on, up to ten. If you lose count start again at one. Do two or three sets of ten out-breaths.

— SET 94 —

WOW We must not cease from exploration. And the end of all our exploring will be to arrive where we began and to know the place for the first time. – T.S. Eliot

3Rs How was money handled in your family? Did you have an allowance? If you did have an allowance, how much did you get, and did you have to work for it? If you did not have an allowance, how did you ask for or get spending money, or did you not get any? What did you do with any money that you received?

KISS 1. List a verb starting with the letters: "c", "g", "m", "s", and "t".
2. What is the Big Bang?
3. Which month was named for Julius Caesar?

SOS Jan has great hunting ability but does not always tell the truth. If he tells you that he killed a panther, a mountain lion and a puma at the same time, could he be telling the truth.

ICE Peacocks are tired of their look. Create in your mind a new look for them.

TAB Much research over the years indicates that the brain is naturally designed to view anything from a number of different creative angles and perspectives.

Mmm Sensing with Curiosity – Close your eyes and breathe for a few moments. When you open your eyes again, imagine that you are in this space for the very first time as if you are a baby or an alien from another planet. Everything is new and unfamiliar. Explore the space with your senses as if you are curious to discover more about it. Imagine that each thing you see, hear, smell or touch is something you are encountering for the first time. What do you notice?

— SET 95 —

WOW Although the tongue weighs very little, few people are able to hold it. – Anonymous

3Rs Suppose you could live anywhere in the world expense-free. What locale or city would you choose? Why?

KISS 1. What famous novel has as its subtitle "*A Story of the Old House*"?
2. Is it a fact that honey is less fattening than sugar?
3. Where would you find Mount Fuji?

SOS In order to keep fish from tasting flat after capture because they do not move around in the tank, what would be the easiest way to keep the fish swimming?

ICE List things that can be flipped.

TAB There is a word for the feeling that a word is on the tip of your tongue. It's . . . uhm . . . "anomia."

Mmm Tongue Meditation – Lightly touch the tip of your tongue to the roof of your mouth as if you were about to say the letter "T." The whole mouth and jaw should be relaxed. Allow the "body" of the tongue to rest in the lower jaw. Let the jaw be loose and open. The lips can be closed gently or slightly parted. Close your eyes and focus on the sensation of contact between the tongue and the roof of the mouth for several breath cycles.

— SET 96 —

WOW Originality is nothing but judicious imitation. – Voltaire

3Rs How was your name chosen? What is the story behind it? Who chose the name and why? Would you rather have had a different name? What and why? What is the story behind your last name?

KISS 1. In what country was Johann Sebastian Bach born?

2. Which has more muscles, a caterpillar or a human being?

3. What does GNP stand for?

SOS Corrie was driving in her car when it shifted gear by itself. Why wasn't she worried?

ICE The following are common sayings with the ending listed in parentheses. Replace the part in parenthesis to create new alternative endings: Busy as a (bee) ________; Stubborn as a (mule); Arrogant as a (king).

TAB Your brain's cerebrum is divided into two hemispheres. The right hemisphere deals especially with attention, rhymes, poetry, tunes, music, awe, inspiration, emotions, creativity, etc. The left hemisphere deals more often with sounds, words, meanings, logic, analysis, synthesis, active reflection, application, etc.

Mmm Scalp Massage – Place the fingertips of both hands along either side of the crown of your head just above the center of your forehead. Pressing down firmly wriggle your fingers to massage the scalp. Work your way back along the middle part of the head to the base of the skull. Repeat massaging in rows from front to back until you have done the entire scalp.

— SET 97 —

WOW I was a freethinker before I knew how to think. – George Bernard Shaw

3Rs If you had won 100 million dollars in the lottery early in your life, how would you have used the money? Why?

KISS 1. What part of speech is each word in this sentence? "WOW! The brown dog jumped quickly over my fence and gate."

2. List as many gemstones as you can.

3. In colonial times, what was the basic ingredient of soap?

SOS A genie came to Mike's house and Mike was granted his wish. Mike was shocked when he found a hundred deer in his back yard. Explain.

ICE The state you live in is having a contest. You need to come up with an original new motto for your state. What is it?

TAB Memory involves a number of abilities. You need to make a number of perceptual associations, and also continually work to recall and use what you are learning. Failure to do so results in forgetting half of what you learned within 30 minutes, and the rest gradually fading and disappearing over time.

Mmm Seated Meditation: Water Reflecting — Sit in a position of comfort with your back upright. Close your eyes. On an in-breath begin to visualize yourself as a still body of water, clear and calm. Imagine the sensation of your liquid body as still water with light reflecting off the surface leaving the water's calm and stillness. Then as you exhale, visualize the surface of the water within you reflecting things clearly and calmly. As you inhale say in your mind, "Breathing in, I see myself as still water." Then as you exhale say, "Breathing out, I reflect all that is." Continue for at least 10 breath cycles.[48]

—— SET 98 ——

WOW Courage doesn't always roar. Sometimes courage is the quiet voice at the end of the day saying "I will try again tomorrow." – Mary Anne Radmacher

3Rs If you had the money access to buy any famous artwork in the world, which would you choose? Why?

KISS 1. What are the opening words to *A Tale of Two Cities* by Charles Dickens?
2. What is the next number for each number set? 14, 15, 17, 20, __.
3. What is the "Mile High City"?

SOS Is it possible to pick up a piece of rope with one end in each hand and tie a knot in the rope without letting go of either end of the rope? If so, how?

ICE Don't assume. Think! Jennifer appeared to be sleeping. When she woke up and saw the masked man, she knew she would be alright. Explain.

TAB Approximately one in five people in the U.S. suffer from damage to the nervous system. That is about 50 million people in all.[49]

---

48 Nhat Hanh, Thich. (2009). The Blooming of a Lotus. (Revised). Boston: Beacon Press.

49 National Institute of Neurological Disorders and Stroke, Brain Basics: Know Your Brain (April 28, 2014) at http://www.ninds.nih.gov/disorders/brain_basics/know_your_brain.htm

Mmm Making Circles – Walk around the room in circles. Make circles with your arms and legs. too. Make large circles and small circles. High circles and low circles.

— SET 99 —

WOW Some see things as they are and say "Why?" I dream things that never were, and say, "Why not?" – George Bernard Shaw

3Rs How well did you know your grandparents (or other older people such as uncles and aunts) when growing up? Describe your relationships with them. Did you have favorites? What are some of those special memories?

KISS 1. Who was the "Godmother of Rock and Roll"?

2. Is it a fact that it is legal for a customer to remove the mattress tags from a mattress purchased?

3. What did Alfred Nobel, for whom the Nobel Prizes were named, invent?

SOS Find a one word answer to the following so that the last two letters of each answer are also the first two letters of the next answer. When dried it is a raisin: Permanently frozen earth: Place where pigs are kept: A severe tropical storm: The beginning of something: And so forth.

ICE A publishing company wants to publish your memoir for a large sum of money. All they ask in return is for three or more titles. What will you call your book?

TAB Contrary to popular assumptions, extremely creative people often have a method to approaching a creative problem. Creative aids such as the SCAMPER technique help stimulate the brain to generate more unique ideas.[50]

Mmm The Bunny Hop – If you know the song you can hum or sing along with the movement. Stand in a comfortable stance. If you have fellow bunny hoppers stand in a line with each person's hands on the hips of the person in front of them. If you are alone, just put your hands on your own hips. Start with the right foot. Pick up the foot and touch the heel down out to the side. Return the foot back to center. Again put the heel out to the side and bring it back to the center. Repeat with the left foot: Heel out, center, heel out, center. Hop like a bunny on both feet: forward once, backward once, forward one-two-three. Repeat at least five times.

---

50 http://www.creativethinkingwith.com/SCAMPER.html

— SET 100 —

WOW Only those who see the invisible can do the impossible. – Bernard Lown

3Rs Suppose you could have a free, three-week vacation each year to any place in the world. Where would you go and why?

KISS 1. Use the word "fancy" in a sentence as a noun, verb and adjective.
2. Which fish in South America is one of the most vicious and dangerous fish in the world?
3. Bali and Java are islands in what nation?

SOS Find a one-word answer to the following so that the last two letters of each answer are also the first two letters of the next answer. Not stale: humiliation: Unkind: Addition: Not including.

ICE Tim and Bob were playing with a little birdie. Tim hit it very hard. It landed near Bob. The crowd cheered. Explain.

TAB A 2014 study led by neurologist Leslie Vosshall of Rockefeller University in New York City estimates that the human nose and brain are capable of distinguishing a trillion different scents from one another.[51]

Mmm Eye Crunches – Close your eyes and squeeze them tight for a count of five. Release and repeat 5 times. Next, do the same opening your eyes as wide as you can. Now keeping your head facing forward, look with both eyes to the right as if there is something just outside of your view that you want to see without drawing any attention. Hold for a count of five, then return your gaze to the front. Do the same looking left, then down, then up above your head. For each, hold for a count of five before returning gaze to center, and repeat 5 times.

— SET 101 —

WOW One who asks a question is a fool for five minutes; one who does not ask a question remains a fool forever. – Chinese Proverb

3Rs Laws are not easy to change, but if you could change (or enact) one law, what would it be? Why?

KISS 1. Who kept a diary while hiding with her family in an Amsterdam attic during World War II?
2. What gas do most scientists believe causes temperatures in the atmosphere to rise: carbon dioxide, helium, nitrogen or radon?
3. What is an MP?

---

51 http://news.sciencemag.org/biology/2014/03/human-nose-can-detect-trillion-smells

SOS Mississippi – can you spell it without using any "s"?

ICE List as many words, compound words, or paired words as you can using color words. Be creative.

TAB The two hemispheres of the brain are intimately interconnected and work together. For example, in processing speech, the left hemisphere specializes in distinguishing sounds and determining words and syntax, while the right hemisphere tunes in to the emotional or relational aspects of language communicated in the rhythm, accent, and tone of voice.[52]

Mmm Standing Meditation: Reaching to the Sky – Stand with your feet in a narrow to hip-width stance. Sense the feet on the ground and the vertical line of your body. Breathe, and sense a strong connection to the earth like a magnet. Then on an out-breath, visualize yourself growing taller like a plant reaching toward the sunlight with the crown of the head reaching up beyond the limits of your physical body. When you are ready to end the meditation, pat your belly a few times to reground.

— SET 102 —

WOW I don't have to attend every argument to which I am invited. – Anonymous

3Rs Did you ever give a name to a special toy, stuffed animal, or other inanimate object? What happened to that toy or object?

KISS 1. How many beats are in "measure in ¾ time"?
2. What is considered a vacuum in science?
3. What are the Swiss Guards most known for guarding?

SOS What do all of the following have in common: shoe, loaf of bread, and sock?

ICE Name items with labels.

TAB A 2013 study at Harvard concludes that drinking two cups of cocoa a day may assist cognitive health because chocolate produces an increased blood flow to the brain.[53]

Mmm Dish Washing Meditation – Mindfully wash the dishes by hand today. Bring as much attention as you can to the sensations of the dishwashing process. Fully sense the water as you fill the sink. Sense your arm and hand reaching for each dish. Feel the weight and texture of each dish as you wash it. Sense the soapy water and the sponge or wash cloth in your hand.

---

52 Zimmer, Carl. http://discovermagazine.com/2012/apr/07-brain-connections-may-be-key

53 http://www.sciencedaily.com/releases/2013/08/130807204447.htm

Notice the shape and movements of scrubbing and wiping and rinsing each dish, etc.

— SET 103 —

WOW The secret of patience is to do something else in the meantime. – Spanish proverb

3Rs Of all of those in your family, who do you think had/has the warmest personality and biggest smile? Why?

KISS 1. Correct the double negative in the following sentence: She doesn't have nobody to mow her lawn.

2. Which of these is a major concern about the overuse of antibiotics: Antibiotics are expensive. It can lead to antibiotics-resistant bacteria. People will become addicted to antibiotics?

3. What percentage of the earth's surface is covered with water?

SOS Chris was bragging about the animals he owned. Chris said, "I have all pigs but two, all cows but two, and all horses but two." How many animals does Chris own?

ICE You have been hired to design a new seal for your town. What will it look like? Why?

TAB The brain of Albert Einstein weighed 11.4 ounces, compared to the average human brain weight of about 3 pounds.[54]

Mmm Pushing a Boat – Throughout this exercise, keep the muscles of the hands and arms activated and move as if pushing them though a great force. Hold your hands out in front of you with the fingers together and the thumbs away to the side so one hand forms an "L" shape and the other forms a reverse "L". Maintaining the "L" shape, bring the hands to your sides. Take a solid stance with knees slightly bent. Then as if resisting a great force, bend the elbows to bring the L-shaped hands up to the armpits. Touch the heels of your hands to the ribs. Twist the wrists and forearms so that the palms now face away from you; the elbows and upper arms will come up and point out to the sides just below shoulder height. Focusing on the palms of the hands, imagine that you are pressing on the backside of a large boat. Push the heavy boat away from you until your arms are fully extended. Hold for several breaths. Then, turn your palms toward each other and strongly use your shoulders and arms to "pull the boat back,"

54 https://faculty.washington.edu/chudler/ein.html

returning the hands first to their position by the armpits, and then down to your sides again. Repeat.

— SET 104 —

WOW The flower that follows the sun does so even on cloudy days. – Robert Leighton

3Rs Think about friends from your past. What were their names and what did you especially like about them?

KISS 1. What American woman won a Pulitzer Prize for her novel titled *The Good Earth*? (She later won a Nobel Prize for Literature for other works.)

2. What adult fish has both eyes on one side of its head?

3. Who began the American Institute of Public Opinion (polls) in 1935?

SOS Fill in the blanks with homonyms (words that sound the same, but are spelled differently): The ghost of Blackbeard sails the seven ________. Any sailor who _______ the ghost ship, may _________ his heart in fear.

ICE Which would you choose: Every contest you come in second, or you come in last four times but win every fifth contest? Why?

TAB It will help you to remember something if you can associate it with a rhyme and a simple rhythm. The brain likes hearing slogans that rhyme, knowledge that has been used with great success in advertising.

Mmm Eensy Weensy Spider – There's nothing like a second childhood moment. Ω Touch the index finger of one hand to the thumb of the opposite hand. Rotate the hands around the connected thumb and finger to touch the other thumb to the other index finger (eensy-weensy spider-style). Release the first thumb and index finger connection, and rotate back the other way around, keeping the newly connected thumb and index finger in contact. Repeat several times. Reciting the poem is optional. If this brings up fond memories of childhood or times with children and grandchildren, feel free to sing.

— SET 105 —

WOW Vitality shows in not only the ability to persist but the ability to start over. – F. Scott Fitzgerald

3Rs Think about a time you had to forgive someone. What was the situation? How did it make you feel? For what things in your life was it important to be forgiven?

KISS 1. In a music score, what does the 8 in 6/8 time mean?
2. Does "nanotechnology" deal with things that are extremely: cold, hot, large or small?
3. What two states border eight other states?

SOS If seven people each shake hands only once with each of the others, how many total handshakes will there have been?

ICE If a movie were being made of your life, who would you cast to play you and your family and friends?

TAB In addition to neurons, which "do the thinking," the brain also contains glial cells. Glial cells provide support functions to the neurons, such as supplying nutrients and developing insulation.

Mmm Earth Meditation – Sit or lie down on the earth. Contemplate how the earth supports you through gravity, maintaining an atmosphere and regular livable temperature, producing food, etc.

— SET 106 —

WOW A fundamental law of the mind is: We act in accordance with what we believe to be true. – Anonymous

3Rs Of all of those in your family, who do you think was the funniest? Why?

KISS 1. Change the word "communicate" to a noun.
2. What is the name for what is left over when doing a division problem?
3. Who is the governor of your state?

SOS Dave owned a construction outfit and there was stealing going on by the employees. Josh was a suspect. Every night he would leave pulling a wagon behind him. Security checked each time and found that nothing in the wagon was being stolen. What was Josh stealing?

ICE How many new uses can you think of for a single pillowcase?

TAB It has been estimated that there are approximately a trillion glial cells in your brain. They are needed by all of the neurons in your brain to speed up their ability to transmit signals.[55]

Mmm In the Swim: Breaststroke – Do a swimmer's breaststroke. Bring the palms together in front of the breastbone with fingers closed and elbows bent. Keeping the palms in contact, straighten the elbows to push the hands forward in front of you. Turn the palms out and push the hands and arms

55 http://www.discoverymagazine.com/2009/sep/10-dark-matter -of-the-human-brain/

away from each other out to the sides of the body. Then rotate the hands up under the upper arms to return to the starting position. Repeat.

— SET 107 —

WOW Dwell in possibility. – Emily Dickinson

3Rs Think about a time you deceived someone. Why did you do it? How did the deceit affect you and those who knew you?

KISS 1. Name the word meaning a Greek goddess, a part of the eye, and a type of flower.

2. Is it true or false that one should have at least one hot meal a day because hot food is more nourishing?

3. What did the following men have in common: Alexander Graham Bell, Beethoven, Edison, and President Herbert Hoover?

SOS What single word has four e's and five s's?

ICE List reasons for a person to fake fainting.

TAB Our brains have rhythm. Neuroscientist Nathan Urban describes the rhythmic nature of brain cells firing as "little clocks" with "intrinsic frequency." Some cells fire fast and some fire slow.[56]

Mmm Rhythm Work: Syllable Clap – Clap on the syllables and pause on the periods to create the following rhythm: Clap. Clappa clap. Clappa clap. Clap, clap. Repeat and increase speed as you get it.

— SET 108 —

WOW Don't let what you cannot do interfere with what you can do. – John Wooden

3Rs Think about a time your feelings were hurt. What were the circumstances? Would that hurt your feelings today?

KISS 1. What is a plié?

2. What is the difference between white rice and wild rice?

3. Name five small countries.

SOS How can you make eight 8's equal 1000?

ICE Remember Rapunzel in the fairy tale, the one who let down her long hair so her rescuer could climb up to her. How could Rapunzel have rescued herself?

---

56 http://www.npr.org/sections/health-shots/2014/06/17/322915700/your-brains-got-rhythm-and-syncs-when-you-think

TAB Research suggests that during childhood, the brain makes more synapses than it needs. It later scraps those that experience shows are not needed. It has been estimated that from early childhood until puberty, synapses are being scrapped at the rate of one hundred thousand synapses per second as new and more complex constellations of synapses are created and utilized by the brain. A 2014 Columbia University study suggests that autistic children's brains do not do enough scrapping, which results in too many synapses.[57]

Mmm Eensy Weensy Spider: All Fingers – Do the eensy weensy spider movement. Touch an index finger to the opposite thumb, and. Rotate the hands around the connection and to touch the other thumb and index finger. But on the second round, pass over the index finger to connect the thumb to the middle finger instead. Continue in this way walking the thumbs down to the pinky finger and back up to the index fingers.

—— SET 109 ——

WOW A journey of a thousand miles must begin with a single step. – Lao-Tzu

3Rs Did you go to a school banquet, formal, prom or other special event? Why or why not? If so, where was it held and who did you go with? What did you wear? What were the theme and decorations? What time did you get home? What was the experience like, and what special memories do you still have of the event?

KISS 1. Spell the word that is Native American for shoes made from animal hide.
2. What is the lightest element found naturally on Earth?
3. What event was a major impetus for the U.S. to enter World War II?

SOS If you put a coin in an empty bottle and insert a cork into the neck of the bottle, how can you get the coin out without taking out the cork or breaking the bottle?

ICE What are some things that stretch?

TAB Learning physically changes the brain. Every new experience we encounter actually alters the brain's electrochemical wiring.[58]

Mmm Walking Meditation: Heel Roll Ball Lift – Practice the walking meditation. Once you can maintain mindful awareness of the sensation of your foot

57 https://www.autismspeaks.org/science/science-news/brain-study-finds-evidence-autism-involves-too-many-synapses

58 http://bigpictureeducation.com/can-learning-physically-alter-brain

stepping on the earth, see if you can go deeper into your awareness. Notice when your heel first touches the ground. Then notice as your weight shifts from the back foot to the front foot as the foot rolls forward to the ball of the foot. Then notice when the ball of the back foot presses and lifts off the ground. In your mind, label each part of the process as you experience it: "Heel . . . Roll . . . Ball . . . Lift . . ." You will probably want to walk quite slowly.

— SET 110 —

WOW Thank God every morning when you get up that you have something to do which must be done whether you like it or not. – Charles Kingsley

3Rs Think of the insect pests you experienced throughout your life. Which was the most annoying? Why?

KISS 1. The following is a quote from the Pablo Neruda poem "The Lemon." In this quote, is the comparison with a cathedral a simile or a metaphor? "Cutting the lemon the knife leaves a little cathedral: alcoves unguessed by the eye"

2. The moon is primarily made up of what substance?

3. About how many miles is it from the eastern-most coast to the western-most coast of the continental U.S.?

SOS Make as many words as you can of at least three letters each from the word "confidential".

ICE The following are common sayings with the ending listed in parentheses. Replace the part in parenthesis to create new alternative endings: You catch more flies with (honey than vinegar). All work and no play (makes Jack a dull boy). Fools rush in (where angels fear to tread). Slow and steady (wins the race).

TAB The frontal lobe is the largest area of the brain, and is located in the front of the brain behind your forehead. The primary functions of the frontal lobe are to plan, organize information, and regulate emotions and behavior. This area of the brain is not fully developed until people are in their 20s.

Mmm Rhythm Work: Syllable Clap/Slap/Stomp – Clap, stomp and slap your thighs to create the following rhythm: Stomp stompa slap slap. Slap slappa clappity. Clap clappa clapity. Stomp Stomp. Slap Slap. Clap Clap. Repeat and increase speed as you get it.

— SET 111 —

WOW It is always good to be a little kinder than necessary. – James M. Barrie

3Rs Think about the life you have lived; what would be the title of your autobiography? What kind of film would it make, and what should be the title? Who should write the script, and who should direct? Of living actors, who would you choose to play yourself in the film? Why?

KISS 1. In what country was ballet first developed?

2. Which type of solar radiation does sunscreen protect the skin from: Infrared, Microwaves, Ultraviolet, or X-rays?

3. How many presidents have been impeached?

SOS Why are manhole covers round rather than square?

ICE Which is strongest: ideas, knowledge, or dreams? Why?

TAB For most people, high levels of activity in the left pre-frontal cortex correlate to positive emotions such as happiness, enthusiasm, and high energy. High levels of activity in the opposite side correlate to experiences of distressing emotions, such as anxiety and sadness. A 2013 study found these opposing emotions share some common neural building blocks.[59]

Mmm Pre-Frontal Meditation – Sit in a position of comfort with your back upright, and place your hands on your forehead. Close your eyes and bring your attention to your breath. After a few breaths, begin to focus on and visualize the area of your pre-frontal cortex. Imagine that you can actually sense the pre-frontal cortex of your own brain, which is behind your forehead and above your eyes. Once that image is clear for you, play with moving your focus back and forth from the right pre-frontal cortex to the left pre-frontal cortex to balanced in between. Possible images you can try are a light getting brighter or dimmer on one side and the other, sounds getting louder or quieter, or water or sand pouring from one side to the other. Use whatever metaphor or image works for you. How are the sensation of the right side and left side different for you? Which side seems stronger to you? Now use the imagery to begin to strengthen the sensation of the left pre-frontal cortex which is correlated with more positive emotional states and dim down the sensation of the right pre-frontal cortex.

---

59 http://www.psycholigicalscience.org/index.php/publicaions/observer/obsonline/fear-happiness-and-sadness-share-common-building-blocks.html

— SET 112 —

WOW Life isn't about waiting for the storm to pass. It's about learning to dance in the rain. – Vivian Greene

3Rs Did you go to college, tech school or some other training after high school? Why? If so, where did you go and what attracted you there? What was your major? Why? How did your going to school or not relate to your career?

KISS 1. Which of the words that follow is the head of a school: Principal, Principality, or Principle?

2. Is it true or false that snakes bite with their tongue?

3. From what country did we get these foods: casserole and croissant?

SOS Take a word for something you might get sweet or dill, and add a letter of the alphabet (on the front or back) to get a high-pitched band instrument.

ICE List at least four famous pairs.

TAB Synesthesia is the neurological term for when the brain automatically connects together sensations that other people experience separately. For example, words may be connected to visual images (colors, pictures, shapes) or to some combination of other senses such as smells, tastes, touch, etc.

Mmm Floor Cleaning Dance – Take some time today cleaning the floor. Make the experience into a dance. Bring rhythm and flow to your movement. Glide around the room. Imagine that the broom, mop, and/or vacuum cleaner is your Fred Astaire or Ginger Rogers. Sashay, swivel, dip and twirl.

— SET 113 —

WOW Those who wish to secure the good of others have already secured their own. – Confucius

3Rs What would a song about you be titled, and who would you choose to compose and to sing it? Why?

KISS 1. In the following quote from the traditional Scots song and poem by Robert Burns is the comparison with a rose a simile or a metaphor? "My love is like a red, red rose."

2. What rock is toothpaste made of?

3. What country has the largest coal reserve?

SOS Make as many three- or four-letter words from the word "relaxation" as you can.

ICE How many things can you think of that can be folded?

TAB If something you are trying to recall does not come to mind right away, do not let it upset you. Remind yourself that you do remember the information, but will just recall it a little later than you wanted. Usually, if you remain calm and relaxed, the information you are trying to retrieve will come to you a short time later.

Mmm Breathing Meditation: Pause Between Breaths – Close your eyes, and observe the breath. Notice that there is a brief, subtle pause at the peak of each in-breath and each out-breath. Focus your mind on that pause only. Do this for at least ten breath cycles.

— SET 114 —

WOW A problem well-stated is a problem half-solved. – Charles Franklin Kettering

3Rs Think about your best friends. How are they alike and how are they different? Share some of your memories of those friends. What do you most appreciate about them?

KISS 1. What country is the Samba from?
2. Can you count to 139 by 9's?
3. Which country's flag is closest to that of the U.S.?

SOS Josh did the same experiment every day for a month. It took 80 minutes on Mondays and the rest of the week days it took one hour and 20 minutes. Why?

ICE Create your own symbol of power.

TAB Studies on rats suggest that antioxidants in grapes used in red wine (resveratrol from the skin and proanthocyanidin from the seed) may protect against problems with blood flow to the brain, which could prevent stroke and Alzheimer's.[60]

Mmm Parting the Clouds – Stand in a stable shoulder-width stance. Cross the arms at the wrists directly in front of your belly with palms facing in. First pierce the clouds. As you inhale, bend the elbows and lift the arms up in front of the body. Keep the wrists connected and the palms facing into the body, by allowing the wrists to pivot around each other as you lift the arms. Once the hands are over your head, turn the wrists out. Exhale, and push the hands to the side "parting the clouds." Continue to push the arms out

---

60 Morgan, Claudine. *Health News & Views at* http://news.health.com/2013/02/20/is-red-wine-good-for-you/

and downward in a big circle until the wrists cross and you are back in the starting position. Repeat in one fluid motion following the breath.

— SET 115 —

WOW The race goes not always to the swift, but those who keep on running. – Anonymous

3Rs Think back to when you took your driver's test. How did you feel? What are your driving experiences? If you never learned to drive, why not? What are your experiences of other people's driving?

KISS 1. "Predator" is to "hawk" as 'glutton" is to what?
2. Is it faster to blink our eyes open or closed?
3. Which three states in the U.S. have the most letters in their full names?

SOS Rearrange the letters within each set of letters to form animal names: nails, reed, shore.

ICE You are going back for your school class reunion and have been asked to suggest a theme for the Homecoming luncheon and your class's Homecoming Parade float. What will you suggest?

TAB According to the Brain and Behavior Research Foundation, one fifth of adolescents suffer from mental illnesses that affect them on into adulthood.[61]

Mmm Acupressure Sun Points – Pressing on these acupressure points is a recommended memory support as reported in a Prevention Magazine publication on natural healing. To find the Sun Points, follow the line of your eyebrows until you get to the soft depression in your temple about a half an inch out. Sit with your elbows on a desk or table and gently press into the Sun Points with the heel of your hands. Close your eyes and breathe deeply for a minute or so before releasing the pressure.[62]

— SET 116 —

WOW It is one of my sources of happiness never to desire knowledge of other people's business. – Dolley Madison

3Rs When you were younger, suppose you were told that you would have an unlimited expense account for a day at any store of your choice to buy

61 https://www.bbrfoundation.org/

62 Dellemore, Doug, et al. (1995) *New Choices in Natural Healing.* Ed. Bill Gottlieb. Emmaus, PA: Rodale Press.

whatever you wanted. What store would you have chosen, what things would you have bought, and for whom? Why?

KISS 1. What literary device was John Kennedy using when he said," Ask not what your country can do for you, but what you can do for your country"?
2. What animal was named athlete of the year in 1973?
3. Who was the only U.S. president to serve non-consecutive terms as the 22nd and 24th president of the U.S.?

SOS It is twenty-six minutes to one. The year is 1978 and the date is May 6. What is interesting about this?

ICE Make a list of best kept secrets.

TAB In a 2014 study, scientists from The Scripps Research Institute found that moving forward, as opposed to backwards, trains the brain to perceive the world normally. They also found that based on complex relationship between neurons in the eye and the order in which we see things helps the brain calibrate how we perceive time.

Mmm Walking Backwards – Carefully walk around the house backwards. Be sure to have a clear path before you start and look behind you as needed.

— SET 117 —

WOW Even if you are on the right track, you will get run over if you just sit there. – Will Rogers

3Rs During your lifetime, what do you perceive to be the most unfortunate and regrettable thing that occurred in U. S. History? What do remember about that event?

KISS 1. What is a potter's oven called?
2. Is it possible for an airplane to fly backwards?
3. Did John Hancock sign the U.S. Constitution?

SOS How much more is there in 20 four-gallon cans each half full than in 24 gallon cans each half empty?

ICE The following are common sayings with the ending listed in parentheses. Replace the part in parenthesis to create new alternative endings: "It's not over 'til (it's over)." "People who live in glass houses (shouldn't throw stones)." "A rolling stone (gathers no moss)." "You can't judge a book (by the cover)."

TAB In reflexology, the tips of the toes and the top segment of the fingers are associated with the brain.

Mmm Tennis Ball Reflexology – This exercise is best done by a wall or with a stable piece of furniture to help with balance. Get a tennis ball and place it on the floor near your foot. Keeping the majority of your weight on one foot, raise the other foot and place it on the tennis ball. Gently and carefully press the foot on the tennis ball and roll it under the foot to massage and stimulate the sole of the foot. Repeat using the other foot.

— SET 118 —

WOW Two wolves fight in each person's heart. One wolf is a vengeful, angry and violent one. The other wolf is a loving and compassionate one. The one that will win is the one that you feed. – Cherokee parable

3Rs What are some of your favorite holiday experiences? What made those experiences special?

KISS 1. Can you think of four or more meanings for "bow"?
2. Who theorized that for each action there is an equal and opposite reaction?
3. What is the only U.S. state named for another country?

SOS How many words can you make by adding three letters within each of the following sets of letters: t_ _ _e, r_ _ _d, b_ _ _y, m_ _ _t?

ICE Your mission, if you choose to accept it, is to really keep people quiet while in the library. What will be your plan?

TAB A person's short-term memory is fully developed at about eight years of age. Continued repetition of a short-term memory eventually leads to long-term retention of it.

Mmm Compassion Meditation: School Age –Close your eyes, relax and place your hands on your heart. On the next breath, invite an image of yourself as an elementary school-aged child. See your younger self in front of you as you were then—happy or sad, active or passive, troubled or happy-go-lucky. Smile to your younger self. In your mind give that child a hug. Send the child you were gentle and loving compassion.

— SET 119 —

WOW One day your life will flash before your eyes. Make sure it's worth watching. – Gerard Way

3Rs Throughout your life, who was your favorite news anchor? Why? What was most distinguishing about her/him?

KISS 1. What literary device does Emily Dickenson use to describe the flowers, birds, and shadows in the following quote from "Have You Got a Brook in Your Little Heart"? "Where bashful flowers blow, And blushing birds go down to drink, And shadows tremble so?" Hint: They have emotions like people.
2. Which sports use each of the following terms: free throw, bunt, rebound, sack?
3. From which countries did we get: lasagna, tortilla, and teriyaki?

SOS Don't assume! Think! Jean's friends always greeted her with a wave and a "Hi Jean," but Jean always wondered if they thought of her as one who didn't wash her hands or shower. Explain.

ICE Would you choose to be able to fly or be able to be invisible? Why?

TAB In the brain, the supporting glia cells actually outnumber the "thinking" cells by at least 3 to 1.[63]

Mmm Arm Float – Lie on your back in a comfortable position. Relax and tune into the sensation of your hands, wrists, and arms. Allow your arms to rise up in the air above you as if they were seaweed floating under water. Gently explore the space above you with your arms by opening and closing the elbow, rotating the shoulder joint, and/or alternately pushing the arms away from your body and pulling them back into your body, as if they were caught in a current of water. Play with flexing and rotating your wrists, too. Allow your eyes to follow your hands.

— SET 120 —

WOW It isn't that they cannot see the solution. It is that they cannot see the problem. – G. K. Chesterton

3Rs Visualize home(s) you lived in growing up. What was the decor, room placement, furniture, etc. like? Have you ever been back? What home was your favorite? Why? What are your special memories there?

KISS 1. What century was photography invented?
2. What do you call people who study animals?
3. Which states are referred to as the Aloha State, Grand Canyon State, and Bluegrass State?

SOS Before Mt. Everest was discovered, what was the tallest mountain in the world?

---

63 Purves D, Augustine GJ, Fitzpatrick D, et al., editors. Neuroscience. 2nd ed. Sunderland (MA): Sinauer Associates; 2001.

ICE If you could decide on one petty thing that should be illegal, what would you choose?

TAB Learning to play an instrument appears to strengthen the brain's ability to capture the depth and richness of speech sounds.

Mmm Big Body Drum – Imagine your body is a drum set. Snap, clap, slap, stomp to create your own rhythm solo.

— SET 121 —

WOW I can live two months on a good compliment. – Mark Twain

3Rs Were you ever teased/bullied? Why or why not? If you were teased, what were you teased about and how did you react? Did you ever tease anyone? If so, who and why?

KISS 1. What is a three-letter verb in the past tense that spelled backwards is also a three-letter verb in the past tense?

2. When salt is added to water, does the water boil at a higher temperature, a lower temperature, or the same temperature?

3. List words associated with Social Studies that start with "c", "g", "m", "s" and "t".

SOS How many birth days does the average person have?

ICE Name some strange food combinations.

TAB In 2012, researchers at Duke University, King's College in London and University of Otago in New Zealand found that teenagers who were dependent on marijuana before age 18 and who continued using it into adulthood lost an average of eight I.Q. points by age 38.[64]

Mmm Cross Body Tug-o-War – Lie down with your legs extended and your arms stretched out above your head. Imagine you are the rope in a tug-o-war contest. One team is pulling on your arms and one team is pulling on your legs. After a while, switch to just the right side of the body. Then the left side only. Then do the opposite legs and arms.

— SET 122 —

WOW Life is what happens to you when you're making other plans. – Betty Talmadge

---

64 http://www.drugabuse.gov/news-events/nida-notes/2013/08/early-onset-regular-cannabis-use-linked -to-iq-decline

3Rs Think of your various family members. What do you appreciate most about each?

KISS 1. Who wrote : The line "A rose is a rose is a rose"? *The Jungle Book*? *The Great Gatsby*?
2. What are parallel lines?
3. Where is the U.S. Tomb of the Unknown Soldier?

SOS For each set, put the same word before or after each word in the set to make new words: (1) Stock, super, place, meat; (2) Hair, class, short, throat; (3) House, moon, red, reading.

ICE The answer is 29? What was the question? List at least five different thoughts.

TAB With elaborate meditation training, some people such as advanced yogis can develop the ability to consciously and directly control functions of the autonomic nervous system such as slowing their heart rate or changing their body temperature. These functions are almost completely involuntary for the average person.

Mmm Breathing Meditation: Lengthened Inhale – Observe your breath. After a few breaths, exhale completely and begin to consciously lengthen the inhale. Let the out-breath be normal, and then inhale quietly and more slowly. Do not strain. Continue for at least ten breath cycles with normal inhales and longer, slower exhales. Then return to a normal breath before getting up.

— SET 123 —

WOW When you have to make a choice and you don't make it, that itself is a choice. – William James

3Rs What are some activities you would like to do in the future that you have never experienced before? How have your past memories affected this selection, and how could you best accomplish something from that "bucket list"?

KISS 1. In what medium did artist Dorothea Lange work? Hint: She was famous for her Depression era work.
2. There is one bone in our body that does not connect with any other bones. What is that bone?
3. Name the country where you would find Edinburgh, Liverpool, London, and the Thames River.

SOS What nationalities do you associate with these pairs: (1) Dressing and roulette; (2) Shepherd and measles; (3) Oven and treat; (4) Goulash and rhapsody?

ICE Make up a sentence using all the letters of the alphabet and using the least number of words.

TAB Research at both the University of Hong Kong and Wellesley College suggests that acupuncture can help to reduce symptoms of patients with Alzheimer's. Study participants showed "improvement in memory, attention, and verbal and motor skills such as ability to name an object, follow verbal and written commands, and write a sentence."[65]

Mmm Part the Wild Horse's Mane –Bring one hand in front of your heart with the palm facing up. Then bring the other hand, with palm facing down a few inches above the first hand, close but not touching. On an exhale, pull the hands to the side, across and away from one another. Imagine that the horse's mane is between your two hands and your hands are combing through the mane. Turn your head to follow the upper hand. Allow the elbows to unbend and stretch the arms out so that the upper arm points up above the shoulder and the lower arm points down to the earth. As you inhale, lift the bottom arm up and lower the upper arm down in big arcs out to the side of the body. Continue to circle the arms bending the elbows and drawing the hands back into the original position with palms facing each other in front of the heart, close but not touching. Exhale and repeat parting the horse's mane. Keep the motion fluid and in tune with the breath.

—— SET 124 ——

WOW It is better to keep your mouth closed and let people think you are a fool than to open your mouth and remove all doubt. – Mark Twain

3Rs How would people have described you as a young person? How would they describe you now? How would you explain any changes in how people describe you? How would you explain any similarities?

KISS 1. Which is dry land, desert or dessert?

2. What animal can only travel two-to-three feet a minute and is one of the slowest creatures on earth?

3. Who was a well-known head of the Bureau of Investigation (later known as the FBI) under President Coolidge?

---

65 http://www.acupuncture-online.com/alzheimers.htm

SOS Start with the word "Pup" and change one letter at a time to get to the word "Dog", making real words at each step. Pup _____ _____ Dog.

ICE You want to say something original on your voice mail message. What will you say?

TAB The simple act of tapping your fingers requires millions of nerve cells in the brain to work in tandem with perfect timing. Imagine how much is required for complex thinking and analysis.

Mmm Active Fingers – Starting with the thumb and working through the fingers one at a time on both hands, explore the various ways each finger can move. What sensations and movements are similar with each finger? What sensations and movements are different with each finger?

— SET 125 —

WOW Ask not what your brain can do for you, but what you can do for your brain. – JFK (modified by Renie Lenning)

3Rs Tell some stories about your parents/grandparents? Which is your favorite such story? Who shared them with you?

KISS 1. What title character killed his father and married his mother in Greek tragedy?

2. What element makes up both coal and diamonds?

3. In what state is the geographic center of the contiguous U.S.? Of North America?

SOS What words end in "ster"?

ICE Create as many silly "math" problems as you can; e.g., 2 balls + 2 balls = 1 walk in baseball.

TAB Eating breakfast helps! In one study, students who skipped breakfast did less well on tests of memory and attention that day. And students who regularly eat breakfast generally have higher test scores than students who don't eat breakfast.

Mmm Contemplating an Empty Dish – After you finish one of your meals today, stop and contemplate your empty dish. Acknowledge the empty dish in front of you and the food it contained that is now within you. As you inhale, say to yourself, "My dish is empty." As you exhale, say, "My hunger is satisfied." Repeat 4-5 times.

— SET 126 —

WOW Failure is only the opportunity to begin again more intellectually. – Henry Ford

3Rs What are the most fascinating things you know about your heritage? What are your memories pertaining to this? Who are some of your interesting ancestors that you know about? What made them especially interesting to you?

KISS 1. Ansel Adams was famous for what type of photography?

2. List words associated with math starting with C, G, M, S, and T.

3. What bird did Benjamin Franklin want to make the National Bird of the U.S.?

SOS What do these have in common: brain, fingerprint, snowflake, and spots on a giraffe?

ICE What could you use if you were wrapping gifts and you ran out of transparent tape? List at least six possibilities.

TAB If your diet includes healthy portions of produce, fish, nuts, and vinaigrette-type dressings, a Mayo Clinic study found you could cut your risk of Alzheimer's disease by 42 percent.[66]

Mmm In the Swim: Flutter Kick Back – Lie on your back on a bed so that the legs extend off the bed. Stretch the legs out straight and point the toes. Do a flutter kick by alternately raising and lowering the legs without bending the knees. See how fast you can go and for how long. Try for at least one minute.

— SET 127 —

WOW If you are not afraid to face the music, you may someday become the leader of the band. – Anonymous

3Rs Tell of your best and worst memories of picnics? Where did you go? What did you eat? What did you do?

KISS 1. Which of the following means "in any case": "any way" or "anyway"?

2. Would you rather be food deprived or sleep deprived for a month?

3. By volume of materials used, what's the largest single human-made structure on earth?

SOS Denise is buying something for her house. The price of 1 is 12 cents, the price of 44 is 24 cents, and the price of 144 is 36 cents. What is Denise buying?

---

66 http://www.usatoday.com/story/news/nation/2012/10/17/carb-diet-alzheimers/1637481/

ICE Which has more fun, an adjective or a noun? Why? Think outside the box.

TAB Studies show that brain cells communicate more effectively when their electrical firing is rhythmically synchronized.[67]

Mmm Rhythm Work: Syllable Clap/Slap/Stomp – Clap, stomp and slap your thighs to create the following rhythm: Clappity clappa clap. Slappity slappa slap. Stompity stompa stompity stompa. Stomp Clap Slap. Repeat and increase speed as you get it.

— SET 128 —

WOW My mission in life is not merely to survive, but to thrive; and to do so with some passion, some compassion, some humor, and some style. – Maya Angelou

3Rs List titles of some of your favorite books? Why did you choose them? What kinds of books are they? What is your absolute favorite novel? Why? How about your favorite non-fiction book?

KISS 1. What is satire?

2. Which wingless insect can jump one hundred times its height and two hundred times its length?

3. Identify these states: First State; Keystone State; Lone Star State.

SOS How many words can you make by inserting three letters within each of the four sets of letters that follow: d_ _ _m; s_ _ _t; p_ _ _n; w_ _ _t?

ICE List what you would put into a time capsule.

TAB In 2013, researchers at Emory University found concrete evidence that a gene in humans called "oxytocin receptor," previously known to influence mother-infant bonding and pair bonding within gender, is also important for one's ability to recognize/remember faces.[68]

Mmm Compassion Meditation: Mother –Close your eyes, and place your hands on your heart. On the next breath, invite a memory of your mother. See her in front of you as you remember her. Next see her as she might have been at age five. What was she like as a young child? Smile to your mother's younger self, give her a hug and send her gentle, loving compassion.

---

67 http://www.npr.org/sections/health-shots/2014/06/17/322915700/your-brains-got-rhythm-and-syncs-when-you-think

68 http://www.nih.gov/researchmatters/january2014/01132014oxytocin.htm

— SET 129 —

WOW The time to repair the roof is when the sun is shining. – John F. Kennedy

3Rs What are things other people do that make you happy or sad? Why?

KISS 1. What was the "arts and crafts movement" in architecture?

2. Why do things often break more easily when they are cold?

3. Of the Americans arrested, what are most of them arrested for?

SOS Oscar is 40 and Chris is 13. How many years ago was Oscar four times as old as Chris?

ICE Would you rather be an ant or a bee in a cartoon? Why?

TAB Noted Russian neuropsychologist Alexander Luria studied the extraordinary memory of Solomon Shereshevsky. Shereshevsky's memories were so strong he could recount thousands of them in vivid detail years later. He reported that he remembered everything, including numbers, through visual pictures that his brain automatically created and connected to the information. The only way he could get rid of a memory was to visualize covering over that particular picture with a large sheet.[69]

Mmm The Phoenix Spreads Its Wings – Throughout this exercise, keep the muscles of the hands and arms activated and move as if pushing them though a great force. Hold your hands out in front of you with the fingers together and the thumbs away to the side so one hand forms an "L" shape and the other forms a reverse "L". Maintaining the "L" shape, bring the hands to your sides. Take a solid stance with knees slightly bent. Keeping the upper arms tucked in close to the body, bend the elbows to bring the L-shaped hands up to the armpits. From there, slowly bring the arms across the body so that they cross at wrists (without touching) in front of the breastbone as if the back of the hands were framing your face. Hold the hands stiffly with fingers pointing to the sky as you press out with the outside edges of the pinkie fingers to open the arms out to the sides like wings. Repeat two times.

— SET 130 —

WOW It isn't what you have, or who you are, or where you are, or what you're doing that makes you happy or unhappy. It is what you think about. – Dale Carnegie

---

69 http://peakmemory.me/2013/12/07/the -vast-memory-of-solomon-shereshevsky

3Rs Of the various disputes in the world, which one is the most important to solve? Why?

KISS 1. What do these word mean: Subservient? Rescind? Contiguous?
2. How do you divide fractions?
3. Which state has the most cacti?

SOS What common word contains double C, double S, and double L? Can you think of a second such word?

ICE Describe an imaginary "cronkoplat." What is it? What does it do? What does it look like? Sound like? Smell like?

TAB It has been estimated that if all of the neurons in a person's brain were strung end to end, they would stretch from the earth to the moon and back.[70]

Mmm Twist It – Put on some music and do the twist. Turn your hips in one direction and your torso in the opposite.

— SET 131 —

WOW None of us is as smart as all of us. – Kenneth H. Blanchard

3Rs What are things you would not have found in your house fifty years ago? How have life and the world changed in those fifty years because of having those things? Think about two ways your life is more difficult now than fifty years ago, and two ways your life is easier now than fifty years ago.

KISS 1. Name as many of the major gods and goddesses from Greek mythology as you can.
2. What is the term for the move used to dislodge something from the throat of someone who is choking?
3. What are the first words of the U.S. Constitution?

SOS Small peaches are eight cents each and large peaches are 13 cents each. How many of each can you buy for $1.00?

ICE "My trees are missing." Who said this, to whom, and why?

TAB Memories that overlap and are shared among people who have something meaningful in common are called collective memories.

Mmm Standing Meditation: Sensing Gravity – Stand with your feet in a hip-width stance. Sense the feet on the ground and the vertical line of your body. Then bring your awareness to the pull of gravity on your body. For every moment of your life, the earth's gravity holds you close and keeps you from flying

70 https://www.ck12.org/book/Human-Biology-Nervous-System/4.1/

off into space. Sense the earth beneath your feet as a giant magnet. You do not need to make any effort; the earth does all the work. Let yourself relax and feel the earth's pull all the way to the center of the planet.

— SET 132 —

WOW Great minds discuss ideas; average minds discuss events; and small minds discuss people! – Eleanor Roosevelt

3Rs What are your memories of a group you were part of when you were young (such as scouts, 4-H, church group, band/choir etc.)? How did your experiences in that group affect you as an adult?

KISS 1. Name an American religious group famous for their simple furniture design.
2. In the sky, which color stars are the hottest: black, blue, orange, yellow, red, or white?
3. What place are the kings and queens of England not allowed to go?

SOS Your car is facing north, driving on a straight road. After driving four miles in a straight line, without turning the car, you find that you are south of where you started. How is this possible?

ICE Create a sensible and long sentence with all of the words starting with the letter "T".

TAB "Mnemonics," coined from the name "Mnemosyne" the Greek Goddess of memory, consists of rhymes, synonyms, sayings, special tricks, etc. intended to help you remember anything. For example, the Great Lakes can be remembered by the way the first letter of each lake spells "HOMES".

Mmm Breathing Meditation: Lengthened Exhale – Observe your breath. After a few breaths, consciously begin to lengthen the exhale. Let the in-breath be normal, and then exhale quietly and more slowly. Do not strain. Continue for at least ten breath cycles with normal inhales and longer, slower exhales. Then return to a normal breath before getting up.

— SET 133 —

WOW There is a past that is gone forever, but there is a future which is still our own. – F. W. Robertson

3Rs What are you proud of yourself for doing? What is the most important thing you have done? If you were to get an award for doing something, what would you want it to be?

KISS 1. The answer for each of the following four items applies to a word that has “nation” in it: A flower; Well lit; Quit your job; Strong displeasure due to a perceived affront

2. What green stone is prized by the Chinese for its beauty and medicinal properties?

3. Where is each of these located: Big Ben; Colosseum; Eiffel Tower; Golden Gate Bridge?

SOS Hannah, Bradyn, Aspen and Jackson work as a trucker, teacher, accountant, and engineer. Aspen is either the accountant or the engineer, and Hannah is neither of those. Jackson is either the teacher or the accountant, and Bradyn is neither of those. The engineer is not Aspen. Which person has which job?

ICE You are given ten thousand oranges at your house. They must go to a minimum of four different uses and you get a bonus for coming up with the most original use. What will you do with them?

TAB Astroglia are star-shaped glial cells that help nourish neurons, remove dead neurons, and hold neurons in place.

Mmm Dead Bug – Lie on your back in a comfortable position with your knees bent and your feet on the floor. On an in-breath, allow your feet and arms to rise up in the air above you. Now shake your arms and legs in the air as if you were an upside down beetle.

—— SET 134 ——

WOW If you have built castles in the air, your work need not be lost; that is where they should be. Now put the foundations under them. – Henry David Thoreau

3Rs What are your thoughts about religion? Why?

KISS 1. What happens to the boy who cried wolf in Sergei Prokofiev’s *Peter and the Wolf*?

2. True or false: Lasers work by focusing sound waves.

3. What item invented in China in the 1500’s do we still use today? In 1938 nylon bristles were added.

SOS Put the same word in front or behind each word within each of the following sets to make a compound word or phrase: (1) head, ice, shoulder; (2) red, pepper, dog; and (3) house, street, moon, switch.

ICE “Where are the volcano pads?” Who said this, and to whom?

TAB Research by an international team of scientists suggests that creativity increases with a comfortable level of background noise, a slightly messy desk, and the color blue predominant in your surroundings. However, too much interferes with and inhibits creativity.[71]

Mmm Folding – Get out a towel. Fold it up. Now unfold it, and fold it up in a different way. Fold the towel in as many different ways as you can think of. Do you always fold your towels in the same way?

— SET 135 —

WOW The road to the heart is the ear. – Voltaire

3Rs Have you ever been lost? How old were you and where were you going? Were you alone? How did you eventually find your way? What advice would you have for someone who is lost?

KISS 1. What period was Art Nouveau, and what does Nouveau Riche mean?
2. When a person dies, what is the last sense to go? What is the first to go?
3. Name the country where you would find: Bonn, Danube River, and Hamburg.

SOS What nationalities do you associate with each of the following pairs: Toast and fries; Pine and tape; Massage and meatballs; Walnut and muffin?

ICE List as many novel uses of a paper clip as you can.

TAB Music involves the whole brain. Just listening to music has favorable effects on brain functioning as long as it is not too loud or jarring.[72]

Mmm Listening Meditation: Follow the Musician – Put on some music. Rather than listening to it as a whole, choose one instrument and listen for when that instrument plays and when it stops. Play the song again and listen for a different instrument.

— SET 136 —

WOW Fear is never a reason for quitting; it is only an excuse. – Norman Vincent Peale

3Rs What are your dreams most often about? Describe a significant dream or nightmare you have had. How did you feel about the dream? Was there any relationship to events happening in the day or days before the dream? Do you have any recurring dreams?

---

71 http://www.sci-news.com/othersciences/anthropology/article00313.html

72 http://www.sci-news.com/othersciences/anthropology/article00313.html

KISS 1. The answer for each of the following four items is a single word that has cat in it: Lists sale Items; Plant that cats love; Class of things; Behind home plate.

2. How many pairs of legs does a lobster have?

3. What continent on the Earth is not owned by any country?

SOS A woman had only six potatoes for her ten children. How did she make sure each child got an equal amount of the potatoes?

ICE Think of things you can eat that are black and white.

TAB Current neuroscience indicates that the brain does not distinguish between thoughts and emotions. Both involve interactions across the whole brain.

Mmm Triangle Pose – Stand with your feet wide apart. Turn your right foot 90 degrees out to point to the side wall. Turn the left foot in just slightly. Put your arms out to the sides at shoulder level with palms facing down. Keeping the arms level and the feet stable, lean from the waist to the right as if someone were lightly pulling on your right arm. Now keeping the arms and legs straight, bend sideways at the waist so that your left arm points up toward the sky while the right hand points down to the earth. Allow the right hand to rest on the leg wherever it falls—above the knee, on the calf, ankle, foot, or floor. Hold for a few breathes. Then on an inhale, lift the right hand and slowly unbend the waist to come up. Repeat on the other side.

— SET 137 —

WOW An aim in life is the only fortune worth finding; and it is not to be found in foreign lands, but in the heart itself. – Robert Louis Stevenson

3Rs What were your favorite programs on the radio? What type of music did you like? Why?

KISS 1. What is the moral of the Aesop's fable "The Tortoise and Hare"?

2. Why does ice form on a bridge before the rest of the road?

3. What do all these have in common: Berlin, China, and Jericho?

SOS What is full of holes yet holds water?

ICE You are on the Council for keeping your city litter-free. What will be your recommendation?

TAB Brains tend to forget names rather than remember them. To help remember a name you must listen carefully and create a "mental name tag" for your brain to associate with the name. It can also help to visualize something unique that connects with the name, to repeat the name several times over a period of time, and to write it down for later review.

Mmm Sense Suppression – the goal of this exercise is to withdraw from sensory awareness in order to direct attention internally and away from the external world. According to *Yoga for Dummies,* this exercise can be used effectively to manage pain and symptoms of physical discomfort. Sit in a comfortable position with the spine upright. You will place the five fingers of each hand on your head and face to close off the senses of sound, sight, and smell. Start by placing the pinkie fingers on the lower lip, and the ring fingers on the upper lip. Rest the middle fingers over the nostrils. Close your eyes and place the index fingers over your lashes to hold the eye softly closed. Finally place the thumbs over your ear, closing out sound. Once you have the fingers in position, take a deep breath and hold it for as long as you can. Focus your inner vision on the inside of your forehead between your eyebrows.

— SET 138 —

WOW If your lips can speak a word of encouragement to a weary soul, you have talent. – Eva J. Cummings

3Rs Did you have any household pets; yours or others? What were their names? How did you interact with them?

KISS 1. Name some famous architects.

2. How quickly can you find the answer to this problem: 25 x 5 x 3,659 x 0 = ?

3. Name two African countries that start with "Z".

SOS Use the same three letters to fill in the blanks to create legitimate words from the following: ex____, en____, re____.

ICE Use the letters of your name to write a silly sentence.

TAB Be careful in making judgments about people's potential cognitive abilities. For example, Walt Disney was once fired by a newspaper editor because he had "no good ideas."[73]

Mmm Meditation: Gift to Younger Self – In this meditation you will visualize offering something to yourself at an earlier time in your life. Close your eyes and place your hands on your heart. After a several breaths, begin to visualize yourself at a younger age, as a child, a young person, or even as

73 http://www.uky.edu/~eushe2/Pajares/OnFailingG.html

an adult in the past. Allow whatever image comes and trust that it is the right one. See that younger self in sitting in front of you right now. Look the younger you in the eye and smile. Ask what gift your younger self would like from you now. Accept whatever answer comes. It can be an image, words, a quality, or a symbol. Whatever gift came to mind, offer it lovingly to your younger self.

— SET 139 —

WOW If money is your hope for independence you will never have it. The only real security in this world is a reserve of knowledge, experience and ability. – Henry Ford

3Rs What are your feelings about computers and technology? How important do you think computers are? Have you been a person who likes to learn new things? Does that include learning to use new technology?

KISS 1. The answers to the following all contain the word "bell": Bag carrying hotel worker; Hemmingway novel; Person who financed Columbus.

2. What is the thigh bone technically called?

3. What do Princess Anne, Roman Emperor Nero, Benjamin Spock, and George Patton have in common?

SOS What day of the year has 25 hours in it?

ICE You are buying a house and find out the seller is moving out because the house really is haunted. What will you do?

TAB University of Virginia researchers found that the human brain is wired to connect with others so strongly through empathy that it responds to what they experience as if it is happening to us.[74]

Mmm Mindful Tracking: Conversations – Mentally tracking our thoughts, words, feelings or actions can help to create more mindfulness and is a good mental workout. For the purposes of this exercise, do not alter your choices or behaviors; simply observe without judgment. Choose a conversation (in-person or by phone) to track. Notice how much time you spend speaking compared to how much time you spend listening. Other things to track in a conversation can include how frequently you interrupt or how often your mind wanders when you are supposedly listening. What do you notice?

---

74 http://news.virginia.edu/content/human-brains-are-hardwired-empathy-friendship-study-shows

— SET 140 —

WOW The noble secret of laughing at oneself is the greatest humor of all. – Anonymous

3Rs What are your memories of floods, tornados, droughts, earthquakes or another type of natural disaster? If you have not had such personal experience, how do you visualize it from TV or newspaper accounts? What natural disaster during your lifetime has been the most serious? Why?

KISS 1. In Roman mythology, Mercury was god of _____.

2. About how many eggs does an average hen lay in a week?

3. Identify the city for each airport: O'Hare; Heathrow; John F. Kennedy; Charles De Gaulle.

SOS Johnny was asked what kind of fruit trees he had. He said, "All but two are apple trees, all but two are cherry trees, and all but two are peach trees." How many trees does Johnny have?

ICE A porcupine is in your kitchen cupboard. How can you get it out without getting stuck with those prickly quills? List as many ways as you can.

TAB Genuine laughter releases endorphins and increases oxygen to the brain. It increases motivation, retention, and deeper levels of thought.

Mmm Disco Dance – Imagine you have been transported back to the nineteen seventies, and do your best *Saturday Night Fever* impression. Bell bottoms are optional!

— SET 141 —

WOW None but ourselves can free our minds. – Bob Marley

3Rs Have you ever been stopped by a patrol/police car, or received a traffic ticket(s)? What was the situation? How did you react? If this has not happened to you, how do you think you would react?

KISS 1. Who painted American Gothic? Hint: the Farmer holds a pitchfork and the stern woman is his daughter, not his wife.

2. How does a mercury thermometer work?

3. Which country's national flag has a maple leaf?

SOS Tomorrow will be three days after the day before Sunday. What day is today?

ICE List situations in which 40 is the answer.

TAB People's temperament can shift through mindfulness and meditation, according to a recent study at the University of Wisconsin at Madison. The study found that four months after participation in an 8-week meditation training, meditation participants' EEGs showed increased activation in the left (positive emotion side) of the prefrontal cortex compared to before they did the training (and compared to a control group).[75]

Mmm Seated Meditation: Space Free — Close your eyes. On your next inhale begin to visualize yourself as space, expansive and free. Imagine the sensation of space between your cells extending out into the universe. Then as you exhale, visualize the sensation of freedom in space within you. As you inhale say in your mind, "Breathing in, I see myself as space." Then as you exhale say, "Breathing out, I feel free." Continue for at least 10 breath cycles.[76]

— SET 142 —

WOW Keep my thoughts positive, Thoughts become my words. Keep my words positive. Words become my behavior. Keep my behaviors positive. Behaviors become my habits. Keep my habits positive. Habits become my values. Keep my values positive. Values become my destiny. – Gandhi

3Rs What are your most important talents and abilities? Why are they important? Were you good at them as a child?

KISS 1. What U.S. city would you guess is one of the most often misspelled?
2. What happens in a solar eclipse?
3. What was the name of the first Pilgrim ship?

SOS A man from Boston screamed loudly for over an hour and woke up his neighbors. Rather than being upset, the neighbors got up, and the man became a hero. Who is the man and what did he yell?

ICE What would be the worst song title ever?

TAB Protein helps form new brain cells to replace those that die off; it also produces brain chemicals that contribute to one's alertness and ability to analyze.

Mmm Snow Angels – Lie down on your back, with legs extended out and hands at your side. Practice making Snow Angels. Slide your legs along the floor to a full open position; at the same time, slide the arms away from the torso like angel wings. Then slide the legs and arms back to closed position. Repeat several times.

---

75 Goldman, Daniel. (2003). *Destructive Emotions, How Can We Overcome them? A Scientific Dialogue with the Dalai Lama.* Narrated by New York: Bantam Books, p. 75.

76 Nhat Hanh, Thich. (2009). The Blooming of a Lotus. (Revised). Boston: Beacon Press.

— SET 143 —

WOW You can't buy happiness but you can buy books, and that's kind of the same thing. – Anonymous

3Rs List your top ten interests? What do those interests have in common?

KISS 1. In Roman mythology, Venus was goddess of _____.

2. What are the purposes of eyebrows?

3. Is Los Angeles or Reno, Nevada located furthest west?

SOS What do the words in each of the two sets that follow have in common with one another: (1) Ice skate, lawn mower, propeller, razor; (2) House, piano, treasure chest, typewriter?

ICE Think of other names for tic-tac-toe or the cat and mouse game.

TAB Reading is a very complex, difficult, and dynamic activity for the brain that is more demanding neuro-biologically than the processes of speaking or interpreting drawings, paintings, photos or other images. Dylan Barmmer states, "Even as you're reading this . . . parts of your brain that have evolved over time for other functions, such as vision and language, are connecting in a specific neural pathway for reading. Look at an MRI scan of the brain during reading, and you'll see an abundance of activity."[77]

Mmm A Different Read – Read your magazine, newspaper, book or email in a different order today. For a real challenge, try reading upside-down.

— SET 144 —

WOW Whatever we are waiting for – peace of mind, contentment, grace, the inner awareness of simple abundance – it will surely come to us, but only when we are ready to receive it with an open and grateful heart. – Sarah Ban Breathnach

3Rs Have you ever been a guest on the radio or TV? On which game show would it be the most exciting for you to be a contestant? Why?

KISS 1. Thomas Jefferson's home Monticello influenced many government buildings in the United States. What is the architectural style of Monticello?

2. Which of the following animals has the longest average lifespan: Cow, Chimpanzee, or Box Turtle?

3. In 1700, what three European countries had the most territory in what is now the U.S.?

---

77 http://www.reneweveryday.com/the-act-of-reading-has-powerful-positive-effects-for-your-brain/

SOS The English word "startling" allows you to eliminate a letter one at a time and each time still have a word; all the way to a one-letter word. Demonstrate that this is true.

ICE You are chaperoning kids on a school bus. There is a big delay because roads are closed. How would you entertain the kids for an hour?

TAB Listening to music activates many areas of the brain, from brain stem and cerebellum to the cortex of the temporal lobes to the hippocampus and lower frontal lobes.[78]

Mmm Listening Meditation: New Sounds – Play music that is in a different style than you usually listen to. For example, if you listen to jazz, listen to a country song; if you listen to rock; listen to a classical song, etc. Close your eyes and listen deeply to the song.

—— SET 145 ——

WOW Those who wish to secure the good of others have already secured their own. – Confucius

3Rs What are some of your winter memories from throughout your life? Which ones are your favorites, and why?

KISS 1. Translate the following Spanish phrase into English: Mi casa es su casa.
2. What is the main difference between iron and steel?
3. List the four countries that make up the United Kingdom.

SOS Anna grabbed a T-shirt and being in a hurry put it on inside out. Her left arm was in the right sleeve. Where would the label be?

ICE List five creative uses of dust.

TAB The hippocampus is a structure located in the temporal lobe. It deals with learning, remembering and subjective emotions.

Mmm Hippocampus Meditation –Visualize your hippocampus. Focus your attention deep within the center of your skull behind the eye sockets. Imagine that you can actually sense each side of the hippocampus as curled, seahorse shapes curving slightly down from back to front on either side of the middle of your brain. What do they feel like to you? How do the sensations of the right side and left side feel different for you, or do they? Which side seems stronger to you? Once the image is clear, play with altering the image in ways that might strengthen or nourish your

---

78 Levitin, Daniel J. (2007). *This Is Your Brain on Music.* New York: Penguin.

hippocampus. Possible images you can try are: sensing the hippocampus expanding and getting larger, sensing them as lights getting brighter, or seeing them as like plants being given fresh water and sunlight. Tell your hippocampus "thanks for the memories" and for helping you to continue to learn and grow throughout your lifetime.

—— SET 146 ——

WOW Kindness is love with its work boots on. – Anonymous

3Rs Do you have any bad habits? How have you tried to ignore one or more of those bad habits? How have you tried to fix them? Do others know?

KISS 1. In Roman mythology, Mars was god of _____.
2. If you flip a coin, what is the probability that it will be heads?
3. In economics, what does "opportunity cost" mean?

SOS Find a one-word answer to the following so that the last two letters of each answer are also the first two letters of the next answer. A happy face: Not fatty: Argentinean mountain range: An approximation: An octopus has these.

ICE You have been hired to develop new toothpaste flavors that will stand out from all the others. What flavors will you suggest?

TAB While we sleep the brain produces the chemical 4EBP2, which contributes to normal memory functioning. In studies, sleep-deprived mice show lower amounts of the chemical and demonstrate signs of memory problems. When they receive a dose of the chemical before sleep deprivation, their memory functions normally even without sleep.[79]

Mmm Snow Angel Opposite Sides – Lie down in a comfortable position on your back, with legs extended out and hands at your side. Practice making Snow Angels by sliding your legs and arms along the floor. This time instead of using all four limbs at once, only use one leg and one arm at a time.

—— SET 147 ——

WOW Breathe. Let go. And remind yourself that this very moment is the only one you know you have for sure. – Oprah Winfrey

3Rs What children's songs and ditties do you remember from when you were a child? What were the words and melody? Did you say any rhymes when you were skipping, jumping rope, playing hide and seek, etc.?

---

79 http://www.sfn.org/~/media/SfN/Documents/Press%20Releases/2014/Sleep_PressPacket.sshx

KISS 1. What does monochromatic mean?
2. Where is the smallest bone in the body?
3. What American expression is used most often throughout the world?

SOS What do you put in a toaster?

ICE Make up new names for cereals.

TAB Approximately 100,000 miles of so-called "white matter" connect the various parts of your brain. That's "enough to circle the earth four times."[80]

Mmm Breathing Meditation: Lengthened Inhale & Exhale – Observe your breath. After a few breaths, begin to consciously lengthen each in-breath and out-breath. Let each inhale and each exhale lengthen and deepen. Do not strain. Continue for at least ten breath cycles with normal inhales and longer, slower exhales. Then return to a normal breath before getting up.

— SET 148 —

WOW I cannot do everything, but I can do something. One person can make an important difference. – Helen Keller

3Rs Where were you and what were you doing on 9/11? How did you first hear about the event? What do you remember about your thoughts during the event?

KISS 1. What word is a noun in the following sentence: My brain is fit!
2. What is the name given to the joining of two plants so they will grow as one plant? Hint: It is often done with fruit trees
3. From what country did we get these foods: Bologna, salami, lasagna, and spaghetti?

SOS How is it possible that since 1938, SSN 078-00-112 appeared thousands of times on tax returns?

ICE List as many reasons as you can for a scream.

TAB Memorizing the lyrics to songs can strengthen the mind and help one learn more effectively.

Mmm Song and Dance – Sing a song you know. Make up new gestures to go with it, and do them while you sing.

— SET 149 —

WOW No one respects a talent that is concealed. – Erasmus

80 Simmer, Carl (February 2014). Secrets of the brain. *National Geographic*, 34-39.

3Rs If you could run any company/organization in the world, what would be the most exciting to run? Why?

KISS 1. In Roman mythology, Neptune was god of _____.

2. What is a mother lode?

3. What was the leading cause of U.S. troop deaths during the Spanish American War?

SOS The math class Denise is in has 25 students, and they all took a test yesterday. Twenty-four students scored lower on the test than Denise. Where did Denise place in his class on the test?

ICE Is a principal or a principle stronger? Why?

TAB Two studies at Wellesley College indicate that acupuncture can help to relieve anxiety and stress, promote better energy level, improve mood, and can improve the lives of people with Alzheimer's.[81]

Mmm Generating Internal Force – This is a Qi Gong exercise used to build up qi or chi, so rather than pushing with the muscles, relax the body. The intention is for the necessary strength to come from the *mind*. Look at the palms of your hands, and find the line on your palm that curves around the fleshy part of the hand below the thumb. Now close the fingers into a loose fist, and notice where on that line the middle finger touches. This place on each hand is roughly the acupuncture point called "P-8." In this exercise you will be imagining these P-8 points on each hand pushing together. Now stand with the feet about shoulder-width apart and knees slightly bent. Keep the spine upright, but allow the pelvis to turn up and forward slightly as if you were sitting on a high stool. Bring the palms of the hands together in front of the heart with finger-tips pointing up. Close your eyes and touch the tip of the tongue to the roof of your mouth as if you were about to say the letter "t." In your mind, push the two points at the center of each palm (P-8) strongly towards one another. Do this for at least one minute.

— SET 150 —

WOW Nothing is really work unless you would rather be doing something else. – J.M. Barrie

3Rs When you were 10-years old, what did you and your friends in school most like to do together? What special memories of them do you have?

81 http://www.alzheimers.ne/11-19-14-acupuncture-for-alzheimers

KISS 1. What is a fresco?
2. Why don't we treat colds with antibiotics?
3. Who is considered the author of the Declaration of Independence?

SOS Use all the letters of the alphabet to make the following words complete: _ro_ _; _e_ _at; _ _ala; _a_k; _orc_p_ne; _a_z; _uie_; _u_ca; e_tr_; _io_in; _a_ _ful; _ _rtle.

ICE Get some paper and something to write with. Draw something out of the letter M.

TAB Different areas of the brain respond to language depending on whether we are seeing a word, listening to a word, or saying a word, so reading aloud activates more of the brain than reading silently.[82]

Mmm Dress Differently – When you get dressed or undressed today, change something about the way you do it. For example if you usually put your shirt on first, put your pants on first. If you stand up to put your pants on, sit down or lie down to do it. If you usually put both socks on before you put on shoes, put both sock and shoe on one side and then do the other, etc.

— SET 151 —

WOW No one can make you feel inferior without your consent. – Eleanor Roosevelt

3Rs What day in your life would you most like to live over? Why?

KISS 1. What word is written the most in the English language?
2. In what three sports does the winner cross the finish line backwards?
3. Where do you find these words, "Of the people, by the people and for the people"?

SOS As you drive under an overpass, the load is too high and you get stuck. What can you do?

ICE You are eating lunch at a fast food place with the President of the United States. You spill your soda on the table and it spills all over the President. What do you say/do?

TAB Everyone forgets sometimes. Occasional memory failures, such as temporarily forgetting a word, are normal. Contributing factors include information overload and the tendency to filter out less important details.

82 Katz, Lawrence C. and Manning Rubin. *Keep Your Brain Alive*. New York: Workman, 1999. p. 50.

Mmm Walking Knee Hold – Start by marching around the space. Gradually work to lift your knee up higher with each step. After several more steps, hold you knee in the air for 1-3 seconds longer before setting it back down again. Take a few more normal steps and then hold the opposite knee up for 1-3 seconds longer. For more of a challenge, hold on every step and/or hold for a longer time.

— SET 152 —

WOW The actions of people are the best interpreters of their thoughts. – John Locke

3Rs How did you spend your weekends as you were growing up? How much fun was it? Did you pretty much do the same thing every weekend? Did the activities involve other people or did you mostly do things by yourself?

KISS 1. In Greek mythology, who was Zeus?
2. What animals have the sharpest eyesight?
3. Which of these was invented first: TV, lie detector, or pop-up toaster?

SOS The first letter of each word in the following descriptions are also the same as the initials of the person described. Name the famous person being defined in the following: 1) Joyous Chef; 2) Prolific Painter; 3) Major Mime.

ICE How can you connect the following: taco, harp and lizard?

TAB Barry Komisaruk and Nan Wise, at Rutgers University, conducted MRI experiments demonstrating that orgasms increase blood flow to all parts of the brain—bringing nutrients and oxygenation along, too.[83]

Mmm Bathing Meditation – Today when you shower or take a bath, bring as much mindfulness attention as you can to the experience. Fully sense the water as you start to run it. Sense the sensation of the water on your skin. Sense your arm and hand as you reach for the soap or shampoo. Notice the weight and texture of the soap and shampoo. Sense the soap suds in your hand and on your body. Notice the shape and movements of scrubbing and wiping and rinsing, etc.

— SET 153 —

WOW If everyone is thinking alike then somebody isn't thinking. – General George Patton

3Rs What was the most important invention in history? Why?

---

83 http://www.huffingtonpost.com/2013/08/05/orgasms-good-for-you-study_n_3708222.html.

KISS 1. What is pointillism?

2. What is plastic made from?

3. From what countries did we get apricots, spaghetti, and the omelet?

SOS How can you make the letters "L" + "I" equal four?

ICE Pretend that you could star in a TV show. In what show would you like to star? Why?

TAB The results of a 2013 study at Emory University, suggest that reading a novel may have more positive effects on your brain than other types of reading. (https://www.psychologytoday.com/blog/the-athletes-way/201401/reading-fiction-improves-brain-connectivity-and-function)

Mmm Cross Body: Supine Elbow to Knee – Lie down on your back. As you inhale, bend one of your knees and lift it up, and try to touch it with opposite elbow. Release as you exhale. Repeat ten time alternating legs.

— SET 154 —

WOW Most of the time we don't communicate, we just take turns talking. – Robert Anthony

3Rs What do you forget to do most often? Is it important? How could you better remember?

KISS 1. Spell backwards the word for the appliance in your kitchen that keeps things cold.

2. Reduce these fractions: 76/95 and 85/102.

3. Name some of the major world religions.

SOS Forward I am heavy; backwards I am not. What am I?

ICE What would you bring with you if you were going to spend a month alone in a small submarine at the bottom of the ocean?

TAB Research indicates that the potassium-packed banana contains fiber and three natural sugars—sucrose, fructose and glucose. This combination provides an instant, sustained and substantial boost of energy that can assist learning by making students more alert. Bananas are also high in B vitamins that help calm the nervous system.

Mmm Samba Step – Start with feet together. Step the left foot forward. Bring the right foot up to join it. Step the left foot in place. Step the right foot behind you. Bring the left to join it. Step the right foot in place. Repeat with music and your own arm movements.

— SET 155 —

WOW The problem is never how to get new, innovative thoughts into your mind, but how to get the old ones out. – Dee Hock

3Rs How did you spend recess time in grade school? What are your most distinctive recess time memories?

KISS 1. What Greek goddess was the city of Athens named for, and what gift did she give the city?

2. On the average, which mammal lives the longest?

3. Which state has more than half of the coastline of the entire U.S.?

SOS What kind of woodworking is done in homes, offices, schools, etc.?

ICE List as many as you can of unique or unusual places someone could sleep.

TAB Dr. *Sandra Bond,* Chief Director of the Center for Brain Health at The University of Texas at Dallas), suggests taking a 5-minute break every half hour rather than overtaxing the brain by working non-stop on a mentally challenging activity. This gives the brain time to recover from fatigue and allows room for new ideas to come.[84]

Mmm Retaining Breath In – With this breath technique, you will experiment with consciously extending the pause between the in-breath and out-breath. Do not alter the pattern of your breathing right away: just observe it. Notice the brief pause after the in-breath before you exhale. When you are ready, play with holding that pause after the in-breath briefly. Do not overdo it. Inhale. Hold. Exhale. Return to a normal breath for a few breaths, then repeat.

— SET 156 —

WOW There's nothing wrong in making a mistake—as long as you don't follow up with encores. – Anonymous

3Rs What do you like to learn about? Why?

KISS 1. Which is the most ornate style of Greek column? Doric, Ionic, or Corinthian?

2. Which animal cannot jump?

3. What car is named for an elected president of the U.S.?

SOS Johnny's a magician and weighs 190 pounds. He wants to cross a pedestrian bridge with a weight restriction of 200 pounds. He is carrying three gold pieces that put him eight ounces over the limit. What did Johnny do?

---

84 http://www.blog.citrixonline.com/training-your-brain-to-thrive-from-9-to-5.

ICE Think of things that snap or include "snap".

TAB The Foundation for Critical Thinking uses the term "activated ignorance" to refer to information we learn and actively use that is in fact false, though we mistakenly believe it is true. It is important to continually question and re-evaluate what we "know."[85]

Mmm Retaining Breath Out – With this breath technique, you will experiment with consciously extending the pause after the out-breath. Again observe the breath first, noticing the brief pause after the out-breath. When you are ready, play with holding that pause after the in-breath briefly. Do not overdo it. Exhale. Hold. Inhale. Return to a normal breath for a few breaths, then repeat.

— SET 157 —

WOW Behold the turtle! It makes progress only when it sticks its neck out.
– James B. Conant

3Rs What do you most/least love and appreciate about nature? In what ways could you come to enjoy nature more?

KISS 1. Which word of the following is not a homonym: flower, four, hour, and tree?

2. On a computer keyboard, which symbol is on the "4" key?

3. Name some significant figures associated with this world religion: Buddhism.

SOS The answers to the following each contain "jack": Handyman; Nursery rhyme; Cutting instrument in one's pocket; Person of cold weather?

ICE One Saturday afternoon when you come back from running errands, you discover your friendly neighbor has cut down all the healthy bushes between your two properties that you had kept neatly trimmed. What will you do? What will be your approach?

TAB In a study at the University of Michigan, a participant who spent time walking in a serene, natural environment of trees and plants showed improved attention and increased short-term memory scores.[86]

---

85 http://www.criticalthinking.org/pages/critical-thinking-distinguishing-between-inert-information-activated-ignorance-activated-knowledge/488

86 Carper, Jean. *100 Simple Things You Can Do to Prevent Alzheimer's and Age-related Memory Loss.* NY: Little Brown, 2010. p. 201.

Mmm Crawling – Get down on your hands and knees. Letting the eyes lead, look around and above you for several breaths. Imagine you are a curious baby and crawl around to explore the room or environment.

— SET 158 —

WOW Courage is what it takes to stand up and speak. Courage is also what it takes to sit down and listen. – Winston Churchill

3Rs What did your parents do for a living? Were you involved? Did you consider following in their footsteps?

KISS 1. What is the difference between an autobiography and a biography?
2. Where on Earth would you weigh one percent less?
3. What state grows the most apples?

SOS Although it is always before you, what is it you can never see?

ICE It is your first time at an auction and you are not sure of your options. You want to buy a _____ and so you bid on them and you get the bid. When you go to pick up and pay for them you discover you have bought an ugly antique lamp. What can you do?

TAB Traumatic brain injury (TBI) can be serious and even fatal. According to the Center for Disease Control, TBI is an injury "caused by a bump, blow or jolt to the head or a penetrating head injury that disrupts the normal function of the brain." The effects of traumatic brain injury range from temporary to long term and "include impaired thinking or memory, movement, sensation (e.g., vision or hearing), or emotional functioning (e.g., personality changes, depression)."[87]

Mmm Power Stance: Hands on Hips – Stand with your feet in a solid shoulder-width stance. On an inhale, put your hands on your hips. Imagine that you have been asked to take a stand for your own self-worth. Breathe normally, and stay focused on your sensation. According to a 2015, Reader's Digest article, research in social psychology indicates that 2 minutes of holding this pose can reduce stress and increase one's sense of power.

— SET 159 —

WOW The only people with whom you should try to get even are those who have helped you. – John E. Southard

---

87 http://www.cdc.gov/TraumaticBrainInjury/index.html

3Rs What do you remember about going to a rummage sale, garage sale, estate sale, flea market or auction? What did you buy? Did it turn out to be a treasure, a good deal or did you regret your purchase? Why?

KISS 1. What is significant about the Globe Theatre?

2. What is the normal resting heart rate for most adults?

3. Name some significant figures associated with this world religion: Christianity.

SOS Which animal with a mask can be removed from the following and leave a color: ORACAGENCRONO.

ICE What is the prickliest thing in the world? Be creative.

TAB Kindness and helping others stimulate the brain to release endorphins such as serotonin. Endorphins are the brain chemicals that create the energized "runner's high" type of state. Serotonin, in particular, produces feelings of satisfaction and wellbeing. So it does pay to be nice!

Mmm Meditation: Gift to a Helpful Person – For this meditation chose someone who guided you in your life that you wish to express to. This could be a parent, a teacher, a spiritual counselor, a friend. Close your eyes, and place your hands on your heart. After a few breaths, visualize that person as if that person were sitting in front of you right now. Look the person in the eye and smile. Tell the person how his or her guidance was a gift to you. Now imagine what kind of gift you would want to give that person as an expression of your appreciation. It can be something material or symbolic. See the gift in your hands, and then offer the gift to the person.

—— SET 160 ——

WOW Learning is a treasure that will follow its owner everywhere. – Chinese Proverb

3Rs What do you remember about a time something of yours was lost or stolen? What issues did that bring up for you? What item(s) was lost or stolen? How special was the item(s) to you? How did you resolve the loss in your mind? Was the item(s) ever found or returned?

KISS 1. Name the different times to capitalize a word.

2. Is it true or false that snakes charm their prey?

3. What large U.S. city has more people of Polish ancestry than any city in the world other than Warsaw, Poland?

SOS What is impossible to hold for more than several minutes but is lighter than a feather?

ICE The following are common sayings with the ending listed in parentheses. Replace the part in parenthesis to create new alternative endings: No pain (no gain). If you can't stand the heat (get out of the kitchen). If wishes were horses (then beggars would ride). Great minds think (alike).

TAB Although information in the brain often travels at different speeds, transmission can reach speeds as fast as 120 meters/sec., which is the equivalent of 268 miles/hr.[88]

Mmm Nose "Workout" – Try to wiggle your nose, Can you do it? See how many different ways you can move and activate your nose.

— SET 161 —

WOW I will speak ill of no [one] and speak all the good I know of everybody. – Ben Franklin

3Rs Other than your own family, which family throughout history would it have been most interesting to have been a part of? Why?

KISS 1. Who were Odin, Thor, Loki, Freyja and Hel?

2. When rain falls through a layer of super-cold air, does it become snow, hail, or sleet?

3. How many red stripes are on the U.S. flag?

SOS What goes up and down without actually moving?

ICE Where would be a good place to hide presents in your home? Be creative.

TAB Scientists at the University of North Carolina were able to stimulate the brain toward more creativity by physically increasing electrical activity in the brain.[89]

Mmm Foot Rub – Give yourself a foot massage or exchange foot rubs with someone else. Pay close attention to the sensations of your foot and whole body.

— SET 162 —

WOW Your time may be limited, but your imagination is not. – Anonymous

3Rs What do you like to do by yourself? What do you usually like to do with others?

---

88 http://lvescience.com/51376-how-long-fast-does-a-thought-travel.html

89 http://www.huffingtonpost.com/2015/04/17/brain -stimulation-study_n_7087828.ht

KISS 1. What is iambic pentameter?
2. What is the total number of dots that are on a standard pair of dice?
3. Name some significant figures associated with this world religion: Hinduism.

SOS My father owned a grocery store and he always said, "If people would tell the truth I would sell more." What did my father sell?

ICE You have just won 100 jars of peanut butter. What are some unusual uses for all this peanut butter?

TAB It is good to write down lists of things to remember, because writing things down reinforces what you want to remember in a positive way. However, to practice and strengthen your memory, only check your list once you have completed it.

Mmm Clock Stepping – Imagine you are standing at the center of a giant clock on the floor. Without turning around, step to the following times: 12 o'clock; 3 o'clock; 8 o'clock; 6 o'clock; 9 o'clock; 2 o'clock; Repeat.

— SET 163 —

WOW We cannot change the inevitable. The only thing we can do is play on the one string we have, and that is our attitude. – Charles Swindoll

3Rs What do you wish you had learned more about or understood better when you were younger? Why?

KISS 1. Name ten pronouns, starting with a one-letter pronoun then a two-letter one etc. on up to ten letters.
2. What is considered a normal blood pressure for an adult?
3. What is the only city to be on two continents?

SOS What has eight wheels but has only one passenger?

ICE Create some original reasons to convince someone to get a dog.

TAB The cerebellum comes from the Latin for "little brain." It is located in the back of the brain under the occipital and temporal lobes. Although it does not initiate movement, the cerebellum coordinates input for fine-motor muscular control related to balance, muscle timing, and force. It also performs primary cognitive functions pertaining to language and coordination of trial-and-error motor learning.

Mmm Cerebellum Meditation – Place your hands at the base of your skull, and visualize your cerebellum. Imagine that you can actually see and sense this area of your brain beneath where your hands are resting. What color do you visualize it as? What does it feel like? Once the image is clear for you, play with altering the image in ways that might strengthen or nourish your cerebellum. For example, since this area is associated with balance and movement you could imagine it as a set of scales and see them swinging back and forth until they are in perfect balance. Thank your cerebellum for the ways it helps you to "stay in balance" and function well.

— SET 164 —

WOW The way I see it, if you need both of your hands for whatever it is you're doing, then your brain should probably be in on it, too. – Ellen DeGeneres

3Rs Suppose you could have been a world champion in any sport, what sport would you have chosen? Why?

KISS 1. Name some different genres, or types, of literature.
2. On what parts of the body does a dog perspire?
3. Name some significant figures associated with this world religion: Islam.

SOS In the following set of letters, unscramble and take away something dry to find something wet: TERDASEIRN.

ICE You cannot get the lid off a jar and it is essential that you open it. What can you do?

TAB Dr. *Sandra Bond Chapman* describes multitasking as "asbestos to the brain". The brain functions best by doing one task at a time. When we multitask we can create mental fatigue and actually reduce our efficiency, making a task take as much as four times as long as it might have with mono-tasking.[90]

Mmm Mindful Cooking Meditation: Sensations – As you make one of your meals today, bring as much mindfulness as you can to the sensations of the cooking process. Focus on only one step at a time. Fully sense the arm and hand reaching, to open or close the refrigerator or cupboards. Feel the sensation of the food, dishes, cutting boards, pans, heat of the stove, etc. Notice the rhythm of chopping, stirring, pouring, serving, etc.

— SET 165 —

WOW Blessed are they who expect nothing, for they shall not be disappointed. – Anonymous

3Rs What do you wonder about the most? Why?

---

90 http://blog.citrixonline.com/training-your-brain-to-thrive-from-9-to-5

KISS 1. To what does *deus ex machine* refer? Hint: Think theatrical.
2. How long does it take glass to decompose?
3. What four states are included in the Four Corners of the southwest U.S.?

SOS Make common English words by inserting the same pair of letters within each set, but different pairs of letters across sets, for the three sets of letters that follow: (1) _ _ p _ _ zard; (2) _ _ r _ _ tual; (3) _ _ n _ _urse. What is the pair of letters for each set?

ICE Name as many creative expressions as you can that contain the word "square". Example: A square meal.

TAB When you are dreaming, the areas of the brain associated with vision are activated as are emotion related areas such as the amygdala and prefrontal cortex. Relevant theory and related research suggests there is a strong correlation between the nature of one's emotional states during the day and while dreaming.[91]

Mmm Airplane Arms – Put your arms out at shoulder height like airplane wings. Circle your arms in tiny circles ten times forward and then ten times back. Keeping the arms out, point your fingers to the floor, then up to the ceiling, and repeat 10 times. Circle the wrists in one direction ten times and then repeat in the opposite direction. Take off and "fly" around the room.

— SET 166 —

WOW A conclusion is the place where you got tired of thinking. – Arthur Bloch

3Rs What do you worry or have concerns about? Why? How do you handle stress? How can you improve your stress level? Since stress is hard on the brain how can one stop worrying?

KISS 1. Which expression, if taken literally, means to devour something that beats in your chest?
2. What happens in a lunar eclipse?
3. Which is the state with only one school district?

SOS What makes the following set of words unique: the, he, her, here, there, ere, rein, in, herein?

ICE If silence were something you could see, what would it look like?

TAB The Center for Disease Control reports that on average, more than 50,000 people die each year in connection with traumatic brain injury (TBI). About

91 httb://www.ncbi.nlm.nih.gov/pmc/articles/PMC3336925/

40% of all TBIs are the result of falls and the next highest cause is motor vehicle accidents.[92]

Mmm Foot Reflexology Brain Points – According to reflexology, the brain corresponds to points on the tips of each of the toes. Walk your fingers along the tips of your toes, working from the inside out and back again several times on each side.[93]

— SET 167 —

WOW No person is your friend who demands your silence or denies you your right to grow. – Alice Walker

3Rs Think of a time when you or someone cooked or baked something and it did not taste good. What was the mistake?

KISS 1. What is the significance of the Trojan horse in Virgil's *Aeneid*?

2. Where in the human body is the thyroid gland?

3. Name some significant figures associated with this world religion: Judaism.

SOS Two brothers were fighting so their mother punished them by making them stand on the same piece of paper. They could not see or touch each other. How could this be done?

ICE You are taking a hike and staying on the trail. There is a large colony of ants on the path and cacti on the sides of the trail. How can you avoid stepping on the ants?

TAB Lemons have more sugar than oranges, and are thus better at helping your brain to be more alert.

Mmm Pulling the Golden Ring – Hold your hands out in front of you with the fingers together and the thumbs away to the side so one hand forms an "L" shape and the other forms a reverse "L". Maintaining the "L" shape, bring the hands to your sides. Take a solid stance with knees slightly bent. Then as if resisting a great force, bend the elbows to bring the L-shaped hands up to the armpits. Touch the heels of your hands to the ribs. Keep the upper arms tucked in close to the body. Imagine that there is a heavy golden ring hanging right in front of you. Focus on the thumb and index finger of the left hand, as you extend the left arm out towards the golden

---

92 http://www.cdc.gov/TraumaticBrainInjury/index.html

93 Dellemore, Doug, et al. (1995) New Choices in Natural Healing. Ed. Bill Gottlieb. Emmaus, PA: Rodale Press.

ring. Then turn your thumb down and take hold of the golden ring in an open fist. Once you have a hold on the ring, twist the ring with great effort to return your hand back to thumb-side up. Release the ring and bring the hand back into the L-shape and return it to the armpit. Repeat the steps of grasping the ring with the right hand. To finish return both hands down to your sides.

— SET 168 —

WOW What is originality? It is being one's self and reporting accurately what we see. – Ralph Waldo Emerson

3Rs What embarrassing things have happened to you? Why were they embarrassing to you?

KISS 1. Which familiar Christmas carol of German origin is *Stille Nacht* in its original language?

2. True or false? The barnacle is the discarded home of a marine animal.

3. What state has no natural lakes, only man-made lakes?

SOS What is interesting about these words: repaid, reward, and sloops.

ICE It's your lucky day! What happens?

TAB Be careful in making judgments about people's potential creative abilities. For example, Beethoven's music teacher once said "as a composer, he is hopeless."[94]

Mmm Rhythm Work: Right Left Snap – Snap your fingers to the following rhythm: Right, right, left, right. Left, left, left. Left, left, right, left. Right, right, right. Repeat and increase speed as you get it.

— SET 169 —

WOW A person thinks as well through legs and arms as the brain. – Henry David Thoreau

3Rs What especially kind deeds have you done? What happened that you feel good about?

KISS 1. Does "lie" or "lay" mean to recline?

2. What is a seismograph?

3. Who are the Teamsters?

SOS In the nursery rhyme "Sing a Song of Sixpence" how many bluebirds were baked in the pie?

94 http://www.actsweb.org/articles/article.php?i=229&d=2&c=6

ICE If you were at a garage sale, what especially startling things might you find?

TAB Talking about a creative problem too much can actually inhibit the creative process.[95]

Mmm Spiral Walk: In – Stand at the edge of an open space. Walk in a circle around the perimeter of the space. Once you reach the place where you started, step in slightly and continue to walk just inside of the path you just walked. Continue around in this way, each time walking in a slightly narrower circle until your reach the center and your spiral path fills the whole room.

—— SET 170 ——

WOW A grudge is the heaviest thing to carry. – John Bridgman

3Rs Did you ever roast hot dogs or marshmallows, or make s'mores? Did you ever sleep outside overnight or attend a summer camp? What are your memories of those times? Were you scared to sleep outdoors?

KISS 1. Name some forms of poetry. For example, a sonnet.
2. If a billion follows a million, and a trillion follows a billion, what follows a trillion?
3. Which is the least populated state in the United States?

SOS Rearrange the letters in "elation" to spell a part of the body.

ICE Some towns have unusual names, e.g.: Cut and Shoot, TX; Hot Coffee, MS; Truth or Consequences, NM. Create wacky new names for the towns you have lived in.

TAB Failing to get enough sleep isn't just a bad idea, over time, it can also lead to neurological disorders. Recent research conducted at the University of Rochester shows that while we sleep, the brain removes its waste by-products like beta amyloid. If these waste by-products are not removed, they eventually damage the brain.[96]

Mmm Compassion Meditation: Father – Close your eyes, and place your hands on your heart. On the next breath, see your father (or a father figure) in front of you. Next invite an image of your father at age five. In your mind, what was he like as a young child? Smile to your father's younger self, give him a hug and send him gentle, loving compassion.

---

95 https://www.psychologytoday.com/blog/the-athletes-way/201508/why-does-overthinking-sabotage-the-creative-process

96 www.nih.gov/researchmatters/october2013/10282013clear.htm

— SET 171 —

WOW Keep your face to the sunshine and you cannot see the shadows – Helen Keller

3Rs What explorers do you recall from history, and which one most impressed you? Why? What did that person discover? Would you have liked to have been that person? Why or why not?

KISS 1. Name some arts and crafts.

2. What is hypothermia?

3. Why was the Eisenhower Interstate Highway System required to have one mile in every five miles be straight?

SOS A majority of eggs laid by birds are slightly narrower on one end. How is this useful?

ICE You are a butterfly eavesdropping; what do you hear?

TAB When you learn something new and want to remember it, visualize the location where you learned it and concretely connect that information to the image. Keeping some mementos of that place can also reinforce your memory of that particular learning. If you are trying to remember something, it can also help to return to the place you first learned it.

Mmm Visualization Meditation: Summer – Metaphorically, summer is a time of expansion: plants begin to ripen and thrive. This meditation can acknowledge the season or invite growth in some existing phase or aspect of your life. Close your eyes. As you are ready, visualize yourself or some area of your life as a green field of plants. Imagine how the summer's heat energizes the plants and sense them growing and expanding rapidly as insects buzz and flit around you. In the evenings the stars above twinkle and fireflies light up.

— SET 172 —

WOW If opportunity doesn't knock, build a door. – Milton Berle

3Rs If you could go back and change anything in your life, what would it be? How would things be different in your life now if that changed?

KISS 1. What words have the sound of "c", but not a single "c" in it?

2. What animal can outrun most horses, go without water longer than a camel, and see to the rear without turning its head?

3. What does the Cold War refer to?

SOS Today is Sunday. What is the day that follows the day that comes after the day that's before the day before the day before yesterday?

ICE Describe an imaginary "Zymphast." What is it?

TAB Common wisdom has long held that goldfish have a memory span of only 3 seconds. Not true: In addition to more scientific research, the television show *MythBusters* showed that goldfish could remember their way through an obstacle course for at least a month.[97]

Mmm Fish Mudra – Place one hand palm down and then put the other hand on top of the back of it. The thumbs will now be opposite one another on the outside of the hands. Keep the fingers together to make the body of a fish with the thumbs as the fins. Rotate the thumbs in full circles several times both clockwise and counterclockwise. Pretend your hands are a fish for a minute or so and swim them around the room. Then repeat with the opposite hand on top. (This exercise is also good for arthritis).[98]

— SET 173 —

WOW I can't choose how I feel, but I can choose what I do about it. – Anonymous

3Rs Did you ever go fishing? What are your memories of fishing? What "fish stories" have you heard or told?

KISS 1. Name some famous ancient Greek writers.

2. Which of these products causes sugar to ferment: yeast, salt, or baking soda?

3. Which country contains more than 25% of the world's forest?

SOS Why would a manufacturer selling sardines packed in oil try to squeeze so many fish into each can?

ICE Draw a big "**X**" on a piece of paper. What is it? Be creative!

TAB Animal studies suggest early life environments affect brain development. Being brought up in a nurturing environment seems to promote a greater ability to regulate one's emotions.[99]

Mmm YMCA Dance – Y = arms go up overhead and point outward; M = arms bend in so fingertips touch in front of the breastbone; C = arms curve off to the left

---

97 http://www.discovery.com/tv-shows/mythbbusters/videos/goldfish-memory-minimyth

98 Dellemore, Doug, et al. (1995) New Choices in Natural Healing. Ed. Bill Gottlieb. Emmaus, PA: Rodale Press.

99 http://developingchild.harvard.edu/resources/multimedia/videos/three_core_concepts/brain_architecture/

in a semi-circle; A = Arms go up overhead with finger tips touching above head. Singing is optional. What would the dance of your name look like?

— SET 174 —

WOW If there was nothing wrong in the world, there wouldn't be anything for us to do. – George Bernard Shaw

3Rs What food best describes your character as a child? Why?

KISS 1. *Noh, kabuki,* and *butoh* are theatre forms from what nation?
2. Which has the greatest frequency of waves: radio waves, visible light waves, microwaves, or X-rays?
3. During World War I, did Japan ally with the same side as the U.S. or with same side as the Germans and what other nations fought on that side?

SOS Find a one word answer to the following so that the last two letters of each answer are also the first two letters of the next answer. A Hawaiian dance: The language of Caesar: a unit of measurement: A cheap bright, patterned fabric: Title of the rulers of Russia: Creator of beauty: Celestial body.

ICE In the nursery rhyme, why was little Jack Horner sitting in the corner? Be creative.

TAB 2014 studies at the Georgetown University Medical Center provide new evidence that adolescents at higher risk of alcoholism have reduced and impaired connections in key brain networks linked to impulsivity. The studies also connected impulsivity intake of sugar and DHA (an essential omega-3 fatty acid).[100]

Mmm Spiral Walk: Out – Stand in the center of the room or an open space. Turn in a small circle. Then walk around that circle in a slightly wider circle. Continue around in this way creating a spiral path that fills the whole room.

— SET 175 —

WOW A feeble body weakens the mind. – Jean-Jacques Rousseau

3Rs Try to recall the earliest memory you have? Why do you think you still remember that?

KISS 1. What is the word for "subway" in Swahili and Russian?
2. What does CPR stand for?
3. The source of the Mississippi River is found in what state?

---

100 https://gumc.georgetown.edu/news/Researchers-Find-Common-Factors-in-Teens-at-Risk-for-Alcohol-Abuse

SOS What do lots of people eat before it is born and after it is dead?

ICE Generate a list of brands that are often used as universal names for all products of that type.

TAB Learning a new language changes your brain network both structurally and functionally, according to researchers at Penn State University.[101]

Mmm Clock Arms –Imagine that you are a clock, and your arms are the hands of the clock. Make your arms say the following times: Noon ; 1:30; 6:45; 7: 15; 9:20.

—— SET 176 ——

WOW The only thing worse than being talked about is not being talked about. – Oscar Wilde

3Rs What one thing about your parents would you most liked to have changed? Why?

KISS 1. What does a novel, opera, play, etc. generally always have?
2. Which species of bear is the largest?
3. How many judges are there on the U.S. Supreme Court?

SOS What do all of these words have in common: cotton, hard, rock, bar?

ICE What would be a good topic for a ridiculous "Letter to the Editor" competition?

TAB Research by Dr. Oliver Sacks, professor of neurology at the NYU School of Medicine, indicates that our brains "keep time to music, involuntarily, even when not consciously paying attention to it."[102]

Mmm Rhythm Work: Snap a Song – Think of a song you know different from one you have used before. Instead of singing it, snap your finger to create the rhythm of the song.

—— SET 177 ——

WOW The one who says it cannot be done should not interrupt the one doing it. – George Bernard Shaw

3Rs What former possession of yours broke that you wish you still had? Why was it so important? Could it be replaced?

---

101 http://news.psu.edu/story/334349/2014/11/12/research/learning-languages-workout-brains-both-young-and-old

102 http://www.livestrong.com/article/157461-how-music-affects-the-human-brain/

KISS 1. Name some famous operas.
2. What chemical compound is known as the universal solvent?
3. For what are Cesar Chavez and Dolores Heurta best known?

SOS The sign reads "If you don't see what you want you have come to the right place." What is the business?

ICE You are curator of a museum. What unique exhibit will you create?

TAB Depression and Post Traumatic Stress Disorder are associated with abnormal shrinkage in the hippocampus.[103]

Mmm Cooling Breath – Stick your tongue out. Now roll your tongue into a tube shape as best you can. For your next inhale, draw a full breath of air in through your tongue like drinking from a straw. Then pull your tongue back in and close your mouth. Tuck your chin and hold your breath for a bit. When you are ready, exhale and repeat. This breath can be cooling on a hot summer day!

— SET 178 —

WOW There are better things ahead than any we leave behind. – C. S. Lewis

3Rs Prices have changed. What did gas, bread, shoes, etc. cost when you were young? What about wages/salaries; how did they compare to today? What are your feelings about prices/wages over time?

KISS 1. Punctuate the following phrase so you have three sentences: What was isn't what is what was was what is is.
2. What mathematical symbol can you put between 2 and 3 to make a number greater than 2 but less than 3?
3. In what state is there the most land area of Indian Reservations?

SOS Take a Medieval European fighter and add a letter of the alphabet (on the front or back) to get something that sounds like coming together.

ICE Give uses for a single staple.

TAB Research suggests that people whose brains recover more quickly from agitated emotional states also seem to have better ability to voluntarily control their emotions, have lower levels of cortisol (stress hormone), and higher immune functions.[104]

---

103 http://www.ncbi.nih.gov/pmc/articles/PMC3182008/

104 http://www.today.com/id/42367193/ns/today-today_books/t/its-always-personal-coping-emotions-stress-work/

Mmm Mindful Dusting Meditation: Loving Effort – Dust your home today with as much mindfulness and loving intention as you can. When you touch any object or piece of furniture, contemplate how it contributes to your home space. As you interact with each object or piece of furniture, let your dusting be a loving caress. Let each of your movements show how you care for the elements that make up your environment on a daily basis. See the physical energy you put into dusting and polishing as radiating out to infuse your home environment with love, peace, goodwill, and/or any other qualities you would like to be part of the experience of your home for you and others.

— SET 179 —

WOW The value and interest of life is not so much to do conspicuous things . . . as to do ordinary things with the perception of their enormous value. – Teilhard de Chardin

3Rs What hair styles have you had over the years? How has your hair style changed?

KISS 1. In the Robert Frost poem "The Road Not Taken" the narrator comes to a place where "Two roads diverged in a yellow wood." Which road was taken? Hint: " . . . and that has made all the difference".

2. What creature on earth is the biggest threat to people, in that it is responsible for the most deaths of humans each year? Hint: Think small.

3. Name significant members of the American Civil Rights Movement.

SOS A man in a uniform is running home. Suddenly he sees a second man wearing a mask and holding a scary object. He quickly turns around and runs back to where he started. What is happening?

ICE Use your imagination to think of an unusual prize for an unusual contest. What are the rules?

TAB Laughter releases hormones in the brain that reduce stress and improve functioning.

Mmm Laughing – Spend a few minutes laughing. You can "fake it until you make it" with this one. Start with standard laughing sounds: "Ho-ho-ho-ho" "ha-ha-ha-ha" Hee-hee-hee-hee-hee." Silly? Yes! Repeat for 30-60 seconds or until genuine laughter takes over.

— SET 180 —

WOW Education never hurt anybody who was willing to learn after it was obtained. – Anonymous

3Rs What has been the most exciting place, person, or thing you have ever seen in real life? Why was it exciting?

KISS 1. Name painters well-known for self-portraits; and which famous old painter painted more self-portraits, Rembrandt or Van Gogh?

2. What color is a coffee bean when picked?

3. Of the five largest cities in the U.S., which has the greatest seasonal extremes in temperature?

SOS The fire went out and two people fell to the ground. Why? Where were they?

ICE Think of ways you could give an elephant a bath?

TAB The first cervical vertebra in the neck has to bear the weight of the brain. Called the atlas vertebra, it is named for Atlas of Greek mythology, who carried the world on his shoulders.

Mmm Bobble Head – Using your imagination, sense for the top of your spinal cord. The spinal cord itself is part of the nervous system and integrates with your brain. With correct posture, the actual top of spine is nearly level with your eyebrows. Move your head with small, gentle motions to sense the skull floating above and supported by the spine.

— SET 181 —

WOW Tomorrow is the most important thing in life. Comes to us at midnight very clean. It's perfect when it arrives and it puts itself in our hands. It hopes we've learned something from yesterday. – John Wayne

3Rs Describe a school you attended, including your school building, the surrounding playground, the classrooms, etc.

KISS 1. Punctuate the following sentence in two different ways so that the principal and the teacher are alternately the foolish one: the teacher says the principal is a fool

2. What type of oil is used for cooking in submarines because it doesn't smoke unless it is heated above 450 degrees?

3. Name one president of the U.S. who is not *currently* buried in U.S. soil. Tricky!

SOS I am on sale when you buy me or I can be a sign of a parting.

ICE What are some things you can pick up with a spoon but not a fork?

TAB Researchers have found the following minerals—in appropriate doses—important for brain functioning: Calcium, copper, iodine, iron and magnesium, selenium and zinc.

Mmm Spiral Walk: Backing In – Stand at the edge of a clear, open space. Carefully walk backwards in a circle around the perimeter of the space. Continue around, each time walking in a slightly narrower circle to c create a spiral path that fills the whole room.

— SET 182 —

WOW If you are waiting for something to turn up, you might want to start with your own shirt sleeves. – Anonymous

3Rs What have you been praised or rewarded for in your life? What types of people praise you and do not praise you? Why do you think that is the case? How do people praise you now? How do you praise others?

KISS 1. Name some writers associated with Romanticism in the first half of the 1800's?

2. What is moonlight?

3. Where did Martin Luther King give his famous "I Have a Dream" speech?

SOS To whom are you most closely related, your mother or your sister?

ICE List as many three-letter animals as you can.

TAB The parietal lobe is located at the top back of the brain. Among other functions, it integrates information from the senses and processes spatial relations such as eye-hand coordination. The parietal lobe is particularly associated with the sense of touch.

Mmm Parietal Lobe Meditation – Place your hands on top of your head just above and behind your ears. Begin visualizing the parietal lobes of your brain. Imagine that you can actually see and sense that area of your brain beneath where your hands are resting. What color do you visualize them as? What do they feel like? How do you imagine the right side and left side as different, or are they? Which side seems stronger to you? Once the image is clear for you, play with altering the image in ways that might strengthen or nourish your parietal lobes. For example, since this area is associated with touch, you might imagine it with different textures or imagine that you are stroking it like a pet. Thank your parietal lobe for the ways it helps you to "stay in touch" and function well.

— SET 183 —

WOW The true test of character is not how much we know, but how we behave when we don't know. The true test of a [person's] character is what [that person] does when no one is watching. – John Wooden

3Rs What are some of the happiest moments in your life? Where did they take place? What happened?

KISS 1. What percussion instrument is named after its geometric shape?

2. When should you take an emetic?

3. Where is Angel Falls, the world's highest waterfall, located?

SOS What does this code say: "NE1CDB"?

ICE Describe how you would teach a bull to tap dance.

TAB Listening to emotional music activates centers in your brain that respond to "naturally rewarding stimuli" such as food and sex according to studies by neuroscientists, Robert J. Zatorre and Valorie N. Salimpoor.[105]

Mmm Listening Meditation: Sound of Silence – Put on some music, and close your eyes. Rather than listening to the sounds, listen for moments of silence between the sounds.

— SET 184 —

WOW We are what we pretend to be, but we better be very careful what we pretend. – Kurt Vonnegut

3Rs What have you been the "first" in your family to do? How did it happen? Why had no one else done it before?

KISS 1. What is the error in the following sentence: "The zebra will not eat it's food."?

2. Name a plant that must be grown by bulbs rather than seed.

3. Who was King of England during the American Revolution?

SOS Who is the most beautiful woman or man in the world? Why?

ICE When you get home from work you are surprised to find people you know in your living room. What are possible situations for this? Get those creative juices going!

---

105 http://www.nytimes.com/2013/06/09/opinion/sunday/why-music-makes-our-brain-sing.html?_r=0

TAB Paul Ekman of the University of California at San Francisco Medical School has developed a video that can train people to recognize micro-emotions that may cross the face in as little as one twenty-fifth of a second.[106]

Mmm Crawling Backwards – Get down on your hands and knees. Crawl like a baby for a minute or so. Then reverse the movement and crawl backwards.

— SET 185 —

WOW There are two ways of meeting difficulties, you alter the difficulties or you alter yourself to meet them. – Phyllis Bottome

3Rs Describe your teachers. Did you have lots of homework? What did you most appreciate about your teachers?

KISS 1. In the *Legend of Sleepy Hollow*, what was Ichabod Crane's occupation?
2. True or false: The continents on which we live have been moving their location for millions of years and will continue to move in the future.
3. Maine borders which U.S. state?

SOS What does this code say: "URAQT, I M 1 2!"?

ICE Think of what you could fill a room with that would cost the least.

TAB Practicing skills in your mind during sleep can be quite productive.

Mmm Hotdog Roll – Lie down on the floor or a large bed. Roll over first to the right, then to the left, and then over and over in each direction. Imagine you are a hotdog and you want to make sure all four sides cook evenly.

— SET 186 —

WOW The happiest people seem to be those who are producing something; the bored people are those who are consuming much and producing nothing. – William Inge

3Rs What have you most liked and disliked about your job or profession? What would have been the alternate job or profession you would have chosen if circumstances had been different? Why?

KISS 1. Who is the "prima donna" in an opera company?
2. What is the large, easily-seen vein in the side of the neck called?
3. What is an elected official who has been defeated and still must serve called?

SOS What do you call creatures that have four legs and can fly?

---

106 http://www.pauleman.com/micro-expressions/

ICE The answer is: "At noon." What could the question be?

TAB "Remembering words of praise and hugs of appreciation . . . helps to shape your mental image of yourself. Who you are grows out of your past—as you recall it. Day by day you are what you remember."[107]

Mmm Compassion Meditation: Half Your Age – Close your eyes, and place your hands on your heart. On the next breath, invite a memory of yourself at half the age you are now. See your younger self in front of you as you were then. Smile to your younger self. In your mind give that younger self a hug and send the younger you gentle, loving compassion. Repeat seeing yourself at 5-10 year intervals until you reach the age you are now.

— SET 187 —

WOW The two hardest things to handle in life are failure and success. – Anonymous

3Rs What have you wanted to buy and could not? What happened?

KISS 1. What is the error in the following sentence: "The money was equally divided between the girls"?

2. What are the names given to the members of a horse family: father, mother, son and daughter?

3. Who were the following states named for: North/South Carolina, Pennsylvania, Georgia, Virginia?

SOS Where do you often see the fraction 24/31?

ICE Name things that do not change.

TAB A recent European university study found that a patient who was physically, completely blind could still sense another person's gaze; apparently another part of brain perceives non-visual stimuli from the other person's gaze.[108]

Mmm The White Horse Shakes Its Mane – Stand in a shoulder-width stance with your hands crossed at the wrist and hanging down in front of you. Close your mouth and touch the tip of your tongue to the roof of your mouth as if you were about to say the letter "t." As you exhale, slowly roll your spine down so you are hanging over from the waist. As you inhale, draw the arms swiftly up and overhead as you straighten your back up. Once

---

107 Swanson, Dianne. (2001). *Mysterious you; Hmmm? The most interesting book you'll ever read about memory*. NY: Scholastic. p. 38.

108 http://www.medicaldaily.com/blind-mans-brain-still-responds-eye-contact-unhappy-faces-and-averted-gazes-video-246914

you are upright, lower your hands halfway to make a "T" with arms out and palms down. Hold. As you exhale, release the arms and cross them at the wrists in front of you as you roll your spine down to repeat.

— SET 188 —

WOW Genius is the ability to put into effect what is on your mind. – F. Scott Fitzgerald

3Rs What kinds of activities did you do when school was cancelled for weather or other reasons when a child? What did you enjoy or dread most about "school-free" days?

KISS 1. When Walt Whitman wrote "O Captain, My Captain," to whom was he referring?

2. How is glass recycled?

3. North is Germany; south is Italy; east is Austria and Liechtenstein; and west is France. What country am I?

SOS Who was the first person to break all of the Ten Commandments?

ICE What items could you use to reach something if you could not get up from a chair?

TAB There is an interesting case of woman with Urbach-Weithe disease, a disorder that has killed off cells in her amygdala. Although she still experiences other emotions, she does not experience fear in the face of risks or threats to bodily harm.[109]

Mmm Breathing Meditation: Three-Breath Count – Observe your breath. Count the next three in-breaths. Once you get to the third in-breath, start over again at one for the next breath. Do this for 5 sets of 3 in-breaths.

— SET 189 —

WOW Everyone sees what you appear to be, few experience what you really are. – Niccolò Machiavelli

3Rs What historical events happened the year you were born? What effects did they have on your family's life?

KISS 1. In blues music, what is "call and response"?

2. Which three of these numbers will add up to 50: 2, 4, 6, 12, 15, 19, 24, 25, 27, 30?

3. Name some pharaohs/of ancient Egypt.

---

109 http://www.nature.com/news/researchers-scare-fearless-patients-1.12350

SOS The scorecard had X's, a striking performance by the person. What was happening?

ICE Make up how it came about that money began to grow on trees.

TAB A 2014 study at Stanford University found that direct stimulation of a set of nerve cells in the motor cortex of the brain substantially enhanced addiction recovery for mice.[110]

Mmm Puppeteer – Imagine that you are a puppeteer with the strings of a marionette attached to each of your fingers. Make your puppet walk, sit, eat, and dance.

— SET 190 —

WOW If only we'd stop trying to be happy, we could have a pretty good time. – Katherine Anne Porter

3Rs What most often makes you upset? Why? What helps calm you down? Why?

KISS 1. "Boom" is a word imitating natural sound. What do you call such words?
2. What diagnosis is "visible contusion with subcutaneous hemorrhaging below the orbital arch"?
3. In what year was the Suez Canal opened?

SOS Start with the word "Hand" and change one letter at a time to get to the word "Foot", making real words at each step. Hand ____________ Foot.

ICE List reasons for not having a TV.

TAB Some may claim to have a photographic memory, but many scientists believe no such thing exists, even though some people can train their brains to remember things well.

Mmm Spiral Walk: Backing Out – Stand in the center of the room or an open space. Carefully turn and walk backwards in a small circle, gradually widening the circle to create a spiral path that fills the room.

— SET 191 —

WOW Nothing is so strong as gentleness, nothing so gentle as real strength. – Francis de Sales

3Rs What kinds of experiences did you have with music in school? Did you play an instrument? Did you sing? Did you participate in band, vocal music,

---

110 https:med.stanford.edu/news/2014/08/targeted-brain-stimulation-aids-stroke-recovery-in-mice-scienti.html

marching band, piano concert, church choir, etc.? What are your memories of that? What other instrument would you have liked to have played?

KISS 1. What was strange about the 50,000 word novel *Gadsby* by Ernest Wright?

2. To which animal family does a prairie dog belong?

3. Which U.S. President is last when listing them alphabetically?

SOS Name a kind of horse with force.

ICE The answer is "Yes." What are the questions?

TAB Eating dark chocolate releases chemical endorphins to the brain that help reduce anxiety, pain and stress. These endorphins contribute to the same feel-good sensations present in love and courtship. A 2007 study in England found that compared to kissing, chocolate produced a much more intense and longer lasting boost of excitement in all regions of brain for both men and women.[111]

Mmm Chocolate Meditation – Get a small, bite-sized piece of chocolate. Eat the chocolate with mindful awareness to deepen and extend the pleasure. Start by noticing the chocolate's smell, shape, color, and appearance. Put the whole piece of chocolate into your mouth and savor it on your tongue for a moment without chewing. Let the chocolate melt gradually in your mouth and sense the different layers of taste. Notice the changing texture of the chocolate as it melts. Then let the chocolate trickle down your throat and swallow mindfully.

— SET 192 —

WOW We can choose to throw stones, to stumble on them, or to build on them.
– William Arthur Ward

3Rs What is something no longer available in stores you wish you could still purchase? What are creative ways you could still find it or make it yourself? Why do you still appreciate this item?

KISS 1. What does the term "dynamics" refer to in music?

2. What is condensation on the earth's surface called?

3. Many of the great civilizations of the ancient world started in river valleys. Which civilizations are associated with the following rivers: the Tigris-Euphrates, the Nile, the Indus, and the Yellow River?

---

111 http://news.bbc.co.uk/2/hi/health/6558775.stm

SOS What is the missing date in this series: April 5, May 4, June 3, _____, August 1?

ICE Complete the following statements with something completely new: Quiet as a _______; Sly as a ________; Wise as a _______.

TAB Research at the Mayo Clinic found that older persons with slower and unstable patterns of walking had a higher risk of mental decline. This research and other studies suggest that a person's gait can be an early indicator of cognitive impairment.[112]

Mmm Internal Balance – This is a balancing exercise so you may want to do this with a wall or other solid support nearby. Stand with one foot just in front of the other like on a tightrope. Cross your arms over your chest so that each hand is resting on the opposite shoulder. Close your eyes and count to see how long you can comfortably stay balanced in that position. Anything over 48 seconds is a sign of healthy balance.

— SET 193 —

WOW We are what we believe we are. – Benjamin Nathan Cardozo

3Rs What is something you would be good at teaching other people? Why?

KISS 1. Write words that mean the same as "light."

2. Why does a hot air balloon fly?

3. What is the world's tallest obelisk?

SOS I am a woman's name, a flower, and the past tense of pizza dough rising. What am I?

ICE An alien has left his "suitcase" on earth when he escaped. What is in the suitcase?

TAB Scientists at the University of Southampton in England conducted a four-year study of more than 2,000 patients who had suffered cardiac arrests. They found that nearly 40 percent of those who survived described some kind of brain 'awareness' during the time when they were clinically dead before their hearts were restarted.[113]

Mmm Corpse Pose – Corpse pose is the final resting pose in any yoga class. It trains the brain and body to relax. Stretch the legs and arms out. Then

---

112 http://www.nytimes.com/2012/07/17/health/research/signs-of-cognitive-decline-and-alzheimers-are-seen-in-gait.html?pagewanted=all&_r=0

113 http://news.nationalpost.com/health/largest-study-into-near-death-experiences-discovers-awareness-may-continue-even-after-the-brain-shuts-down

extend the legs down away from the torso, in line with the body with the heels close together. Allow the legs and feet to relax and roll out slightly. Place the arms at your sides with palms up. The arms should be just slightly away from the torso. Allow the arms, hands and fingers to relax. Close your eyes and breath, focusing your attention on the weight of the body as if it were sinking or melting into the ground.

—— SET 194 ——

WOW Keep your ideals high enough to inspire you and low enough to encourage you. – Anonymous

3Rs What funny story did you like to hear or tell when you were younger? Do you still think it is funny? Why or why not?

KISS 1. Define "Humanities".
2. How is it possible to tell how far away a thunderstorm is, from where you stand?
3. What is the name of the U.S. track star who won 4 gold medals at the Berlin Olympics in 1936, and Hitler refused to shake his hand?

SOS What do the following have in common: bell; gun; whistle?

ICE How is life like spaghetti?

TAB Research suggests that left-handed people have a greater probability of recovering from strokes and brain damage than right-handed people.[114]

Mmm Chopsticks – Eat with chopsticks. If you already know how to use chopsticks, eat with chopsticks in your non-dominant hand.

—— SET 195 ——

WOW If you don't like it, change it. If you don't want to change it, it can't be that bad. – Anonymous

3Rs What is the worst advice you have ever received? What was the situation? How did it work out? Would this have been good advice for someone else? Have you ever given bad advice to others that you know of? What happened?

KISS 1. What does "break a leg" mean to an actor?
2. What is the world's longest venomous snake?
3. Name three U. S. state capitals which are two words.

---

114 http://helathland.time.com/2013/08/13/happy-left-handers-day-what-science-says-about-handedness/

SOS What kind of apples seem to always be in a bad mood?

ICE What might be a good secret ingredient for a famous cookie recipe?

TAB Richard Davison, at the University of Wisconsin at Madison, found that an increased activity in the positive emotions side of the prefrontal cortex of mediators also correlates to a stronger immune response after getting a flu vaccine.[115]

Mmm Between the Eyes Meditation – Close your eyes, and bring your attention to the area between your eyebrows. Imagine that you can sense the spot on the inside of your skull just above the nose and between your eyebrows. Focus your attention on that spot for several breath cycles. If you feel your mind wondering, gently return to the space inside the skull and between the eyebrows.

— SET 196 —

WOW We could never learn to be brave and patient if there were only joy in the world. – Helen Keller

3Rs What is the closest you had to a "near death" experience, either to yourself or someone else? When, how and where did it happen? How old where you? Was someone with you? What are your thoughts about it now?

KISS 1. What is the possessive of father-in-law?

2. What is a hypothesis?

3. What did the Algonquin Indian tribes call the polished shells used as money?

SOS My lamp is sixteen feet away from my bed. Without using any aid, how can I turn out the lamp and get into bed before the room is dark?

ICE What are some different things that can be hidden under your shoe?

TAB Recent research found that six hours of brain games over 10 weeks played by first-graders attending school irregularly allowed them to catch up with their regularly-attending peers in math and language grades.[116]

Mmm Lateral Neck Stretches – Go slowly and be gentle with the neck throughout this exercise. Do not force the movement, and stop if there is any pain. Sit or stand in a comfortable position with spine upright and the chin parallel to the floor. From this neutral position, gently allow the head to tilt to the

---

115 http://www.ncbi.nlm.nih.gov/pmc/articles/PMC2944261/

116 http://www.theatlantic.com/health/archive/2014/04/new-studies-show-promise-for-brain-training-in-improving-fluid-intelligence/360290/

left. Hold for a breath and then return to neutral. Repeat five times. Then do the same tilting to the right five times.

— SET 197 —

WOW Focusing your life on making a buck shows a certain poverty of imagination. – Barack Obama

3Rs Suppose you fell asleep for fifty years. In what ways do you think the two worlds would be the same and in what ways would they be different? Why? What might be the most important change?

KISS 1. What do Ichabod Crane, The Headless Horseman and Katrina Van Tassel have in common?
2. What is the highest total you can roll with four dice?
3. What happened to the ancient Roman cities of Pompeii and Herculaneum in 79 AD?

SOS Jennifer was making coffee, and her earring fell into the cup. Even though the cup had coffee in it the earing did not get wet. Why?

ICE You just received a gift of a parrot. What unusual things would you teach it to say?

TAB Previous knowledge and experience relevant to new material to be learned can help new learning, but if one is not careful, it can also hinder creativity pertaining to that new learning.

Mmm Holding a Ball of Chi – Stand with the feet about shoulder-width apart and the knees slightly bent. Turn the palms of the hands up with fingers pointing in towards one another, but not touching. Bring the elbows out as if you were holding a baby. Close your eyes and visualize a light and fragile ball in your hands. Focus your attention on the sensation of the ball and the palms of your hands. Hold for at least 10-12 breaths.

— SET 198 —

WOW We cannot discover new oceans until we have the courage to lose sight of shore. – Andre Gide

3Rs What is your first recollection of spending your own money? What were your feelings? What did you buy? How did it affect your later life?

KISS 1. What Chicago architect's "prairie houses" are associated with the Arts and Crafts movement at the turn of the 20th century?
2. What do most people have 23 pairs of?

3. What do these state capitals have in common: Augusta, Boston, Helena, Jackson, Jefferson City, Lansing, and St. Paul? (Tricky!)

SOS How far can a dog run into the woods?

ICE What can you balance on your hand?

TAB Can you read this? 7HIS M355465 53RV35 7O PROV3 HOW OUR MINDS C4N DO 4M4ZING TH1NGS! As long as the basic shape of the letter is there, the brain can often adjust to reading the message, sometimes more quickly than others.

Mmm Leg Writing – Lie down comfortably on your back with your legs out straight. Lift one of your legs off the ground and write your name in the air as if your leg and foot were a giant pencil. Lower the first leg and write your name again with the other side.

— SET 199 —

WOW The mind ought sometimes to be diverted that it may return to better thinking. – Phaedrus

3Rs Describe your experiences of practical jokes. What practical jokes have you played on others? What practical jokes have been played on you by others?

KISS 1. What is the plural of sister-in-law?

2. What North American animal may also be referred to as a "polecat"?

3. What countries originated the following: Syrup and tuna, bologna, and tofu?

SOS A masked man is attacked by a gang of five men with sticks who shoot at him and then leave quickly. He survives but the gang returns again and again. The next night a different gang attacks. What is the man's profession and what is on his feet?

ICE The answer is "round"; what is the question? Think silly!

TAB Research indicates that many successful and noteworthy artists and athletes make a habit of taking mental breaks to refocus attention and encourage creativity."[117]

Mmm Word Meditation: "Healthy Brain" –Imagine hearing the words "Healthy Brain" over and over in your head for one to five minutes. If your mind wanders gently return your attention back to the phrase. You may also say the phrase aloud to help you refocus.

---

117 Jabr Ferris . (October 15, 2013) *Scientific American.* Why your brain needs more downtime. At http://www.scientificamerican.com/article/mental-downtime/

— SET 200 —

WOW The difference between a dream and a goal is a plan. – Anonymous

3Rs What is the most beautiful thing you have ever seen? Where was it? Why was it so beautiful to you?

KISS 1. What is the purpose of a preface in a book?
2. What form of energy is lightening?
3. Which continent receives the least precipitation per square mile?

SOS Decipher the following: TUIwoman'sTION; NOON GOOD; TIjustME. (Example: irighti = right between the eyes)

ICE List excuses for not doing homework? Be creative.

TAB Some brain diseases such as epilepsy, schizophrenia and Parkinson's disease are correlated to abnormal rhythms in the brain. And in the case of Parkinson's disease, external rhythms such as music and dancing seem to reduce symptoms such as tremors and problems with movement.[118]

Mmm Salsa Step Right Side – The basic step of a salsa dance starts with the feet together. Step the left foot in front of you. Step the right foot in place. Step the left foot back into its original position. Pause. Then step the right foot behind you. Step the left foot in place. Step the right foot back into its original position. Pause. Repeat, letting your hips swing as you move. Feel free to add music and add your own arm movements.

— SET 201 —

WOW The best way to forget about your problems is to help others solve theirs. – Anonymous

3Rs What is the most difficult decision you have ever made? What happened? How do you feel about the decision now?

KISS 1. What musical term comes from the Latin word meaning eight?
2. What are the solstices?
3. Which U.S. president served the longest?

SOS When was the beginning of the twenty-first century: 11:59 p.m. December 31, 1999 or 12:00.01 a.m. January 1, 2000?

ICE "Click!" What will people think? When and why was this said?

---

118 http://www.npr.org/sections/health-shots/2014/06/17/322915700/your-brains-got-rhythm-and-syncs-when-you-think

TAB "Cognitive reserve" refers to how well-developed an individual's brain is and how rich and diverse that person's thinking and experience is. Cognitive reserve provides a buffer against the effects of brain diseases. For example, according to David Bennett, M.D., of Chicago's Rush University Medical Center, people with high cognitive reserve can continue to function without symptoms of dementia even if the disease is present in their systems.[119]

Mmm Salsa Step Left Side – Do the salsa step starting with the left foot this time. Step the left foot in front of you. Step the right foot in place. Step the left foot back into its original position. Pause. Then step the right foot behind you. Step the left foot in place. Step the right foot back into its original position.

— SET 202 —

WOW Vision is the art of seeing the invisible. – Jonathan Swift

3Rs What is the most memorable graduation ceremony you ever attended? What things made it so very special? Describe your graduation.

KISS 1. TOPS is to STOP as 6329 is to ___?

2. What does a Sphygmomanometer measure?

3. Which came first, the ball point pen or the pencil with attached eraser?

SOS Johnny was born on December 16, yet his birthday is always in the summer. How can this be?

ICE List three ways a car and a turtle are alike.

TAB A stroke is the result of blood flow to the brain getting stopped by a blockage or hemorrhage, so the brain does not get enough oxygen.

Mmm Mindful Floors Meditation – Take some time today cleaning the floor. Bring as much mindfulness attention as you can to doing this chore. Fully sense your body in motion interacting with the broom, mop, and/or vacuum cleaner. Contemplate how doing the chore is an act of love directed toward yourself, your environment, and/or others.

— SET 203 —

WOW Until you try, you don't know what you can't do. – Henry James

3Rs Have you ever been hurt by an animal, bee/wasp, etc.? Where were you? What were you doing? Was anyone with you? What was done about the situation?

---

119 http://www.hbo.com/alzheimers/science-building-cognitive-reserve.html

KISS 1. What animal does the Little Prince character in the book *The Little Prince* tame?

2. What insect swarms in groups as large as 100 billion? Hint: Farmer's dread them.

3. Compare/contrast two states that begin with the same letter.

SOS The first letter of each word in the following descriptions are also the same as the initials as the person described. 1) Union Side General; 2) Created Snoopy; 3) Humorous Mute.

ICE You have a paper with a rectangle drawn on it. Inside are three circles in the top row and three circles below in the bottom row. List ideas of what the drawing could represent.

TAB According to a long-term study on 5,500 elderly people, healthy teeth and gums correlate to a reduced risk of developing dementia later in life. Study participants who reported brushing their teeth less than once a day demonstrated a 65 percent increased risk of dementia compared to those who brushed every day.[120]

Mmm Non Dominant Tooth Brushing – Brush your teeth with your non-dominant hand.

— SET 204 —

WOW Follow your heart; just remember to take your brain with you. – Anonymous

3Rs What is the most serious prejudice you ever experienced or observed? Why was it serious? Where and when did it occur?

KISS 1. What nationalities do these folk dances represent: Bolero, Mazurka, and Tarantella?

2. Name some types of severe weather.

3. In ancient times strangers shook hands to show that they were what?

SOS What must be true of a herring in order to be labeled a sardine?

ICE What is in the bag? It is soft, liked by kids, and costs about $2.

TAB The Greek philosopher Aristotle believed that the heart, not the brain, was the seat of mental processes. Most people of that time agreed. Thus the phrase "learn by heart."

Mmm Spacious Heart Meditation – Close your eyes, and place your hands on your heart. With each in-breath, sense your heart opening and expanding.

---

120 Sheriff, Natasja. (August 20, 2012). Dental health linked to dementia risk. *Reuters Health*. At http://www.reuters.com/article/2012/08/20/us-dental-health-dementia-idUSBRE87J0RC20120820

With each out-breath see your heart as a clear and open space. As you inhale you can say in your mind, "Breathing in, my heart opens." Then as you exhale say, "Breathing out, my heart feels spacious."

— SET 205 —

WOW The only fools greater than those who "know it all" are the ones who argue with them. – Anonymous

3Rs Which is your all-time favorite movie? Why is it your favorite? Describe the movie? Would you like to see it again sometime?

KISS 1. Think of an animal that talks too much. Hint: Play on words.
2. How fast do the winds travel for a storm to be called a "hurricane"?
3. What continent borders only the Arctic and the Atlantic Oceans?

SOS Fill in the blanks to create hyphenated words. 1) _____- of - _____; 2) _____ - in - _____; 3) _____ - in- the _____.

ICE What would you make with a pile of potatoes?

TAB L-tyrosine is an essential amino acid protein for proper brain function. It is found in almonds, avocados, bananas, cottage cheese, chicken, eggs, fish, lean meat, lima beans, milk, oats, peanuts, pumpkin seeds, sesame seeds, sharp hard cheese, soy products, tofu, turkey, whole grains and yogurt. Nutritionists recommend an average daily L-tyrosine intake of 56g for men and 46g for women.

Mmm Hand Massage – Hold both hands out with the palms up. Place one hand palm up on top of the other palm. Wrap the thumb of the bottom hand around into the palm of the top hand. Starting at the wrist, "walk" the thumb up the palm of the opposite hand pressing and massaging in a line out to the end of the finger. Then switch hands.

— SET 206 —

WOW To err is human, to forgive divine. – Alexander Pope

3Rs Were you ever given any nicknames by others? How and why did the nickname come about? Who still uses the nickname? If few people call you by that nickname anymore, when and why did the nickname change?

KISS 1. What famous novel is about Captain Ahab and a whale?
2. What insect causes sleeping sickness?
3. Which nation controls Greenland?

SOS You are facing west, then turn right, next about face, and finally turn left. Which direction are you now facing?

ICE Name some companies or products that should sell items where their names suggest?

TAB In acupuncture, a patient with symptoms such as "weakened mind, inability to concentrate, and disturbed spirit" would be diagnosed as having "Deficiency of Kidney and Deficiency of Heart Blood or Yin".[121]

Mmm Spacious Heart, Forgiving Self Meditation – Close your eyes and, place your hands on your heart. With each in-breath, sense your heart opening and expanding. With each out-breath see your heart as a clear and open space. As you are ready, invite an image of yourself now or in the past that reflects something you have regrets about. Notice what happens to the sensation of the heart. If needed, breathe and re-invoke the spacious heart again while you look at the image of yourself. Once your heart feels spacious again, tell the image of yourself about the regrets you want to release and that you want to forgive yourself. Then visualize that forgiveness in your hands in some form. As you are ready, offer the forgiveness to yourself.

— SET 207 —

WOW Have a heart that never hardens, and a temper that never tires, and a touch that never hurts. – Charles Dickens

3Rs Think of your favorite color? How does that color make you feel? Which of your possessions are that color? Why do you think that became your favorite color? In what ways does that color describe or not describe you and you personality? Would you paint your house that color?

KISS 1. What is the difference between a sharp and a flat in music?

2. What is considered to be the most intelligent of the domesticated animals?

3. From which countries did we get these: Mayonnaise, pumpernickel, sauerkraut?

SOS Two men were tried for murder; one was found guilty and the other innocent. The law compels that they both be set free. Why?

ICE You see a straight line with a circle on the end. List five things it might be.

TAB Our brain thinks and remembers in color. According to some studies, being surrounded by the color orange leads to increased blood flow to the brain that in turn stimulates mental activity.[122]

---

121 http://acupunctureamerica.com/acupuncture_alzheimer.html

122 http://www.digitalskratch.com/color-psychology.php

Mmm Breathing Meditation: Rainbow Breath – On your next breath, imagine that you can see the breath as it enters and leaves the body. Without judgment or manipulation, notice what color you imagine the air that you breathe in is. Then notice the color it is as you breathe it out. After a few breaths, experiment with visualizing the air in different colors of the rainbow. Breathe in red air, and breathe out purple air. Breathe in orange air, and breathe out yellow air, etc. How do the various color combinations feel? When you find one you like, continue to breathe using that color combination for a while. Allow the in-breath color to penetrate through your whole body, and the out-breath color to flow out of every pore.

— SET 208 —

WOW We must develop and maintain the capacity to forgive. [One] who is devoid of the power to forgive is devoid of the power to love. There is some good in the worst of us and some evil in the best of us. – Martin Luther King, Jr.

3Rs What is your favorite company logo or motto? Why? What is its message?

KISS 1. Can you think of at least three words of five letters or more which do not contain the vowels A, E, I, O and U? Hint: second letter is "y".

2. Which is lighter in weight, milk or cream?

3. What is the name of Florida's most popular orange and Spain's third largest city?

SOS The answers to the following clues all contain the word "pen" in them: 1) A common antibiotic; 2) Arms and legs; 3) A tree that shivers and quakes; 4) A Washington D.C. building.

ICE "How dare you!?' What have you done? Who, when and why was this said?

TAB The June 2017 issue of the *British Medical Journal*, reported on a 30-year study by researchers at the University of Oxford and University College London. The study examined 550 men and women with no alcohol dependence to see how alcohol intake affected their performance on various cognitive tasks. At the end of the study, researchers concluded that even moderate amounts of alcohol can damage the brain and impair cognitive function over time.[123]

Mmm Spacious Heart Forgiving Others Meditation – Close your eyes, and place your hands on your heart. With each in-breath, sense your heart opening and expanding. With each out-breath see your heart as a clear and open

123 http://www.bmj.com/content/357/bmj.j2353

space. As you are ready, invite the image of a person, living or dead, that you have feelings of resentment towards. See the person as if that person were sitting in front of you right now. Notice what happens to the sensation of the heart. If needed, breathe and reinvoke the spacious heart again while you look at the image of that person. Once your heart feels spacious again, tell the person about the resentment you feel and want to release now. Tell the person that you want to forgive them, and visualize that forgiveness in your hands. As you are ready, offer the gift of forgiveness to the person.

—— SET 209 ——

WOW Great are the achievements of those who excel in teamwork. – Anonymous

3Rs In the past, what one gift from you would your parents have most appreciated? Why? Did they ever receive it?

KISS 1. What literary detective is Sir Arthur Conan Doyle famous for creating?
2. What is density?
3. Whom did Sacajawea guide?

SOS How can you physically stand behind your mother while she is standing behind you?

ICE What things can you think of that have handles?

TAB Memory improves when we discuss learning with others.

Mmm Pick Stars, Change Hands – Stand in a shoulder-width stance with the arms hanging comfortably to your sides. Close the mouth and then touch the tip of the tongue to the roof of your mouth as if you were about to say the letter "T." Inhale slowly and raise the right arm up in an arc out to the side and over your head. At the same time, circle the left hand back to rest in the small of your back with the palm out. Exhale and return hands to your sides. Then repeat on the other side.

—— SET 210 ——

WOW Take time to think . . . it is the source of power. – Old English saying

3Rs What is your favorite hobby or activity? How did you first become interested? How often do you practice it? How much more do you know now than earlier?

KISS 1. What are the primary colors?
2. What do all of the following have in common: goal, point, run, set, and touch?
3. From what countries did we get: Hamburger? Tempura?

SOS In a science lab, the professor said all temperatures must be entered into a log. However, when the students said the temperature was minus 40 degrees, the professor didn't care whether it was Celsius or Fahrenheit. Why?

ICE One morning when you walk into your garden you find water all over only one spot. What happened? Think of several possible scenarios.

TAB The greater the ratio of "leftward tilt" toward the positive emotion side of the prefrontal cortex activity, the stronger a person's immune response. Positive thinking helps your immune system.[124]

Mmm Cross Body: Knee to Shoulder – Lie down comfortably on your back with your legs out straight. Bend one knee. Use your hands and arms to hug that knee in close to your body. Then pull that knee gently to the opposite side so it crosses over the belly button and points toward the opposite shoulder. Repeat with the opposite leg.

— SET 211 —

WOW Impossible only means that you haven't found the solution yet. – Anonymous

3Rs Think of a time when you were the most relaxed. Where were you, and was anyone with you?

KISS 1. Which of the following is an infinitive verb: jumped, jumping, to jump, will jump?

2. Do polar bears live in the Arctic or Antarctic?

3. What presidents had the first name James? (4)

SOS Which one of these words does not belong: Aunt, Cousin, Father, Mother, Sister, and Uncle?

ICE How could you make someone move away (as in changing residence)?

TAB Researchers have found that reducing the risk of heart disease, by treating hypertension, high lipids, cholesterol, obesity and Type 2 diabetes, is crucial for brain health.

Mmm Toe "Workout" – Try to pick something up off the floor with your toes.

— SET 212 —

WOW Remember that you are needed. There is at least one important work to be done that will not be done unless you do it. – Charles Allen

---

124 http://www.eubios.info/EJ141ej141j.htm

3Rs Think of your favorite piece of architecture anywhere in the United States or the world? Why did you choose this particular architecture?

KISS 1. Laura Ingalls Wilder is best known for what series of books?
2. What substance weighs more in the liquid state than the solid state?
3. Roman troops were paid with salt. What English word comes from this?

SOS What is the value of one-half of two-thirds of three-quarters of six-sevenths of seven-eighths of eight-ninths of nine-tenths of one thousand?

ICE "Crash!" What are you going to do about it? Who and where was this said?

TAB The Bronx Aging Study identified five leisure activities that lowered the risk of cognitive decline and dementia. In order of benefit, they were: 1) dancing, 2) playing board games, 3) playing musical instruments, 4) doing crossword puzzles, and 5) reading.[125]

Mmm Flamenco – Imagine you are in Spain and do "your" version of a flamenco dance. Stomp those feet! Clack the castanets!

—— SET 213 ——

WOW To ignore the facts does not change the facts. – Andy Rooney

3Rs What is your favorite place to shop? What makes it special/different? Why do you like to go there?

KISS 1. What word is the centerpiece of an arch and for the nickname of Pennsylvania?
2. What is the Roman numeral for 7?
3. In what state was the first oil well drilled (1859)?

SOS Make two different words out of the following letters using all the letters: tueni.

ICE You walk into work and everyone is staring at you. What are three possible situations?

TAB Be careful in making judgments about potential cognitive abilities. For example, all of the following people either did poorly in school or failed in school subjects related to their later fame: Winston Churchill, Thomas Edison, Isaac Newton, Louis Pasteur, and Leo Tolstoy.

Mmm Fire Gazing Meditation – Light a candle or if you have a fireplace and the season is appropriate you can build a bigger fire to gaze at. Dim the lights, and find a place to sit where you will be able to look at the flame easily while maintaining a comfortable upright position. Breathe gently

125 http://www.nejm.org/doi/full/10.1056/NEJMoa022252#t=article

and focus your attention on the flame. If your mind wanders gently return your attention back to the fire.

— SET 214 —

WOW See into life—don't just look at it. – Anne Baxter

3Rs Who was your favorite elected official? What do you remember about him or her? Why did you like her or him?

KISS 1. Punctuate this sentence to show you are not a cannibal: "I say let's eat grandma"

2. What do you call the hollow spaces in the bones around your nose?

3. Which came first, baseball or football?

SOS John F. Kennedy was the youngest person elected to the presidency. How is it that he was the second youngest man to hold this office?

ICE What might be six non-dietary uses of cheese?

TAB A too-messy desk can drain your brainpower, because having too much stuff in your line of sight can make it harder to focus.

Mmm Cross-Body: Upright Elbow to Knee – Take a stable stance with both feet directly below the hip joints. Lift the Left knee up and at the same time bend the Right elbow, so that you can bring the knee and elbow together to touch one another. Repeat on alternating sides.

— SET 215 —

WOW Self-trust is the first secret of success. – Ralph Waldo Emerson

3Rs What was your favorite restaurant growing up? What food did you order? Could you be satisfied eating there the rest of your life?

KISS 1. How did George Orwell choose his title for the book *Nineteen Eighty Four*?

2. Which crop grown in the U.S. is the best source of protein?

3. What nation has the lowest birth rate in the world?

SOS Find a one word answer to the following so that the last two letters of each answer are also the first two letters of the next answer. Ours is the Milky Way: Melodic percussion instrument: Not messy: Type of island formed from coral: Pack animal in the Andes Mountains

ICE What unusual ways could you use a "safety pin"?

TAB The stress caused by frequent jet lag and frequently changing work hours can damage memory and temporal lobe of the brain.[126]

---

126 http://news.berkeley.edu/2-10/11/24/jetlag/

Mmm Neck Stretches Forward and Back – Go slowly and be gentle with the neck throughout this exercise. Sit or stand in a comfortable position with spine upright and the chin parallel to the floor. From this neutral position, gently allow the chin to drop and the head to roll forward. Hold for a breath and then return to neutral. Repeat five times. Then using your eyes, look up toward the ceiling and allow the head to tilt gently back. Hold for a breath and then return to neutral. Repeat five times.

—— SET 216 ——

WOW What seems like only a ripple today . . . can become the wave of the future. – Anonymous

3Rs Name your favorite treat, snack, candy or dessert? Do you prefer sweet or salty? Has this always been your favorite? If not, what other favorites have you had in the past?

KISS 1. What instrument was named because it could be played softly and loudly?

2. What element's characteristics gave it the nickname "quicksilver"?

3. What was Thomas Nast's contribution to the two-party system?

SOS Hannah had an unusual way of pricing in her new clothing store. A vest cost $20, socks cost $25, a tie cost $15 and a blouse cost $30. How much for a pair of underwear?

ICE You are taking a class and begin coughing. What might be six reasons you are purposefully coughing? Be creative.

TAB We learn best through themes, patterns and whole experiences where the context is fully considered and all five senses are involved, rather than focusing solely on the observable facts.

Mmm Drinking Meditation: Follow the Flow – Get a clear glass of water to drink. Start by gazing at the water in the glass. As you look at the water, think about the cycle of water around the world—from oceans, to clouds, to rain and snow, to snow-capped mountains, to clear mountain streams and great rivers returning to the sea. Consider how water sustains all life on the planet—plants, insects, animals, and humans. Slowly sip the water and as you feel it go down your throat, imagine how this glass of water connects you to water in many forms all over the globe.

— SET 217 —

WOW Patting someone on the back is the best way to get a chip off their shoulder. – Anonymous

3Rs What other family that you knew do/did you most appreciate? What was most distinguishing about them? Were there ancestors or family members that you never knew that you appreciate or are curious about? Why?

KISS 1. Count as high as you can in any language other than English.
2. During what months do the solstices happen?
3. What do the letters MADD stand for?

SOS What will happen about 70,000 times a minute in a building with 1,000 people?

ICE List things you cannot hear.

TAB With practice you can train your brain to notify you exactly when a minute (or ten) has passed. Similarly, you can train your brain to wake you up the same time each day.

Mmm Whole Body Clock – Lie down. Imagine that you are a clock and your arms are hour hand and your legs are the minute hand of the clock. Make your body clock say the following times: 12:30, 4:00, 3:25, 8: 55, 11:15.

— SET 218 —

WOW What is a weed? A plant whose virtues have not been discovered. – G. K. Chesterton

3Rs What were your high school mascot and colors? What kinds of uniforms did the various sports players and cheerleaders wear? Who were your school's biggest rivals?

KISS 1. Which character from Greek mythology carries the weight of the world?
2. How do you find the area of a circle?
3. Where is the Nobel Peace Prize awarded? Think Europe.

SOS You have a five-gallon container and a three-gallon container. You need to have one gallon of water. How do you do it?

ICE You cannot sleep. Make a list of things you might try in order to get to sleep?

TAB A recent study suggests that emotions literally color our brain's perceptions. In the study, participants identified the same complex colors differently when they were in different emotional states.[127]

---

127 http://faculty.haas.Berkely.edu/c_lee/manuscript.pdf

Mmm Emotion Observation Meditation – Sit in a comfortable place. Close your eyes and wait. Notice what emotions come to your attention as you wait. Are you happy, sad, bored, irritated, etc.? Examine the emotion like a scientific specimen. What type of emotion is it? Is it about the past, the present or the future? Is it pleasant, unpleasant or neutral? What does it say about your life right now? What does the emotion want from you? Contemplate the answers without judgment. Then let go and redirect your attention to waiting, and notice if the emotion returns or if a new emotion arises. If something new arises examine that emotion, too.

—— SET 219 ——

WOW In the middle of difficulty lies opportunity. – Albert Einstein

3Rs What is your favorite time of the day? Why? Was this also true when you were growing up? Why or why not? What is your best time of the day for thinking? Why? Which hour of the day is the least important/productive for you? Why? Has that always been so?

KISS 1. What colors make black?

2. What are the following: com, edu, org?

3. Joseph Stalin received a scholarship when he was 14 to study for what?

SOS What school happens when the California smog clears? Think Los Angeles.

ICE An ant is making a very important announcement to his community including you. What is the announcement? Are you going to agree?

TAB A University of Texas study found that people remember 10 percent of what they read, 20 percent of what they hear, 30 percent of what they see, 50 percent of what they see and hear; 70 percent of what they say; and 90 percent of what they do and say.[128]

Mmm Word Meditation: Your Name – A common form of concentration meditation involves repeating a word or sound over and over again. For this meditation, you will focus on the sound of your own name. You can choose your first name, last name or full name. Close your eyes. Bring your awareness to your breath. As you feel ready, repeat your name aloud or silently in your head for one to five minutes.

---

128 Metcalf, T. (July 1997). Listening to your clients, *Life Association News*, 92(7), 16 – 18; https://supporting-paa.wikispaces.com/file/view/You+Remember+Approximately.pdf

— SET 220 —

WOW Talk slowly, but think quickly. – Ritu Ghatourey

3Rs What part did imagination have in your childhood play? Who or what did you or your playmates pretend to be? Did you have imaginary friends? What were their names? What were they like?

KISS 1. How does a country's capital differ from its capitol?

2. What are some causes of earthquakes?

3. The three largest cities of Ohio all begin with the same letter. What are the cities?

SOS What do you call a woman who does not have all of her fingers on one hand?

ICE What will a billion bucks buy you?

TAB The brain needs some fat in order to keep its cells young and strong. However, some experts theorize that too much fat also produces "free radicals" that destroy brain cells by the billions.

Mmm Right Angle Walk – Walk around the room at right angles. Always move in straight lines and turn at sharp ninety degree angles, fill the room with large and small square-shaped, rectangular and stair step pathways.

— SET 221 —

WOW It is good to let a little sunshine out as well as in. – Chinese saying

3Rs What is your favorite time of the year? Why? If you had to give up a season, which one would it be? Why?

KISS 1. Which of the following is a poet musician; a troubadour; an illusionist, or a vagabond?

2. Begin with the number of keys on a piano, subtract the number of squares on a chessboard, and subtract the number of hours in a day.

3. What Himalayan goat grows fine hair to make expensive sweaters and garments?

SOS A man came to the doctor with three tongues. How did the doctor remove two of them?

ICE What makes rhinoceroses lovable?

TAB Get out into the sunshine. Research suggests that vitamin D is important for effective functioning of the brain. Vitamin D is a steroid hormone the skin naturally produces through sun exposure. So it is a good idea to spend at least some time outdoors without sunscreen (since it blocks vitamin D production).[129]

Mmm Sun Meditation: Sit or lie down outdoors where you can feel the sun on your skin. Focus on the sensation of the sun on your body, and contemplate how the sun supports your life by providing warmth, light, food, Vitamin D, etc.

— SET 222 —

WOW Life can only be understood backwards, but it must be lived forwards. – Soren Kierkegaard

3Rs What is your most prized possession? Why? Would it be valuable to others? Why or why not?

KISS 1. From which two languages are most English words derived?
2. What edible substance comes from orchids?
3. What is the largest desert in the world?

SOS What four consecutive numbers add up to 94?

ICE Create your own TV show.

TAB The acupuncture point Du 20, known as "one hundred meetings," is located in the center of the top of the head. Traditionally, this point has been used to clear the senses, calm the mind and allow for clarity of thought.

Mmm Acupuncture Head Tap – See if you can stimulate the Du 20 point. Use one or two fingers to lightly tap the center of the top of your head until you feel a centered, calm focus.

— SET 223 —

WOW 'Tis better to understand, than to be understood. – St. Francis of Assisi

3Rs As a child, what was a special toy, blanket, etc. you had? Who gave it to you? What happened to it?

KISS 1. Write sentences with the word "fine", where "fine" has different meaning in each.
2. Swans and elephants are at the local zoo. If there are 30 eyes and 44 feet for these animals, how many are there of each of these two species at the zoo?
3. With which state does Texas share the shortest of its borders?

---

129 http://articles.mercola.com/sites/articles/archive/2014/05/28/vitamin-d-deficiency-signs-symptoms.aspx

SOS Chris and Jennifer each have a different hobby. One collects old coins while the other collects model airplanes that he makes. What does each of them collect?

ICE List as many words/phrases as you can that have the word "run" in them; e.g., homerun.

TAB With the right tools, brainwaves can be seen and heard. So you can hear yourself think after all. ☺

Mmm Waltz Box Step – The basic waltz step creates a box. Start with feet together (in the back left corner of the box). Step the left foot directly in front of you (forming the front left corner). Step the right foot forward and sideways, outside of the left foot, and quickly bring the left to join it (forming the front right corner.) Then step the right foot directly behind you (back right corner). Step the left foot back and sideways, wide of the right foot, and bring the right foot to join it back in the original starting position. Repeat and add music if you wish.

— SET 224 —

WOW Plan for the future because that's where you are going to spend the rest of your life. – Mark Twain

3Rs What is your philosophy on politics? Did you ever think about being a politician? Why, or why not? If so, for what office?

KISS 1. How many lines are in a limerick?

2. Which American biochemist first identified the molecular structure for DNA?

3. What auto maker was called the "Father of Mass Production"?

SOS What is black when you buy it, red when you use it, and gray when you throw it away?

ICE Name things that would fit into a walnut shell?

TAB Researchers at the California Institute of Technology and UCLA conducted a study using celebrity photos to track where and how the brain processes and recognizes faces. They found that a single, particular neuron fired in response to photos of one celebrity, and a different neuron responded only to pictures of another celebrity.[130]

---

130 *National Geographic*, Secrets of the Brain, by Carl Simmer, February 2014, p. 41.

Mmm Face Relaxation Stretch – Place your index fingers just under your eyebrows and push up. At the same time, push down on the cheeks with the thumbs. Hold for about ten seconds and release.

— SET 225 —

WOW A person who is good at making excuses is seldom good at anything else. – Benjamin Franklin

3Rs What kinds of emotional experiences might bring a tear to your eye or cause you to cry? Do you cry easily or are you more reserved? How do you respond when other people cry around you?

KISS 1. List five musical terms that sound the same for both music and baseball.
2. What is Archimedes' Principle?
3. What country has the most llamas?

SOS A fireman slipped off a fifty-foot ladder onto the concrete sidewalk below. Amazingly, he did not get hurt. How could this be?

ICE You are running a business named "Odds and Ends." What do you sell?

TAB A 2017 study by medical school researchers in Singapore found that those who drank brewed tea at least once a day had a 50% lower risk of memory problems. Those who drank green tea reduced their risk by 43%; while those who drank black or oolong tea reduced their risk by 53%. Bottled tea did not have the same effect.[131]

Mmm Drinking Mediation: Sensory Awareness – Get a clear glass of water or tea to drink. Start by gazing at the drink in your glass. Notice its liquid form—flowing, swishing, taking the shape of its container, etc. Sip the water slowly. As you drink, sense the feel and temperature of the water. Swish the water around in your mouth. Sense it against your tongue, teeth, cheeks, roof of the mouth and soft palate. Notice the sensation of drinking—the cup on your lips, the liquid pouring in and filling your mouth, swallowing, and the sensation of it going down your throat.

— SET 226 —

WOW Never cut what you can untie. – Joseph Joubert

3Rs What is the most comfortable place for you to be? Why? What was the most comfortable place to be when you were a child?

---

131 https://www.institutefornaturalhealing.com/2017/05/study-drink-tea-cut-dementia-risk-half/

KISS 1. How do you spell the kind of bird that is most often served "under glass"?
2. For what disease did Edward Jenner develop the first vaccine?
3. What terrible tragedy occurred on April 15, 1912?

SOS Which eight alphabet letters can be put in front of a mirror and are not backwards?

ICE What are some things that cover other things? Be creative!

TAB A 2002 study by researchers at Yale University found that "Thinking Positively About Aging Extends Life More than Exercise and Not Smoking." People with positive self-perceptions about their growing old lived 7.5 years longer than people who felt negative about their growing old.[132]

Mmm Yoga Ear Squat – With your left thumb and index finger pinch your right ear so that the thumb is in the front and the finger is behind the earlobe. Crossing the right arm over the left, pinch the left ear with the right thumb and finger in the same way. Squeeze the earlobes. Inhale through the nose as you do a deep squat while maintaining a straight back. Exhale through the mouth as you come back up. Repeat 10-12 times. An article in *Navigator Fitness* called this the "Super Brain Yoga" move.

— SET 227 —

WOW To the world you might be one person, but to one person you might be the world. – Anonymous

3Rs What kinds of problems have you experienced that were caused by weather? Describe the most serious time you were affected by the weather.

KISS 1. Who is Tom Sawyer's girlfriend in Mark Twain's *Adventures of Tom Sawyer*?
2. What creature eats and digests dirt while working its way to the surface?
3. In what city does Chocolate Avenue intersect with Cocoa Avenue?

SOS What is the center of America and Australia? The answer is the same for both.

ICE You do a number of different odd jobs for a living. Being creative, what odd jobs do you do?

TAB The transfer of information from long-term storage within the brain to conscious memory cannot be consciously controlled by the individual. Instead, it is often provoked by stimuli within the individual's environment.

132 http://news.yale.edu/2002/07/29/thinking-positively-about-aging-extends-life-more-exercise-and-not-smoking.

Mmm Thought Observation Meditation – Close your eyes and wait. Notice what thoughts come to your mind as you wait. Without continuing the thought, examine it like a scientific specimen. What type of thought is it? Is it a new thought or a thought you have frequently? Is it a thought about the past, the present or the future? Is it a pleasant, unpleasant or neutral thought? What does the thought say about you and your habits? What does the thought want from you? Contemplate the answers without judgment. Then let it go and redirect your attention to waiting, until a new thought arises.

— SET 228 —

WOW Indecision is the thief of opportunity. – Jim Rohn

3Rs What kinds of reunions have you attended? What experiences have you had at those reunions, and how enjoyable were they? What were your most and least enjoyable experiences at those reunions, and why? If you do not attend reunions, why not?

KISS 1. What are several musical notes played together called?
2. What is the common shape of DNA?
3. Niagara Falls is between what two Great Lakes?

SOS Dave was carrying a cloth bag filled with feathers. Dianne was carrying three cloth bags of the same size, yet Dave's one bag was heavier than her three bags. Why?

ICE How is a family like a bowl of cereal?

TAB Growing up in poverty can have a negative effect on children's language learning. Research suggests that such children often hear fewer words by the age of five. This means that their brains have a harder time distinguishing between sounds, and because of the reduced stimulation, their brains "make up" distracting, random, brain activity referred to as "neural noise."[133]

Mmm Hand and Finger Stretching – Put one of your arms out in front of you at shoulder height with the palm facing up. With the other hand, gently pull the fingers of the outstretched arm away and down; you should feel a stretch in the arm and wrist. Now one at a time, gently pull each finger away and down. Repeat on the other side.

---

133 http://www.npr.org/blogs/ed/2014/09/10/343681493/this-is-your-brain-this-is-your-brain-on-music

— SET 229 —

WOW Unexpressed ideas are of no more value than kernels in a nut before it has been cracked. – Anonymous

3Rs What was the most trouble you ever got into with your parents? Why did it happen? How did things turn out?

KISS 1. Write words that mean the same as "order".

2. Which of the following do not have the commutative property: addition, subtraction, multiplication, division?

3. What famous patriotic song was written on the back of an envelope during the bombing of a fort?

SOS The electricity has gone off. It is dark, and you need to get a pair of matching socks from your sock drawer. You know that there are eight red and eight blue single socks in the drawer. How many of the single socks will you need to take out to insure that you will have a matching pair?

ICE Think about or draw a circle with two more circles in it? What might it be? List several ideas.

TAB Brain waves are the tiny electrical impulses that move through the brain. Scientists have identified several types of brain waves, including alpha waves, beta waves, delta waves, gamma waves, and theta waves.

Mmm New Flavors – Eat a new fruit or vegetable that you have never tried before. Notice how it is similar and different from foods you are already familiar with.

— SET 230 —

WOW The brain is like a muscle. When it is in use we feel very good. Understanding is joyous. – Carl Sagan

3Rs What new language would you most like to be able to speak fluently? Why?

KISS 1. *The Diary of Anne Frank* was written during what war?

2. What is the most common source of lead poisoning?

3. Is the toe of Italy's boot on the west or east side of the country?

SOS The answers to all of the following questions begin with "cat": What cat is an ancient military weapon that hurled missiles? What cat is a terrible happening? What cat is a clouding of the eye?

ICE You are Pinocchio at a liars club. What is the first lie you tell?

TAB Maintaining visual health decreases risk of dementia by 63%, and treating vision problems can delay or prevent cognitive decline according to research at the University of Michigan Health System.[134]

Mmm Seated Meditation: Present Moment/Wonderful Moment – Close your eyes. On your next inhale call yourself into the present moment. Say in your mind, "Present moment." Then as you exhale, recognize how good it is to be alive in the present moment. Say in your mind, "Wonderful moment." Continue for at least 10 breath cycles. Inhale: "Present moment." Exhale: "Wonderful moment."[135]

—— SET 231 ——

WOW Discovery consists of seeing what everybody has seen and thinking what nobody has thought. – Albert Szent-Gyorgyi

3Rs Think of a classroom when you were growing up. Where did you sit? Who did you sit by?

KISS 1. What is the name of a device that "ticks" in "time" to music?

2. Which of the following reptiles are native to Africa: Cape cobra, crocodile, "leopard tortoise," mamba?

3. Name at least four U.S. presidents who died in office?

SOS The local swimming pool has been closed and will be open soon. Figure out the date from the following clues: It will open in the first week of a month without an "a" in it. It is on a day of the week that has a "u" in it. The month has no "e", but the day of the week contains an "e".

ICE What creative things would you say to encourage a nervous kid on the first day of school?

TAB Eating heavy meals with lots of fats and sugars invites lack of learning, inattention to what others are saying, and difficulty in concentrating.

Mmm Alternately Supporting Heaven and Earth – Stand in a stable shoulder-width stance with your hands palm up in front of your belly. Keeping the left palm up, gently straighten the arm to push the left hand up towards the sky. At the same time, turn the right hand palm down and push it down toward the ground. Imagine that your hands are pushing the heavens up and the earth down. Change hands by reversing the palms and pushing the top hand

---

134 Carper, Jean. *100 Simple Things You Can Do to Prevent Alzheimer's and Age-related Memory Loss.* NY: Little Brown, 2010. p. 119

135 Nhat Hanh, Thich. (2009). The Blooming of a Lotus. (Revised). Boston: Beacon Press.

down and the bottom hand up. Repeat, striving for a fluid movement in balance with the breath.

— SET 232 —

WOW The older I get the more I realize that kindness is synonymous with happiness. – Lionel Barrymore

3Rs Suppose you were invited to set up a charitable foundation of your choice. What group or cause would you choose to benefit from the charity? Why? What would you name it?

KISS 1. Spell the word that is sometimes called the "voice box."

2. An atom consists of three parts. Which two of them are in the nucleus of the atom?

3. What do most people call the Spanish Mission in San Antonio de Valero?

SOS I look flat, but I am deep; hidden realms I shelter. Lives I take, but food I offer. At times I am beautiful. I can be calm, angry and turbulent. I have no heart, but offer pleasures as well as death. No person can live without me, yet people die within me. What am I?

ICE I'm wearing two different socks. Why?

TAB Research by Paul Ekman of the University of California at San Francisco Medical School scientifically validates that we all smile in the same language. The brains of viewers across cultures can correctly identify such basic emotional expressions.[136]

Mmm Walk as if : Professions – Take a few minutes to walk as if you were a person who worked in the following professions. Notice what changes. Walk as if you were: A fire fighter; A tightrope walker; Royalty; A spy; A clown; A model.

— SET 233 —

WOW Your mind will answer most questions if you learn to relax and wait for the answer. – William S. Burroughs

3Rs What bad habit(s) did you have when you were young? Did you overcome it/them?

KISS 1. In the book *Scarlet Letter*, what letter was Hector Prynne forced to wear?

2. What does equinox refer to, and how often does it happen?

3. On which Hawaiian island is Pearl Harbor?

---

136 https://www.paykejnab.com/wp-content/uploads/2013/07/Felt-False-And-Miserable-Smiles.pdf

SOS What has roots that nobody sees, and is taller than trees; up, up it goes, and yet it never grows?

ICE List things you can pull.

TAB Practicing creativity not only strengthens your ability to be creative but also builds up intuition in your brain.

Mmm Seeking Guidance Meditation – For this meditation, you will pose a question and wait for an answer. The purpose is not to ruminate and think of an answer, but to wait and listen for an answer to arise more spontaneously or to accept that the answer may not come for a while. Close your eyes. Bring your awareness to your breath. As you are ready, ask (aloud or in your mind) "What can I do to create a happy and healthy brain?" Then return your attention to your breathing, relax and listen for an answer. Do not try to figure it out, just wait and listen. If your mind wanders or you catch yourself using mental effort to figure it out, ask the question again and return to your breath.

— SET 234 —

WOW The smallest good deed is better than the grandest intention. – Anonymous (However, some sources attribute it to Duguet.)

3Rs Did you ever get physically hurt and need to have stitches or wear a cast growing up? What happened?

KISS 1. What introduces a musical work?
2. What is the heaviest gland in your body?
3. What is the color of mourning in Japan?

SOS Fill in the blanks with homonyms (words that sound the same, but are spelled differently): Ed plans to ________ a biography about the _______ brothers. He hopes to start _______ after the New Year.

ICE How is a supermarket like an art museum?

TAB Linking what is said to an expression or feature on the other person's face, and to something relevant you can visualize, will help you remember what the person said.

Mmm Leg Float – Lie on your back in a comfortable position with your knees bent and your feet on the floor. Relax and tune into the sensation of your legs, ankles, and feet. Allow your legs to rise up in the air above you as if they were seaweed floating under water. Gently explore the space above you with your legs by opening and closing the knees, rotating at the hip joints, and/or alternately pushing the legs away from your body and pulling them back into your body. Play with flexing and pointing your feet, too.

— SET 235 —

WOW If you always do what you have always done, you will always get what you always got. – Anonymous (However, various sources have attributed it to persons/groups such as Abraham Lincoln, Anthony Robbins, Aerosmith, Henry Ford, Mark Twain, Trout Daddy, etc.)

3Rs What were the most important things about life that your parents taught you? Why were they so important?

KISS 1. Name at least eight prepositions.
2. True or false? Fleas are flying insects.
3. New Delhi is the capital of what large country?

SOS What is pronounced like one letter, written with three letters, and belongs to all animals?

ICE You are adding a guest room to your home. What creative features would you emphasize if unlimited money was available for the project?

TAB Professional football players develop memory-related diseases at a rate that is 19 times higher than average.[137]

Mmm Cross Body: Jungle Clearing – Imagine you are walking through a jungle. The grass and vines are very thick. Use your arms and hands to push the thick grass and vines away to clear a path for yourself. Repeat alternating both arms.

— SET 236 —

WOW Don't whine. If you tell people you are a failure, they will believe you. – Anonymous

3Rs What one thing about your life would you have most liked to have changed? Why?

KISS 1. Who wrote *War and Peace*? Who wrote "Pilgrim's Progress"? What English poet wrote *The Canterbury Tales*?
2. What is the basic shape of a baseball diamond?
3. What is the name of the mallet which judges use to restore order?

137 http://www.nytimes.com/2009/09/30/sports/football/30dementia?_r=0

SOS At night they come without being fetched, and by day they are lost without being stolen. What are they?

ICE Which is smarter, a semi-colon or a period? Why?

TAB A study on a group of older men found that after a year on a walking program, the men's hippocampi were larger, and they performed better on cognitive tests. Compared to the typical volume lost to normal atrophy at their age, they had regained two or more years of hippocampal youth.[138]

Mmm All Four Float – Lie on your back in a comfortable position with your knees bent and your feet on the floor. Relax and tune into the sensation of your arms and legs. Allow them all to rise up in the air above you as if they were seaweed floating under water. Gently explore the space above you with your arms and legs by opening and closing the joints, rotating joints, and/or alternately pushing the legs/arms away from the body and pulling them back into your body. Allow your eyes to follow your hands.

— SET 237 —

WOW A person who has no imagination has no wings. – Mohammad Ali

3Rs Is there anything you would like to have changed about your physical appearance? What parts about your physical appearance would you not change at all?

KISS 1. What music uses spoken words against a rhythmic background to bring attention to urban issues?

2. If A=1, B=2, and so on, which day of the week adds up to 100?

3. Which ancient civilizations flourished first: Egyptian, Greek or Roman?

SOS I know a word of letters three. Add two, and fewer there will be. What is the word?

ICE Brainstorm a list of silly things to sell. For example, winter coats for the beach.

TAB An abundance of research indicates that play functions as an important mode for learning, especially as it relates to the development of language skills, math skills, reasoning, and creativity.[139]

Mmm Wings – Imagine you have wings on your back. Feel them as an extension of your shoulder blades. Move and flutter them. What type of wings do

---

138 http://member.aarp.org/health/brain-health/info-02-2011/keep_your_memory_strong_by_walking.html

139 http://www.parentingscience.com/benefits-of-play.html#sthash.GJr4c62a.dpuf

you have? Play with different sizes, shapes and textures. Move round the room. How do the wings affect how you move when you are not flying? Now take off and fly!

— SET 238 —

WOW It is amazing what you can accomplish if you do not care who gets the credit. – Harry Truman

3Rs Think about the most difficult school or work assignment you ever had? What made it so hard? Did you complete the assignment? Were you pleased with the result? How would you have changed the way you attacked the problem if you were facing it again? What kind of impact did the assignment have on you?

KISS 1. Much music from Africa and the Middle East is polyrhythmic. What does polyrhythmic mean.

2. What fruit pits does cyanide come from?

3. What country uses the yen as a unit of money?

SOS What are the following words if you put the same three letters within each: pr _ _ _ se, sp _ _ _ al, sp _ _ _ es?

ICE Two people are laughing. What are they laughing about? Be creative.

TAB Beta brain waves, the fastest of the brain waves, indicate an aroused brain. The brain creates beta waves when you are concentrated on learning or linear thinking, but beta waves can also indicate an anxious or over-excited mind.

Mmm Eating with Your Hands – At one of your meals today, eat something with your hands and fingers that you would normally not eat by hand (i.e. not a sandwich; soup is probably not ideal, either.) You may want to be extra sure to have a napkin on hand ☺. As you eat, mindfully focus on the sensation of the food in your hand. How do you have to move to pick it up, to keep it from making a mess. Notice the sensation of your hand at your lips as the food goes into your mouth. Does the food taste different when you eat by hand?

— SET 239 —

WOW In all affairs it's a healthy thing now and then to hang a question mark on the things you have long taken for granted. – Bertrand Russell

3Rs What part of being an adult do you wish you could get rid of? Why? Which part do you enjoy the most?

KISS 1. In which book can you read about Long John Silver?
2. Do the seeds of a flower grow in the stamen, the petal, or the pistil?
3. What type of highway is only four percent of the nation's total road system but carries 40% of all the traffic?

SOS Mr. and Mrs. Hadley had six daughters and each daughter had one brother. How many people were in the Hadley family?

ICE How is a job hunt like a board game?

TAB Most people have very poor visual memory and can retain an image for only a few seconds.[140]

Mmm Seeing Anew – Often we get into habits of perceiving familiar environments in old ways without noticing subtle changes that are occurring all the time. Close your eyes and breathe for a few moments. When you open your eyes again, intentionally use your senses to see, hear, smell and touch what is different. Imagine that you know that someone or something has made at least ten different changes in the space. Can you find them all? Are there more than ten?

— SET 240 —

WOW The ability to perceive or think differently is more important than the knowledge gained. – David Bohm

3Rs Which individual(s) in your life changed you the most and why? In what ways are you a different person as a result of that person's presence in your life?

KISS 1. What is the only "instrument" in "a cappella" music?
2. What is a tsunami?
3. What is the second largest city in Japan?

SOS Five cars are bumper-to-bumper. How many bumpers are actually touching each other?

ICE List things you can push.

TAB Research demonstrates that the memory of music is so strong that songs and musical tunes from childhood are the last memories Alzheimer's patients lose.

Mmm Rhythm Work: Stomp a Song – Think of a song you know. Instead of singing it, stomp or march out the rhythm of the song.

---

140 Nevid, J. S. (2014). *Essentials of psychology: Concepts and applications*, 4th ed. Independence, KY: Cengage Learning. P. 213

— SET 241 —

WOW Unless both sides win, no agreement can be permanent. – Jimmy Carter

3Rs In which ways was the family you grew up in unique? What did they do that most people would think was different?

KISS 1. What is the antonym of "privileged"?
2. What must air do in order for you to hear a sound?
3. The first five presidents of the U.S. all came from which state?

SOS Seven children arrived at school. They may have walked, biked, or ridden in separate cars. Twenty wheels took the children to school. How might they have come to school?

ICE Think of things that are blank or use the word blank, e.g., blank check.

TAB Alpha brain waves are associated with a calm and relaxed brain. Alpha waves also occur just as you are falling asleep, and when you are dreaming.

Mmm Breastbone Tap – Hold the fingers of one hand together and use them to tap on the center of the breast bone for 15 to 20 seconds as you breathe slowly in through the nose and out of the mouth. Afterward, check in to see if you feel any different than before.

— SET 242 —

WOW We don't see things as they are; we see them as we are. – Anais Nin

3Rs Think about memories of a "gift giving" holiday you celebrated. What kinds of gifts did you give/receive?

KISS 1. What was the character Don Quixote famous for doing?
2. What do you call a piece of glass with flat polished surfaces that can separate white light into the colors of the rainbow?
3. Who founded the American Red Cross?

SOS The answers to the following clues all contain the letters "pine" in them: 1) All vertebrates have one; 2) High mountain area; 3) A tropical fruit.

ICE How could you save Humpty Dumpty or prevent him from falling off the wall?

TAB Uncontrolled diabetes that involves excess sugar in the blood can lead to decreased alertness, depression and reduced mental capabilities in recall, recognizing spatial patterns, and problem solving. Research suggests that people with diabetes have a 65% higher rate of developing Alzheimer's disease than those who do not have diabetes.[141]

---

141 http:www.sciencedaily.com/releases/2008/o4/080430125254.htm

Mmm Seated Twist – Sit on a chair with a back and a stable seat (not squishy). Place feet and knees together with the feet flat on the floor. Keep your shoulders down as you lift the spine erect by lifting the head, ribs, and waist up away from the seat. As you inhale, turn your torso to the right. Keep your hands below shoulder level and twist to your arms back and around towards the back of the chair. If you can, grab hold of the back of the chair or else grab on the seat of the chair wherever your arms reach. Turn your head last to look over your right shoulder. Hold the pose for a few breaths. Exhale as you release. Repeat on the other side.

— SET 243 —

WOW Beware of no one more than yourself; we carry our worst enemies within us. – Charles Haddon Spurgeon

3Rs What personality trait or quality of yours would you give to the world to make it a better place to live? Why?

KISS 1. What do artists mix their paints on?
2. Which one of the following is not really a nut: acorn, peanut, pistachio?
3. What country has the world's largest pyramid? Hint: Not Egypt.

SOS The first letter of each word in the following descriptions are also the same as the initials as the person described: (1) Amazing Crime-writer; (2) Cinema's Brilliant Director; (3) Patriot Rider; (4) Inspiring Dancer.

ICE Create a new or improved crayon.

TAB Trans fats or hydrogenated oil have already developed a bad reputation for raising bad cholesterol and clogging blood vessels. Research at the University of California in San Diego suggests that trans fat may hurt memory as well. Researchers found that the more trans fat participants ate, the less words study they could remember on memory tests.[142]

Mmm Rhythm Work: Left Right Tap – Tap your feet to the following rhythm: Right. Left. Right, right, right. Left, left, left. Right, left, right. Left, right, left. Repeat and increase speed as you get it.

— SET 244 —

WOW Anger is only one letter short of danger! – Anonymous

142 https://www.nlm.nih.gov/medlineplus/news/fullstory_153125.html

3Rs Reminisce about your favorite book(s) when you were a child? Did people read to you when you were a child? When did you learn to read for yourself? Do you like to read? Why or why not?

KISS 1. How many words can you think of that end in "ice"?
2. What revolves around the nucleus of an atom?
3. Where did the Incas build temples covered with gold?

SOS Why did Shakespeare not have a favorite actress?

ICE What could you do to improve a rose?

TAB A 12-year study at Johns Hopkins found mild hearing loss doubled dementia risk, and people with severe hearing loss were five times more likely to develop dementia.143

Mmm Visualization Meditation: A Safe Happy Place – Visualize yourself about to open a door to a room that is your ideal safe, and happy place. As you are ready, open the door. What do you see? Walk around the space and notice its color and dimensions. What objects are in the space? Play with any changes you want to make the space a perfect place for you to enjoy yourself in comfort and safety. Find a comfortable place in the space to sit or lie down. Stay as long as you like, and then go back out the door you came in, knowing that you can return here in your mind whenever you wish.

— SET 245 —

WOW Begin now, not tomorrow, not the next week, but today, to seize the moment and make this day count. Remember, yesterday is gone and tomorrow may never come. – Ellen Kreidman

3Rs Did you have any "pet peeves"? Which one irritated you the most? Why? Describe a time that you experienced that pet peeve. What did you do about it?

KISS 1. How many books are in the *Lord of the Rings* trilogy?
2. What do all of the following terms have in common: area; axiom; factor; function?
3. Where in the U.S. would you find the Painted Desert?

SOS Put the same word before or after each of the words or phrases in the following sets to make common words or phrases: (1) Door, cow, dinner; (2) Office, cardboard, batters; (3) Forest, engine, door.

---

143 http://www.hopkinsmedicine.org/health/healthy_aging/healthy_body/the-hidden-risks-of-hearing-loss.

ICE Where would some original places be to hide love letters?

TAB The next time someone asks you if you have a hole in your brain, you can say yes. We all have four, interconnected fluid-filled cavities in the brain called ventricles that produce and carry cerebral spinal fluid.

Mmm Helium Head – Imagine your head is a helium balloon. Allow it to effortless rise and float toward the sky. Imagine that a light breeze picks up and let the balloon sway gently. Then as the wind increases a bit, gently expand the movement, making bigger swoops and circles until the whole body is fluidly carried on the wind with the rising, head in the lead.

— SET 246 —

WOW It is not for us to forecast the future, but to shape it. – Antoine de Saint-Exupery

3Rs Is there any single athletic event, sport match, or other entertainment event in history that would have been the most exciting for you to see? Why?

KISS 1. What do you call a musical note that is twice the pitch of another note?
2. Put the following tooth types in order from front-to-back in your mouth: bicuspids, canines, incisors, and molars.
3. What furniture company is named after the Revolutionary War hero who led the capture of Fort Ticonderoga?

SOS Three people go to the movies together; two of them are fathers of others in the group and two of them are their sons. How can this be?

ICE List as many as you can of things you might find on the side of the highway.

TAB Delta brain waves, the slowest of the brain waves, are most associated with deep sleep. Abnormal delta waves are correlated with such conditions as Parkinson's disease, schizophrenia, and alcoholism.

Mmm *Rond de Jambe* – You may want to do this one near a wall or sturdy table to help with balance. Find a stable stance with feet fairly close together. Point the right toe, sliding it out along the ground in front of you. Keeping the toe touching the ground, trace a semi-circle with your toes moving out to the right and behind you. Bring the foot back to center, and repeat 5-6 times. Switch to the other foot.

— SET 247 —

WOW Cheerfulness is the atmosphere in which all things thrive. – Jean Paul Richter

3Rs What were the first TV programs you can remember? How did you like them? Did such programs contribute in any way to who you are today? How and why?

KISS 1. Divide the word "geranium" into syllables.
2. Do pandas generally walk on two or four legs?
3. What famous French landmark was originally designed and built as a temporary structure?

SOS The answer for each of the following descriptions has a "break" in it: Work pause; Light jacket; TV ad.

ICE Think of things with a bump(s).

TAB A 2015 neurological study on meditation supported by the National Institutes of Health found that people who participated in meditation training reported experiencing more positive emotions in their daily life after the training than people who did not meditate. The findings suggest that "daily positive affect and cognition are maintained by an upward spiral that might be promoted by mindfulness training."[144]

Mmm Word Meditation: "Happy Brain" – Close your eyes. As you feel ready, visualize hearing (or should we say audio-lize ☺) the words "Happy Brain" over and over in your head for one to five minutes. If your mind wanders gently return your attention back to the phrase. You may also say the phrase aloud to help you refocus.

— SET 248 —

WOW Life is change. Growth is optional. Choose wisely. – Karen Kaiser Clark

3Rs Think about a personal story where you found yourself in the wrong place, like going in the wrong bathroom or classroom? What happened?

KISS 1. What is the name of Tiny Tim's father in Dickens' *A Christmas Carol*?
2. What is the difference between a chemical compound and a mixture?
3. What was the first U.S. National Park?

SOS A man bought a parrot and the salesman truthfully said the parrot would repeat every word it hears. The parrot would not say a word. Why?

ICE What would it be like if it rained jelly beans?

TAB We never forget really. It is not that information is gone so much as it is lost. Problems with memory are more about scanning, finding and retrieving a particular piece of desired information from within the brain.

144 http://www.ncbi.nlm.nih.gov/pmc/articles/PMC4313604/

Mmm Magnet Meditation – This meditation can be helpful when your thoughts are scattered or you find yourself worrying about the future or worrying about the past. Imagine that there is a large magnet inside of you. In your own time, visualize the magnet drawing you back to yourself. Let the magnet draw all aspects of you back from any events or relationships in the past, including thoughts of activities you were involved in earlier in the day, week, etc. Let the magnet draw all aspects of you back from any worries expectations or other thoughts of future activities or relationships as well. Keep the magnet activated until you feel whole and fully concentrated in the present moment.

— SET 249 —

WOW Treat people as if they were what they ought to be, and you help them become what they are capable of being. – Johann Wolfgang von Goethe

3Rs Was your room messy or neat as you were growing up? Can you still visualize it?

KISS 1. What orchestral instrument's name is the Italian word for small?

2. Pollution in the air causes what kind of rain?

3. During the Vietnam War, did the U.S. troops fight alongside the North or South Vietnamese?

SOS If eight thousand eight hundred eight dollars is written $8,808, how would ten thousand ten hundred ten dollars be written?

ICE Choose two unrelated people from different historical periods and make-up an interesting conversation they would/might have.

TAB Studies show that listening to music increases the speed of cognitive recovery in stroke patients and reduces their negative moods and depression.

Mmm Eyebrow Dancing – Put on some kind of music ro make your own. Using just your eyebrows, "dance" to the music. You can play with lifting, lowering, furrowing, one-up one-down, changing speed, etc.

— SET 250 —

WOW Finish each day before you begin the next, and interpose a solid wall of sleep between the two. – Ralph Waldo Emerson

3Rs Is there a past leader of another country who impressed you most? Why? What leader of another country today most impresses you? Why?

KISS 1. What words have "me" hidden in them?

2. What is the only number that cannot be written in Roman numerals?

3. What nation built the Panama Canal?

SOS The six letter word "chesty" can be arranged into another word; what is that word?

ICE "What did you forget on Mars?" Who said this, to whom, and why?

TAB Occasionally mixing up names you use often is nothing to worry about. Since the brain works like a library, people close to you—such as family members—are grouped together for ease of accessibility. It is natural to periodically grab the wrong name.

Mmm "Drunken Sailor" Line Dance Step – Stand with feet about hip-width apart. Lift the right foot and cross it behind the left foot. Step the left foot directly to the left. Then step the right forward and alongside the left again. Repeat 5-6 times. This will move you in a "drunken" line to the left. Repeat to the other side.

— SET 251 —

WOW Take care of your thoughts when you are alone, and take care of your words when you are with people. – Anonymous

3Rs What times in your life have you had the most fun? Of all the people in your life, who have you had the most fun with, and what are some of the things you did together? Think of a specific situation or story that stands out.

KISS 1. Is Venus the goddess of beauty, health, or wealth?

2. What are the top two layers of a tooth called?

3. What is Queen Elizabeth's family name?

SOS What word do the following have in common: Surgeon, Attorney, Five-Star?

ICE A letter was mailed, but never received. It was not for the normal reasons mail gets delayed. Why was the letter never received? Make a list.

TAB Neurotransmitters are the chemical messengers that carry information between brain cells. Dopamine, serotonin, and adrenaline are all examples of neurotransmitters.

Mmm Mindful Tracking: Company/Solitude –For today consciously track to the nearest 15minutes how much time you spend alone and how much time you spend with others. You can write it down or make a mental note and tally up at the end of the day. If you want you can also track time spent with specific groups or individuals.

— SET 252 —

WOW The most important things in life cannot be taught; only learned. – Anonymous

3Rs Visualize the different places you have lived. What was most distinctive about particular addresses or phone numbers you have had in the past?

KISS 1. Which country produces and sells the most pianos?

2. What is special about a cheetah's claws?

3. Which state capital is the only one named after a famous German?

SOS A body was found in the snow and there were no tracks. The cause of death was in an unopened backpack that the victim was wearing. The victim did not die from thirst, cold, or hunger. What was in the pack that caused the death?

ICE List ten special items you would have taken if moving out west in the 1800s?

TAB Recent neuroscience research at Harvard indicates meditation and mindfulness training can cause neuroplasticity (the brain's ability to **change** as a result of experience). These changes in the structure of the brain became noticeable on an MRI after only eight weeks of meditation practice.[145]

Mmm Compassion Meditation: Teenager – Close your eyes, and place your hands on your heart. On the next breath, invite an image of yourself as a teenager. See your younger self in front of you as you were then—happy or sad, active or passive, troubled or happy-go-lucky. Smile to your younger self. In your mind give that teenager a hug. Send the teenager your gentle, loving compassion.

— SET 253 —

WOW Time has a wonderful way of showing us what really matters. – Margaret Peters

3Rs Recall about your first job outside your home. Where did you work? What did you do and what were you paid? What are some of your memories of that and other jobs (including volunteer work) that you have experienced?

145 http://www.ncbi.nlm.nih/pmc/articles/PMC4313604/

KISS 1. Which word does the current president spell incorrectly?

2. What is the only metal that does not rust even if it is buried in the ground for thousands of years?

3. What mountain range is the longest in the world?

SOS Sue is a sculptor who makes heavy sculptures and delivers them to her clients. Within 24 hours most of the sculptures disappear. Sue is not upset with the disappearance of the sculptures. Why is she not upset, and what happened to the sculptures?

ICE Think of creative ways to get through the checkout at a store more quickly.

TAB Alzheimer's does not happen overnight. It may develop over decades, and various factors (such as physical condition, education, diet, exercise, and relationships) can influence when and if it develops for any individual. Recent research suggests that even childhood events and brain training can increase or decrease the likelihood of Alzheimer's many years later.

Mmm Whole Body Broken Clock – Lie down. Imagine that you are a clock and your arms are the hour hand and your legs are the minute hand of the clock. This time, however, your clock is cuckoo and always moves the hands in a counter clockwise direction. Make your body clock say the following times: 1:30, 2:40, 10:15, 7:05, 5:35.

— SET 254 —

WOW We are all born with a grab bag of gifts and gaps – Bill O'Reilly

3Rs What was one of the nicest things someone ever told you? Who said it and why? What made it special?

KISS 1. What major task does Beowulf accomplish in the epic Anglo-Saxon poem, *Beowulf*?

2. What is the primary cause of ocean tides?

3. What present-day U.S. State capital was once the capital of a kingdom?

SOS Fill in the blanks with homonyms (words that sound the same, but are spelled differently): Colin bruised the bottom of his ________. I hope it will ________ soon, or else ________ have to miss his tennis match.

ICE "How rutpol does this bergo get before it diproks?" What does this made up sentence mean? Be creative!

TAB A recent MRI study indicates that acupuncture treatments can prevent loss of brain cells in the hippocampus.[146]

Mmm Pressing Down Qi – In Eastern martial arts and acupuncture, qi or chi refers to the life force energy. In this Qi Gong exercise the energy is being pressed down to be stored in the lower belly. Stand in a shoulder-width stance. Inhale deeply and slowly. At the same time raise the hands up overhead so that the fingers point to the sky. Imagine drawing energy up through the body. Pause and hold your breath for a few seconds at the top of the movement. Then exhale through the mouth and lower the arms to the level of your belly button, bending the elbows and turning the palms down to "press" the chi into the lower belly. Repeat 4-5 times.

— SET 255 —

WOW A common mistake that people make when trying to design something completely foolproof is to underestimate the ingenuity of complete fools. – Douglas Adams

3Rs Think about the most valuable thing you ever learned? Why? Did you learn it at home, in school, or in life?

KISS 1. Where would you find an arpeggio?
2. What two contrasting colors usually have the strongest visual impact?
3. What ocean lies between Africa and Australia?

SOS Neither the manufacturer nor the buyer want it, and the user doesn't see it. What can this be?

ICE Three people are stranded on an uninhabited island. They have only a soda pop bottle and the clothes on their backs. How can they use the bottle?

TAB Learning to play an instrument seems to improve children's language processing skills. Based on her research, neurobiologist Nina Kraus of Northwestern University argues that learning music improves the brain's ability to process pitch, timing and timbre which in turn helps children distinguish consonants and vowels more clearly and make sense of them more swiftly.[147]

---

146 http://www.healthcmi.com/Acupuncture-Continuing-Education-News/1281-acupuncture-mri-scan-shows-alzheimer-s-disease-benefit

147 http://www.npr.org/blogs/ed/2014/09/10/343681493/this-is-your-brain-this-is-your-brain-on-music

Mmm Listening Meditation: Move with the Musician – Put on some familiar music. Choose one instrument and listen for when that instrument plays and when it stops. Now, play the song again. This time, move some part of your body whenever your chosen instrument is playing. Freeze whenever that instrument is silent.

— SET 256 —

WOW It is in the whole process of meeting and solving problems that life has meaning. – M. Scott Peck

3Rs Did you have favorite subjects in school? What were they? What subject did you like the least? What was your most difficult subject in school?

KISS 1. "Etc." is the abbreviation for a word. What is that word?

2. Are beavers marsupials, pinnipeds, or rodents?

3. What are the five qualifications a person must meet to become President of the U.S.?

SOS Which is the true beginning of eternity, the end of time, and the end of every peace?

ICE You receive a package that is shaped like a baseball. What is it? List at least five different thoughts.

TAB Conscious breathing is an excellent tool for *indirectly* influencing involuntary functions of the brain such as blood pressure and other stress responses. This is because for the average person, the breath is the only aspect of the autonomic nervous system that can directly and consciously be controlled. (Although if you consciously hold your breath for too long, you will pass out and the autonomic nervous system will take over again.)

Mmm Evening Out the Breath – For this breath technique, you will experiment with consciously evening out the breath and making each part of the inhale and exhale equal and smooth. To start simply observe and notice. Notice the rhythm and flow of your natural breath. Do some parts of the breath seem stronger or weaker, faster or slower, ragged or wheezy, tenser or easier? As you are ready, begin to play with shaping the breath gently. How can you make the breath more regular? Where the breath is rough, make it smooth. Do not over-effort this. The best path will be to relax more and allow the breath to flow with only the gentle mental suggestion of smoothness and evenness. If you feel yourself getting tense or lightheaded, return to a normal breath and just observe again.

— SET 257 —

WOW A gossip is one who talks to you about others; a bore is one who talks to you about her/himself; and a friend is one who talks to you about yourself. – Lisa Kirk

3Rs What was the most heroic thing you have ever done? How was it heroic? How did others respond to your heroism?

KISS 1. In Aesop's fable "Fox and the Grapes," what did the Fox say about the grapes when he couldn't reach them?
2. True or false: Electrons are smaller than atoms.
3. Who was the first American woman medical doctor?

SOS How would you rearrange the letters in the words "new door" to make one word? There is only one correct answer.

ICE Choose three unrelated things; then combine the items to make something new.

TAB Practitioners of Aryuveda (the traditional medicine of India) treat memory problems with the spice saffron according to a *Prevention Magazine* publication. The saffron is drunk after heating it in a cup of milk with a bit of gotu kola powder.[148]

Mmm Mountain Pose – Bring both feet together so that the big toes are touching, and the inside of the heels are as close to touching as you can comfortably get. Straighten the knees without locking them. Without force or tension, extend the spine and feel the entire ribcage gently yearning to go higher. Imagine that your head is attached to a cord in the sky that is gently pulling up. Do your best to ensure that both sides of the body are reaching up equally. Focus on balancing the weight of the body evenly on both feet and press equally into the balls and heels of each foot. Breathe and hold the pose for a minute or so.

— SET 258 —

WOW Learning is like riding a bicycle. You don't fall off unless you stop pedaling. – Claude Pepper

3Rs Did you have any significant childhood diseases? If so, what diseases? Did you miss lots of school? If not, what do you believe accounted for your good health?

---

148 Dellemore, Doug, et al. (1995) *New Choices in Natural Healing.* Ed. Bill Gottlieb. Emmaus, PA: Rodale Press.

KISS 1. What follows this lyric: "All I want is a room somewhere. . ."?
2. How many edges does a cube have?
3. What are the two halves that the Earth is divided into called?

SOS Take something a superhero wears, and add a letter of the alphabet (on the front) to get a jailbreak.

ICE A spell has been cast on your friends and family, turning everyone into different animals. What animals are they? Why did you choose those animals?

TAB Brain training can assist at-risk drivers to be safer by improving such things as field of vision and visual scanning, eye-hand coordination, and focus. For teen drivers, divided attention is often the greatest weakness. Whereas for older drivers, attention to signs in the peripheral field of vision is commonly a greater need. Video games and other such eye-hand coordination devices can be useful in such training.[149]

Mmm On the Periphery –Find the edge of your peripheral vision. Bring the index fingers up in front of you and look at them. Then without moving your head, gradually pull the fingers away from each other and out to the side until they are barely in your line of sight. Play with the range of your peripheral vision by moving your hand in and out of view. Drop your hands and maintain focus on what you see in your peripheral vision. Experiment with moving your head and/or body, but keeping your focus out on the periphery of your vision.

—— SET 259 ——

WOW When you help someone up a hill, you're that much nearer the top yourself. – Anonymous

3Rs Relive in your mind your most memorable family vacation? Where did you go and what did you do? What was especially fun, silly or a problem during that vacation? Why was it so very memorable?

KISS 1. Make a list of homographs. Examples: wind blows, wind an antique clock.
2. Give the wrong answer! Which part of the body is a word for punctuation?
3. What were Europeans primarily looking for when exploring during the fifteenth century?

SOS Which is worth more, a pound of $20 pure gold coins or half a pound of $40 gold coins?

---

149 AAA's *Westways Magazine*. (October 2014).

ICE How is a judge like a cell phone?

TAB A 2012 study at Georgetown University suggests that different parts of the brain are activated when learning a new musical sequence from remembering the song after it's learned. One of the scientists doing the research notes, "The motor system contains brain structures that nature invented to decode sequences, so to learn a melody, the auditory system hijacks the motor system."[150]

Mmm Rhythm Work: Syllables All Four – Clap, stomp, snap, and slap (your thighs) to create the following rhythm: Clapadilly, Clapadilly, Stomp, stomp, stomp. Stompidilly, Stompidilly, Slappa, Snap, Snap. Repeat and increase speed as you get it.

—— SET 260 ——

WOW A wise person hears one word and understands two. – Jewish Proverb

3Rs Did you learn to ride a bike? If so, how old were you, and who taught you? Can you still visualize that bike?

KISS 1. If you were a poet writing in verse, what would you notice about the words Bomb, comb, and tomb?

2. True or false? The ordinary bat cannot take off from a level place; it must have some slight elevation from which it can thrust itself into the air.

3. In which country would you find the city of Istanbul?

SOS If the Vice-President of the U.S. and the Speaker of the U.S. House of Representatives should die at the same time, who then becomes President?

ICE List things that are buried. Be creative.

TAB Research shows that people of all ages do better on cognitive tests if they are socially active.

Mmm Meditation: Visit to a Wise Teacher –Close your eyes, and place your hands on your heart. After a few breaths, invite a wise teacher to come and visit with you in your mind. This could be a real person you know, a fictional character, a mythical or historical figure, or a spiritual being (like an angel). If you want, you can plan to invite a specific teacher in advance or you can send a more open invitation in your mind and just see who shows up. Visualize this wise teacher as if the person were sitting in front of you right now. Notice how your teacher appears in terms of dress, age, posture, etc.

---

150 http://www.georgetown.edu/news/music-brain-research-2012.html

Look the person in the eye and smile. Carry on a conversation with this teacher for a while. Ask a question and imagine your teacher's response.

— SET 261 —

WOW There are no unimportant jobs, no unimportant people, and no unimportant acts of kindness. – H. Jackson Brown, Jr.

3Rs Who was/is your favorite fictional character? Why? Would you have liked to have lived that character's life? Why or why not?

KISS 1. Name the U.S. presidents painted by Gilbert Stuart.

2. A popular saying claims that lightning never strikes twice in the same place. Is that true or false?

3. What is the sudden overthrow of a government called?

SOS While camping, my friend felt something moving in his pocket as he walked. He reached into his pocket and found something with a head and tail, but no legs. What was it?

ICE What would happen if adjectives took over the world?

TAB A six-year study of people over fifty found that people who were socially isolated experienced more memory loss than people who were in long-term relationships and/or who maintained connections with friends, family and neighbors.[151]

Mmm Mime in a Bubble – Imagine you are inside of a bubble. Making sure to include front, sides, back, above and below, use your hands push the edges of the bubble away from you. Remember to cross the hands across the midline of the body, too. When you are ready, break free of the bubble.

— SET 262 —

WOW I don't think much of a [person] who is not wiser [today than] yesterday. – Abraham Lincoln

3Rs Describe your neighborhood. What are some happy memories of your neighborhood?

KISS 1. List six suffixes.

2. What are constellations?

3. What is the difference between libel and slander?

---

151 http://consumer.healthday.com/senior-citizen-information-31/misc-aging-news-10/active-social-life-helps-keep-aging-mind-sharp-615987.html

SOS These five words have two things in common: fish, foxtrot, jitterbug, monkey, and pony. What are those two things that they have in common?

ICE How is a person like a bridge? Be creative.

TAB Careful listening and visualization of what is being said (especially if the visualizing is in color) improves a person's ability to learn and remember what is being expressed.

Mmm Healing Hands – Rub your palms together until they are quite warm. Then place your warm palms on any places of your body where you feel sore or tired.

— SET 263 —

WOW A person who never made a mistake never made a discovery. – Samuel Smiles

3Rs In which areas of your life did you most want success? Why were those areas more important than the others? How did you define success?

KISS 1. What is a decanter?

2. What type of burn is most serious: first degree, second degree, or third degree

3. What state is called the Beehive State?

SOS The following descriptions can be rephrased to create rhyming word pairs (Example: chubby feline = fat cat). 1) Hilarious rabbit; 2) Piggy shop; 3) Shopping dance.

ICE There once was a different prompt here, but now it is missing. What happened?

TAB Fear of mistakes and excessive focus on the problem can actually hinder your brain's creativity. Instead, look past the problems to the possibilities and let go of standards of perfection.

Mmm Hula – Imagine you are in Hawai'i and do "your" version of a hula dance. Move those hips!

— SET 264 —

WOW Challenges make you discover things about yourself that you never really knew. They [are] . . . what make you go beyond the norm. – Cicely Tyson

3Rs What would make today more special for you? Picture that happening in your mind. What could you do to make that happen?

KISS 1. Who was the artist who first thought of the helicopter?
2. Platypuses have characteristics of birds and mammals. How are they like birds?
3. First introduced in France, the concept of Daylight Savings Time was invented by an American. Who was he?

SOS My sister put a nail in a tree to mark her height. After 15 years she returned to the nail and found it was at the same height. How is this possible?

ICE Name things that go bump in the night.

TAB Prolonged stress can kill cells in the hippocampus, the part of the brain that's critical for memory. Thankfully, we're able to grow new neurons in this area again, even as adults.

Mmm Adrenal Cool Down Meditation – This meditation is intended to reduce stress by inviting the adrenal glands to ease up. After a few breaths, reach behind you and touch your back about where your ribs end. This is where your kidneys are. Begin to focus on and visualize your adrenal glands. They sit on top of your bean-shaped kidneys like small, peaked stocking caps. Visualize each of the adrenal glands as water faucets that are releasing adrenaline into the blood stream. How much flow is coming out of the faucets? Turn the taps of the faucets down until the faucets are dripping just the right amount for your body to function at an optimal level of relaxed ease.[152]

— SET 265 —

WOW It is never too late to be what you might have been. – George Eliot

3Rs Explain your worst report card grade in school. What was the subject? Who was the teacher? Why the low grade?

KISS 1. Make a list of adjectives that are said to encourage someone.
2. What do you call the center of the atom?
3. What do these have in common: Mount Everest, Pacific Ocean, and Angel Falls?

SOS Changing only one letter at a time, go from "fire" to "mint".

ICE List things that should never be put in water.

---

152 Achterberg, Jeanne, Barbara Dossy and Leslie Kokmeir. (1994) *Ritual and Healing: Using Imagery for Health and Wellness.* New York: Bantam.

TAB Former World Memory Champion Ben Pridmore took only 5 minutes to memorize the dates of 96 historical events. Among other things, he also memorized a shuffled deck of playing cards in just 24.68 seconds.[153]

Mmm Creepy Crawlers – With your hands out in front of you wriggle your fingers like little worms or snakes. Be sure to include your thumb as well as all the fingers. Be aware of the sensation of each moving fingers. Move the fingers with palms up and down.[154]

—— SET 266 ——

WOW Today well-lived makes every yesterday a dream of happiness and every tomorrow a vision of hope. – Francis Gray

3Rs How would you spend an extra hour a day? Why?

KISS 1. What does the word valedictorian mean?

2. How many tomorrows are there in three weeks?

3. What was the occupation practiced by the fathers of most U.S. presidents?

SOS The first letters of which five consecutive months spell a man's name?

ICE How is a lawyer like a pair of lungs? Be creative.

TAB Lucid dreaming refers to a dream state in which you know that you are dreaming. The person's brain is in the REM sleep cycle where dreaming occurs, and simultaneously the conscious mind is active and aware. Some people can enter a lucid dreaming state naturally. And a recent study demonstrated that a low-level gamma wave can artificially induce lucid dreaming.[155]

Mmm Visualization Meditation: Autumn – Metaphorically, autumn is a time of completions: harvest and falling leaves. This meditation can be used to reflect on the season or to acknowledge or invite completion of some phase or aspect of your life. As you are ready, visualize yourself or some area of your life that you are bringing to closure as a leaf hanging from a tree. Let your breath be the breeze gently blowing and stirring the leaf on its branch. Imagine the cooling of the wind and the leaf drying and changing colors. Let your exhale be a sigh as the leaf lets go of the connection to the familiar home base it has known and freefalls down to the earth below. Imagine how that leaf will be transformed into new soil nourishing the tree from which it came and the new leaves that will come in the spring.

---

153 http://memorise.org/tag/ben-pridmore

154 Rosas, Debbie and Carlos Rosas. (2004). The Nia Technique. New York: Broadway Books.

155 http://io9.com/lucid-dreaming-can-be-induced-by zapping-brains-with-ga-157623

— SET 267 —

WOW If you're not stubborn you'll give up on an experiment too soon, and if you're not flexible, you'll pound your head against the wall and you won't see a different solution to the problem you're trying to solve. – Jeff Bezos

3Rs What would you like people to say about you in your eulogy? How would you like to be remembered?

KISS 1. What is another name for a B- sharp?

2. Tear a sheet of paper into exactly 13 pieces about the same size.

3. In which war did Ulysses Grant and Robert E. Lee fight on the *same* side?

SOS The first two letters are male, the first three are female, the first four letters make a great man; the whole word refers to a great woman. What is the word?

ICE What are some things people blow on, in, or up?

TAB The brain of a six-month-old baby is half its adult weight. By the age of 2 ½, the brain is three-fourths of its adult weight, and at age 5, the brain is nine-tenths of its adult weight.[156]

Mmm Healing Hands: For Tired Eyes – Rub your palms together until they are quite warm. Then gently place your warm palms over your eyes for about a minute. Also try this with opposite hands over each eye.

— SET 268 —

WOW I have not failed. I've just found 10,000 ways that won't work. – Thomas Edison

3Rs Which U.S. presidents were your favorite and why? If you had an opportunity to serve in their administration, what role would you have chosen? Why?

KISS 1. Write or say the pledge allegiance as fast as you can.

2. How many stomachs (or stomach compartments) does a cow have?

3. What country occupies the largest island in the Indian Ocean, off the coast of Africa?

SOS Which word does not belong in the following list: dad, level, pop, racecar, and worm? Why?

ICE If you could invite any six people who are alive that you don't already know personally to a dinner party, who would you invite? What topics would you bring up for conversation?

---

156 https://faculty.Washington.edu/chudler/dev.html

TAB More often than not, creative people are very persistent, even when they receive rejection or skepticism from others.[157]

Mmm Mouth Dancing – Put on some music. Using just your mouth, "dance" to the music. You can play with opening closing, tight lips, loose lips, smiling, scowling, snarling, frowning, kissing, pouting, twisting, tongue in and out, teeth clicking, and biting etc.

— SET 269 —

WOW The Earth has music for those who listen. – George Santana

3Rs Think about things you would you most like to change (remodel) regarding your current home, if anything? Why or why not?

KISS 1. What reference book gives lots of synonyms? Hint: Not the dictionary.
2. What do you call giant sections of the earth that slide over one another?
3. Which Native Americans lived in long houses?

SOS Start with the word "Dry" and change one letter at a time to get to the word "Wet", making real words at each step. Dry ____ ____ ____ ____ Wet.

ICE How is a pillow like a puddle?

TAB Neurological research generally contradicts the commonly held belief that we only use 10% or a small percentage of the brain. According to neurologist Barry Gordon at Johns Hopkins School of Medicine, "[W]e use virtually every part of the brain, and [most of] the brain is active almost all the time."[158]

Mmm Listening Meditation: Nature – Go outdoors to a natural environment that you enjoy. Settle into a comfortable relaxed position and close your eyes. Bring your attention to your breath for a few moments to quiet your mind. Then listen to the sounds of nature around you. What do you hear? The sounds of nature may be layered. Some may be more noticeable and some more subtle or you may even notice the sound of silence around you.

— SET 270 —

WOW We act as though comfort and luxury were the chief requirements of life, when all that we need to make us really happy is something to be enthusiastic about. – Charles Kingsley

---

157 http://www.theatlantic.com/magazine/archive/2014/07/secrets-of-the-creative-brain/372299/

158 http://hub.jhu.edu/2014/07/24/busting-a-brain-myth

3Rs Describe the biggest surprise you have ever had? How did it happen? Did it make you happy? Who was involved? Have you ever surprised someone else? If so, what were the circumstances in this case?

KISS 1. In what country did European theatre begin?

2. Radar can determine an object's distance away and the direction it is traveling. What else is radar used to determine that you might have personal experience with?

3. What mighty river carved the Grand Canyon?

SOS What do a circle, a college graduation, and a thermometer have in common?

ICE You are hosting a debate for the election of "Historical Figure of the Millennium." Which candidates will be participating in the debate?

TAB Research has found the following to be important in appropriate doses for effective functioning of the brain: Vitamin A; the Vitamin B-complex of B1 (thiamine), B2 (riboflavin), B5 (pantothenic acid), B6 (pyridoxine), B7 (biotin), Vitamin C, Vitamin D, and Vitamin E. Of special importance is Vitamin B-12, to help protect against brain volume loss in the elderly."[159]

Mmm Curled Roll – Lie down in a fetal position (on one side with arms and legs pulled into the body). Relax and bring your attention to your breath for a few breaths. Then on an in-breath gently allow the top arm and leg to rise slightly and pull the rest of the body to roll onto your back. As you exhale, complete the roll to lie on the other side of your body. Do your best to make this one continuous rolling motion with the natural breath. Rest on this side if you want. Then as you feel ready, allow the next inhale to pull the "new" top arm and leg to reverse the motion back to the original side. Repeat for several breath cycles.

— SET 271 —

WOW The significant problems we face cannot be solved at the same level of thinking we were at when we created them. – Albert Einstein

3Rs List important traditions in your family when growing up? Which are still traditions in your life now? Why?

KISS 1. When do you capitalize mother and father?

2. What is the first thing to do to treat a minor burn?

3. The papyrus plant contributed to the origin of what everyday material?

---

159 http://www.webmd.com/brain/news/20080908/vitamin-b12-boasts-brain-benefits

SOS Twenty percent of the residents in a town have unlisted phone numbers. At random you choose 100 names from the phone book. What is the expected number of people selected who will have unlisted numbers.

ICE How are the police like a deck of cards?

TAB A good night's rest is a key to learning and memory. While you sleep, the brain solidifies memories from the day by moving certain memories from short-term to long-term memory.[160]

Mmm Microcosmic Orbit Meditation – This meditation technique visualizes the flow of chi or life force circulating in orbit around two major acupuncture meridians: The "Governing Vessel" and the "Conception Vessel." The Governing Vessel goes from the perineum, up the spine, over the head to the roof of the mouth. The Conception Vessel goes from the perineum up the front of the body to the roof of the mouth. Close your eyes and relax the body. When you are ready, touch the tip of your tongue to the roof of your mouth. This connects the two meridians. Now imagine that you can sense the energy of your body: You can see it as a color, sense it as a temperature, or whatever works for you. Imagine that energy now orbiting though the two meridians. Start at the perineum (or at the "root of your spine") and visualize the energy traveling up the spine, over the head, down the nose to the roof of your mouth. Then the energy travels through the tongue, down the throat, past the belly button, back to the perineum. Keep circulating the energy for 1-3 minutes.

— SET 272 —

WOW It is what it is; but it will become what you make it. – Abraham Lincoln

3Rs When did you find it most difficult to sleep growing up? Did you get plenty of sleep? How many hours of sleep do you generally get every night? What helps you to go to sleep?

KISS 1. What does the word "hyperbole" mean?

2. What is the primary diet for each of the following "picky eater" animals: silk worms, pandas, and koalas?

3. On which side did West Virginia fight during the U.S. Civil War?

SOS Decipher each of the following: TOWTHROWEL; TIJUSTME; I AM/MYSELF; HIJKLMNO. (Example: irighti = right between the eyes)

---

160 http://www.newsweek.com/how-improve-your-memory-sleep-68745

ICE List things that turn red.

TAB Your brainwaves will entrain or adapt to follow an external rhythm of sound pulses or flashing lights if it is set to a speed that matches one of the normal brainwave frequencies. For example, certain specially-designed music can be used to encourage alpha brainwaves for relaxation, or delta brainwaves to help you sleep.[161]

Mmm Rhythm Work: Clap a Song – Think of a song you know. Instead of singing it, clap it.

— SET 273 —

WOW [A] mind, once stretched by a new idea, never regains its original dimension. – Oliver Wendell Holmes

3Rs Remember some happy moments of being outdoors. When were you the happiest? Why? Where were you?

KISS 1. Which hand is usually used to play the bass clef on keyboard instruments?
2. How many pairs of shoes would you need for three spiders, four bees, and four flies?
3. The American Continental Divide follows the Rocky Mountains in North America and the Andes in South America. True or false?

SOS Gus is between 40 and 60. His age is even, and combining the digits gives you 7. How old is Gus?

ICE You just got a job making up fortunes for a fortune cookie factory. List some of the fortunes you would write?

TAB In several scientific studies, yoga's alternate nostril breathing technique (see below) has proven to be beneficial to the brain. It balances right and left sides of the brain, releases tension, and has demonstrated a measurable improvement on test scores, when done right before the test.[162]

Mmm Alternate Nostril Breathing – (You may want to blow your nose before this one ☺) Place the index and middle finger of one hand on your forehead, just between the eyebrows. Keep the pinky and ring finger together and use them to close the nostril on that (pinky/ring) side. Breath in through the opposite, open nostril. Now use the thumb to close the open nostril, and at the same time open the pinky/ring nostril. Breathe out through the now open pinky/ring side, and then breath in through the same nostril.

---

161 http://sedonanomalies.weebly.com/schumann-resonance.html
162 https://www.ncbi.nlm.nih.gov/pmc/articles/PMC4800515/

Then close the Pinky/ring nostril, and open the thumb side. Breathe out and in again through the thumb side. Repeat, altering nostrils—breathing out, then in, then closing/switching sides.

— SET 274 —

WOW When someone does something good, applaud! You will make two people happy. – Samuel Goldwyn

3Rs What were some of your favorite card games, board games or other games when growing up? What did you like about them? What are your favorites today?

KISS 1. Which punctuation marks are used the most?
2. (2 + 4 – 6) x 20 = ?
3. What is the 16th Century rebirth of ideas, culture and political thought in Europe called?

SOS A jewelry store was robbed and the jewels were found in some nearby plants. The detectives kept surveillance on the only two possible suspects. They were confident they would be able to arrest the guilty party without any further investigation, but they waited two days longer to make an arrest. Why?

ICE If you were a bird and there were no grass, leaves or twigs, what would you make your nest out of?

TAB According to researchers at Stanford University, dancing is an excellent way to increase neural connectivity because it simultaneously activates multiple brain functions simultaneously. In particular, dancing stimulates musical, kinesthetic, rational, and emotional functions.[163]

Mmm Cha-Cha Rhythm – The basic rhythm of the cha-cha is: *One. Two. Cha-cha-cha.* Dance around the room doing the cha-cha rhythm.

— SET 275 —

WOW You can't give a hug without getting one in return. – Anonymous

3Rs When is your birthday? How do you celebrate it now and in the past? What birthday do you remember as the best? Why? Is there another way you'd like to celebrate your birthday? How?

KISS 1. Come up with the word that fits the category and fits between the pair alphabetically: Comet, _______, Donner; Van Buren, ________, Wilson; Africa, ________, Asia.

163 http://socialdance.stanford.edu/syllabi/smarter.htm

2. What are the long organs that help you digest your food?
3. What U.S. state was named by the Spanish for its beautiful colors?

SOS The earth weighs approximately six sextillion tons (who weighed it?). How much more would it weigh, if one were to build a wall circling the equator, using the heaviest materials on the planet?

ICE Which is softest: kindness, love, or understanding? Why?

TAB A recent study in England found that images of social support calm and alter the brain's stress response so that the amygdala does not fire off as reactively to perceived threats.[164]

Mmm Image of Support Meditation – Find or create an image with people showing affection, love, or social support in some way. Find a comfortable place and position where you can easily see the image. Consciously breathe and gaze at the image for at least 3 minutes.

—— SET 276 ——

WOW We always have time for the things we put first. What do you put first? – Anonymous

3Rs What is the most unique thing in your home? Describe it. When someone visits your home, what do you feel most proud to show them? Why? Describe the item.

KISS 1. Who was the lead female star of *The Sound of Music*?
2. What dinosaur has a name meaning "three-horned face"?
3. What does the U.S. Supreme Court do the first Monday of each October?

SOS Tim could light a match under water. Explain.

ICE Use the following places in sentences that you create: Delaware, Hawaii, Iowa, Iran, and Tennessee. For example, Washington – The laundry weighed a Washing ton.

TAB A 2009 study found that participants who spent 30 minutes a day for six weeks learning to juggle showed increased white matter in their brains based on MRI scans. This neuroplasticity was true for participating new jugglers regardless of the actual level of juggling skill they achieved.[165]

Mmm Juggling – Try your hand at juggling. Start by tossing one object back and forth between two hands. (A good thing to start with is scarves or hankies,

---

164 http://psychcentral.com/news/2014/11/10/brains-threat-response-calmed-by-observing-love-and-support/77173.html

165 https://www.sciencedaily.com/releases/2009/10/091016114055.htm

because they don't fall as fast as balls.) If you can handle one, then add a second and then a third.

—— SET 277 ——

WOW To the mind that is still, the whole universe surrenders. – Lao Tzu

3Rs What were some times when you were unkind or naughty to a friend or sibling when you were growing up? Did you mean it? What happened?

KISS 1. List five alliterative names. Begin with the same letter and sound, e.g., Peter Pan.

2. What is the process called in which plants use sunlight to create food?

3. Where did the Boxer Rebellion happen?

SOS Find a one word answer to the following so that the last two letters of each answer are also the first two letters of the next answer. Slithering reptile: lock and ____: Fringe around the peepers: Pour down rain: Explode like a volcano: arctic bird: Heavenly being.

ICE Give unique possible uses for a sink plug.

TAB A synapse is the small gap between the ends of neurons in the brain. Synapses allow electrical impulse information to pass from one neuron to the next as information makes its way to and/or through the brain. These synapses form a complex and flexible network.

Mmm Between Thoughts Meditation – Count the time between your thoughts.

—— SET 278 ——

WOW Shoot for the moon. Even if you miss it, you will land among the stars. – Les Brown

3Rs When were there times you went to a new place that you did not know anybody? How did you feel? When you meet people, what is the first thing you generally want to know? Why?

KISS 1. Who wrote, "The face that launched a thousand ships"?

2. What is another name for Aurora Borealis?

3. Spell the capital of Iraq.

SOS Using only the letters SETISDHOMT, make a 1-letter word, a 2-letter word, a 3-letter word, etc. up to 10-letter word.

ICE List things that are spread.

TAB Research at the University of Iowa indicates that even after specific memories are gone, emotions connected to those memories are somehow retained.

This suggests that a visit or telephone call to a friend with dementia or Alzheimer's disease can have important positive effects on the person even though the visit/phone call is soon forgotten.

Mmm A Rhinoceros Gazes at the Moon – Stand in a shoulder-width stance with your hands on your hips. Close mouth and touch the tip of the tongue to the roof of your mouth as if you were about to say the letter "t." Imagine that the moon is up behind you, and you are a rhinoceros. As you inhale, twist and turn to point your big rhino horn at the moon. Exhale and return to center. Repeat 10 times alternating which shoulder you look over.

— SET 279 —

WOW In matters of style, swim with the current; in matters of principle, stand like a rock. – Thomas Jefferson

3Rs What were your jobs or chores in your family growing up? Were you paid? Which chores did you like and not like doing? What happened if you didn't do them? How could you get out of doing those chores?

KISS 1. What does *acoustic* refer to in music? Think acoustic guitar.

2. How many kidneys do most people have?

3. What nation did the U.S. buy Alaska from in 1876?

SOS If you take a regular die and know just the top number, you can guess the bottom number. How?

ICE How is a desert like a dessert?

TAB Neurotransmitters can be classified by their tendency to either excite or calm action in the neuron. For example, GABA is a calming neurotransmitter that reduces anxiety, while epinephrine, also known as adrenaline, is a stimulating neurotransmitter.

Mmm Hands Sensation Meditation – Bring the palms of your hands together in front of your heart with fingertips pointing up. Close your eyes. Without pressing, bring your awareness to the sensation of the hands and fingers where they touch one another. Sense which hand is touching and which hand is being touched. Can you sense the right hand touching the left hand? Can you sense the left hand touching the right hand? Are these sensations different? Can you sense both hands as simultaneously "doing the touching"? As simultaneously "being touched"?

— SET 280 —

WOW Never confuse activity with action. – F. Scott Fitzgerald

3Rs Where have you travelled? What are your memories of those travels? What do you do to pass the time when you are on a bus, train, plane, etc.? What is your favorite place to visit? Why is it your favorite? Would you have liked to live there? What is your least favorite place to travel?

KISS 1. What do these British words mean: lorry; petrol; queue?
2. Which birds lay the smallest eggs, and which lay the largest?
3. In what city were the first Olympic Games?

SOS Anyone can tell the score of any sports game even before it starts. How is this possible?

ICE You are in a formal wedding of a friend, and the heel of your shoe comes off while you are walking down the aisle. What could you do? Be creative!

TAB Memories triggered by scent or aroma form stronger, more intense emotional connections than the other senses. Smell is best able to influence brain activity because the olfactory bulbs within the brain directly connect to the areas of the brain that process emotion and learning.

Mmm Compass Points: Arms – If you do not have a compass and do not already know which way north is where you currently are, you can simply pick one direction to be north and define the other directions accordingly. Stand facing north and point out the following combinations of directions:

- Point east with your left hand and southwest with your right hand
- Point south with your left hand and northwest with your right hand
- Point southeast with your left hand and northeast with your right hand
- Point west with your left hand and south with your right hand

— SET 281 —

WOW If you are depressed, you are living in the past. If you are anxious, you are living in the future. If you are at peace you are living in the present. – Lao Tzu

3Rs Which movies that currently do not have a sequel most deserve one? Why? What would you like to see happen in the sequel if it were made?

KISS 1. Invertebrate animals have no ______.
2. True or false? Hailstorms are most common during freezing weather.
3. What is it called when senators talk non-stop to delay the progress of a bill?

SOS Name one eight-letter word that has the letters "kst" in the middle, "in" at the beginning, "and" at the end.

ICE Complete the following statements with something completely new: Clouds are like ___; Trees are like ___; Flowers are like ___. Be original!

TAB Speaking more than one language is good for the brain. New research conducted at Northwestern University found that bilingual speakers process information more efficiently and more easily than those who know a single language. The benefits apparently occur because the bilingual brain is constantly activating both languages and choosing which language to use and which to ignore.[166]

Mmm Compass Points: Arms & Legs – If you do not have a compass and do not already know which way north is where you currently are, you can simply pick one direction to be north and define the other directions accordingly. Point out the following combinations of directions:

- Point west with your left hand, east with your right hand west, with your right leg
- Point southeast with your left leg, northeast with your right hand, west with your left hand
- Point south with your left hand, east with your right hand, northwest with either foot
- Point north with your left hand, southwest with your right leg, east with your right hand

—— SET 282 ——

WOW A good listener is not only popular everywhere but after a while gets to know something. – Wilson Mizner

3Rs What time did you have to go to bed as a child? How strictly was bedtime enforced? How did it make you feel? Did you have a certain time you needed to be home as a young person? Did you ever break the rule? What happened?

KISS 1. Can you spell the word that Mary Poppins thinks sounds quite atrocious?

2. 2 + 4 – 6 x 20 = ?

3. Which ruler conquered the most territory in Europe: Hitler, Napoleon, or Alexander the Great?

---

166 https://www.washingtonpost.com/national/health-science/study-shows-that-people-who-speak-two-languages-have-more-efficient-brains/2014/11/18/e027a27e-6a7c-11e4-9fb4-a622dae742a2_story.html

SOS An ancient invention still used today allows people to see through walls. What is that invention?

ICE Name things that zip or use the word "zip".

TAB At birth each baby has 100 billion brain cells, and by the time people reach adulthood they will have developed one quadrillion pathways/connections in their brains.[167]

Mmm Compassion Meditation: Young Adult –. Close your eyes, and place your hands on your heart. On the next breath, invite an image of yourself as a young adult (early twenties). See your young adult self in front of you. Smile to your young adult self. In your mind give that young adult a hug. Send that young adult your gentle loving compassion.

— SET 283 —

WOW We need time to dream, time to remember, and time to reach the infinite; just time to be. – Gladys Taber

3Rs Which one of your five senses is the most important to you? Why? Describe a favorite time in terms of your number one sense.

KISS 1. List nouns that can be heard but not seen.
2. How many chambers does the human heart have?
3. Which country is the world's leading exporter of bananas and plantains?

SOS A young woman from Texas married nine different men. She did not break any laws. None of the men died or divorced. How was this possible?

ICE List times you should be "standing up."

TAB Theta brainwaves are associated with states of dreaming and creative innovation.

Mmm Opening and Closing the Limbs – Lie on your back in a comfortable position. On an inhale, allow your arms and legs to float up and spread out, opening and expanding the body. Then with your exhale, gently draw your arms and legs back into your body, closing and contracting into a ball. Repeat for at least ten breath cycles.

— SET 284 —

WOW Blessed are the flexible for they shall not be bent out of shape. – Anonymous

---

167 http://www.nais.org/Magazines-Newsletters/ISMagazine/Pages/What-Recent-Brain -Research-Tells-Us-about-Learning.aspx

3Rs Who is your favorite painter, sculptor or photographer of all time? Why? What do you remember about a time you saw that artists work? What is your favorite art work? Why?

KISS 1. Say this tongue twister at least five times: "She sold six shabby sheared sheep."

2. What's the difference between horns and antlers?

3. Greece marches first in the Olympics opening parade; which country marches last?

SOS How would you cut a pie in eight equal slices with only three straight cuts of the knife?

ICE Beauty is in the eyes of the beholder. Think of things that are beautiful in the eyes of your house plant.

TAB Ginko Biloba is an herb that has been used in traditional Chinese medicine to increase blood flow to the brain and improve memory.

Mmm Tied in Knots – Sit comfortably in a chair. Cross your right leg over your left knee. Cross your arms. Then keeping your arms crossed, rest your elbows on your knee and prop your chin in your right palm. Switch positions by crossing your left leg on your right knee and placing your elbow on your knee with arms crossed. Switch at least ten times and try to make the switch faster each time.

— SET 285 —

WOW When [people's] knowledge is not in order, the more of it [they have] the greater will be [their] confusion. – Herbert Spencer

3Rs Based on your past experience, what is the most important problem or issue today that America's founding fathers did not understand or anticipate? How might it best be solved?

KISS 1. Was Claude Monet an Italian conductor, a musician, or a painter?

2. What do the following have in common: The Cocoa Shrub; The Opium Poppy; The Peyote Cactus?

3. The Missouri, Ohio, and Red rivers all flow into the same river. What is that river?

SOS What do these initials stand for: 1) Shakespearean comedy: M. A. A. N.; 2) American Song: S. S. B.; 3) Science Fiction Movie: S.W.

ICE Draw something using four straight lines and three triangles. Come up with as many different ideas as you can.

TAB How you organize thoughts in your mind can positively or negatively affect your brain power and memory.

Mmm Eating Eyes Closed – Chose something to eat that won't be too messy, but will require a fork or spoon. Close your eyes (or put on a blindfold). Eat it all without opening your eyes.

—— SET 286 ——

WOW When you're through changing . . . you're through! – Bruce Barton

3Rs Would you have preferred a different ending to any books you have read? If so, which ones? Why didn't you like the ending, and how would you change it?

KISS 1. What are three of the most common grammar mistakes?

2. Which nautical term is the opposite of windward?

3. True or false? Puerto Ricans are U.S. citizens.

SOS A large crowd of people enter Carole's workplace. The people do not pay for what they take, as long as they take things in a quiet and orderly way, Carole has no problem with this. Where does Carole work and what are people taking?

ICE List things with flashing lights.

TAB According to the Mayo Clinic, there is an increased genetic risk of Alzheimer's for individuals who have a particular form of the Apo lipoprotein E (APOE) gene.[168]

Mmm The Jig Is Up – Imagine you are in Ireland and do "your" version of an Irish jig dance. Hop and kick! Hop and kick!

—— SET 287 ——

WOW After all is said and done, more is said than done. – Aesop

3Rs Would you rather have a lot of friends or a lot of money? Why?

KISS 1. Say this tongue twister at least five times: Cooks cook cupcakes quickly.

2. What is the biggest bone in our body?

3. The U.S. flag has thirteen stripes. What color is the top stripe?

SOS The first letter of each word in the following descriptions are also the same as the initials as the person described. Name the famous person being

168 http://www.mayoclinic.org/diseases-conditions/alzheimers-disease/expert-answers/alzheimers-disease/faq-20057837

defined in the following: 1) Became Astronaut; 2) Faithful Animal-lover; 3) Comical Broad.

ICE Combine characteristics of two very distinct animals and create a "new" animal. Example: rhinocergator or tigaroo. What does it look like and how does it behave?

TAB People identified as creative have developed their abilities to observe and use all of their senses, to take everything in, to consider anything that comes to mind, to set aside judgment about ideas, and to refrain from focusing on patterns.

Mmm Touch Sensation Meditation – Go through the room and touch the various objects and surfaces. As you touch them, close your eyes and bring your mind to the sensation of the object or surface you are touching. Notice shape, temperature, and texture. What different textures can you find in the room? (Do your dusting at the same time!)

— SET 288 —

WOW The true art of memory is the art of attention – Samuel Johnson

3Rs When you were a child, what did you want to be when you grew up? Did you change your mind? Why or why not? Do you wish you had chosen a different career? What would that have been?

KISS 1. Is a piccolo more like a saxophone or a flute?
2. True or false? Parchment paper is made from animal skin.
3. If you drive from Louisiana to Utah, what direction do you go?

SOS Unscramble the following to spell three different countries: LUTORGAP, NEDACIL, WESNED.

ICE If you discovered tiny little people living inside the walls of your house, what would you do?

TAB Can you read the following: Aoccdrnig to rscheearch at Cmabrigde Uinervtisy, it dseno't mtaeter in waht oerdr the ltteres in a wrod are, the olny iproamtnt tihng is taht the frsit and lsat ltteer be in the rghit pclae. [According to research at Cambridge University, it does not matter in what order the letters in a word are. The only important thing is that the first and last letter be in the right place.] Your brain will do the work to decipher it.[169]

Mmm Body Brush Down – Take the flat of one hand and brush down the opposite arm several times as if brushing lint off. Do the same for the rest of the

169 http://www.mrc-cbu.cam.ac.uk/people/matt.davis/cmabridge/

body: other arm, head, down the front and back of the torso, hips and pelvis, both legs and feet.

— SET 289 —

WOW You will find peace not by trying to escape your problems, but by confronting them courageously. You will find peace not in denial, but in victory. – J. Donald Walters

3Rs What are/were you superstitious about? Are there particularly things you think are lucky or unlucky? Are there things you do to prevent bad luck or ensure good luck? Describe a time that your superstition came up? How did this superstition get started?

KISS 1. List five verbs
2. What do you call the process of wind, heat and rain wearing down rock?
3. Which year came first, 200 B.C. or 300 B.C.?

SOS When can you add two to eleven and get one?

ICE Why would an octopus make a good/bad lifeguard at the pool?

TAB A 2014 study by French scientists found that people who work irregular shifts for ten years or more can age the brain by an extra 6.5 years.[170]

Mmm Power Stance: Victory – Stand with your feet in a solid shoulder-width stance. Imagine that you have been asked to take a stand for your own self-worth. On an inhale, raise your arms over your head in a "V" for victory. Breathe normally, and stay focused on your sensation. Sense your breath, your feet on the ground, the vertical line of your body, and the line of your upraised arms. According to a 2015, *Reader's Digest* article, research in social psychology indicates that 2 minutes of holding this pose can reduce stress and increase one's sense of power.

— SET 290 —

WOW For every minute you remain angry, you give up sixty seconds of peace of mind. – Ralph Waldo Emerson

3Rs Which are/were some of your favorite commercials from TV or radio? What was the slogan? If there was a jingle, sing or hum that jingle to yourself. Picture some of the images from the commercial.

---

170 http://www.dailymail.co.uk/health/article-2819162/Long-term-shift-work-ages-brain-leading-impaired-memory-thinking.html

KISS 1. Say this seven times quickly: "Which wrist watches are Swiss wrist watches?"

2. Should you multiply first or divide first in "10x100/20 = 50"?

3. Antarctica and what country are almost entirely covered by glaciers?

SOS What same word appropriately fits in front of each of the following: Front; Ski; Melon; Fall; Tower?

ICE What are some of the first things you would show an alien visiting you from outer space?

TAB Anger, anxiety, depression, fear and stress all negatively affect memory retention.

Mmm Seeing Anger In the Mirror – This activity is based on an experience from when my sister and mother were in an argument. Mom said, "You should see the angry look on your face." There was a mirror on the wall nearby, and they both turned and were startled to see the anger in their own faces. This exercise also demonstrates how our thoughts affect us emotionally. Find a comfortable position in front of a mirror where you can gaze into the eyes of your own reflection. Then close your eyes and think of something that makes you very angry. It can be helpful to think of a recent conflict or a controversial issue that gets you riled up. As clearly as you can, imagine yourself in that provoking situation. This will likely stir up the anger again. When you feel the anger arise strongly in you, open your eyes and look at your reflection. What do you see? Is that how you want to be? Now while you continue to gaze at your reflection, consciously breathe and calm yourself down. What do you see now?

— SET 291 —

WOW Obstacles are those frightful things you see when you take your eyes off your goal. – Henry Ford

3Rs Where were you born? What stories and/or information were you told about your birth? Who shared that information with you?

KISS 1. What is the world's most expensive painting?

2. "Pocket loop", "tented arch", and "plain whorl" are features of what? Hint: Think like a detective.

3. What name was so popular that it was used by the first Roman Emperors?

SOS When you tighten something with your right hand, which way would you turn it if you used your left hand?

ICE Explain the following statement: Roger watered his piano.

TAB Most experts agree that acquiring new skills can open up inactive areas of the brain and increase the number of neural connections. Statistics from "The Seattle Longitudinal Study" found that 66% of older Americans doing brain exercise activities showed significant cognitive improvement.[171]

Mmm Softening Meditation – Close your eyes, and bring your awareness to the sensations of your body. In particular, notice where there are any minor sensations of pain or discomfort. Choose one of these places for the focus of the rest of this meditation. What metaphor or image best describes the pain or discomfort? For example, it could seem like a hot fire or the color red. Now breathe deeply and begin to soften the image in the metaphor. For example, the fire cools and grows smaller or the red fades. Practicing this meditation regularly with minor discomfort and pain can help train the brain to manage more severe pain and discomfort over time.[172]

— SET 292 —

WOW If one is master of one thing and understands one thing well, one has at the same time, insight into and understanding of many things. – Vincent Van Gogh

3Rs Describe the best costume you ever wore? What was the occasion? Was the costume bought, borrowed, rented or homemade? How did other people respond to you when you wore it?

KISS 1. What is the role difference between a hyphen and a dash?
2. Which one of the following plants is a legume: Carrots, peas, or spinach?
3. Alexander Hamilton (a non-president) is on what U.S. paper money?

SOS If a clock takes five seconds to strike 6 o'clock, how many seconds will it take to strike 12 o'clock?

ICE List things one can spray.

TAB Learning is reinforced and may even be introduced during REM sleep periods, the times when dreams can occur, so things learned just before going to bed are remembered better than things learned early in the

---

171 http://jama.jamanetwork.com/article.aspx?articleid=195506

172 Achterberg, Jeanne, Barbara Dossy and Leslie Kokmeir. (1994) *Ritual and Healing: Using Imagery for Health and Wellness.* New York: Bantam.

morning. During this time period, memories are sifted through, some are discarded and others are consolidated and saved.

Mmm Tae Kwando Rolling Arms – Cross your arms at the wrist. Start to roll the forearms and wrist of each arm over one. Your goal is to move the arms as much as possible without losing physical contact between the two sides.

— SET 293 —

WOW To the one who only has a hammer in the toolkit, every problem looks like a nail. – Abraham Maslow

3Rs When you meet someone with different beliefs or opinions than yours, how do you feel? What do you say or do?

KISS 1. Say these tongue twister words at least five times: cinnamon, aluminum, linoleum.

2. What chemical is responsible for the green color of the grass?

3. Which two Central American countries have their names in the name of their capital cities?

SOS The following descriptions can be rephrased to create rhyming word pairs (example: chubby feline = fat cat). 1) Cruel legume; 2) Salmon entrée; 3) Married rodent.

ICE Make up something that connects a pickle, a starfish, and a hockey puck.

TAB For various reasons, the brain can play tricks with our memory. Sometimes what we are convinced that we remember as true is in actuality completely false, only partially true, or a misrepresentation.

Mmm Untangling Meditation – This meditation can be helpful when you are feeling overwhelmed or confused in a situation. Close your eyes. Imagine that all of the conflicting thoughts (especially other people's perspectives that are creating confusion about a given situation) are wound tight around your head like a giant, tangled wad of string. It may be interesting to notice what color the yarn is. As you are ready, unwind and disentangle the yarn from around your head until your feel lighter and freer.

— SET 294 —

WOW Memory, and hope; one looks backward, and the other forward; one is of today, the other of tomorrow. Memory is history recorded in our brain, memory is a painter, it paints pictures of the past and of the day. – Grandma Moses

3Rs What is your biggest regret in life? How did it affect your life? Did you try to change it? What could help you to release this regret now?

KISS 1. What musical term means gradually becoming louder?
2. Hale-Bopp and Halley's are both what?
3. What Italian explorer reached China in 1275? Clue: The same as a modern swimming game.

SOS What countries do the following spell: NIPSA; LAITY; ACDEORU?

ICE In what ways could you get to the top of a flagpole? Think wild and wacky!

TAB Studies on animals indicate that high fructose corn syrup has a negative effect on memory and brain functioning.[173]

Mmm Can You Outsmart Your Foot? – Sit in front of a desk or table. Lift your right leg, and draw clockwise circles in the air with your right foot. Now at the same time, use your right hand to write the number "6" in the air. Did your foot change directions? Try and stop it. Can you do it? Now try it on the opposite side. This time make circles counterclockwise with the left foot and write the number "9" in the air with your left hand.

— SET 295 —

WOW Don't compromise yourself; you are all you've got. – Janis Joplin

3Rs Where have you purchased/obtained furniture after high school? Any favorite pieces? What are the stories of getting those pieces?

KISS 1. How does adding the suffixes "er" or "est" usually change the meaning of a word?
2. Are decibels used to measure length, light, or volume (loudness)?
3. The Taj Mahal is located in Agra. In what country is the Taj Mahal located?

SOS Add the same two letters to each of the following sets to obtain legitimate words: R _ _; _ R _; _ _ R.

ICE Create reasonable reasons for the following ridiculous statement: "The Governor goes up the stairs backwards."

TAB In 2011, Stanford University researchers provided concrete evidence, that ability to recognize faces is so important in humans that a separate area of the brain, called the "fusiform gyrus," is devoted solely to that task. It only processes facial recognition and nothing else.[174]

---

173 http://naturalsociety.com/high-fructose-corn-syrup-damages-learning-abilities-memory/

174 https://med.stanford.edu/news/2012/10/precisely-targeted-electrical-brain-stimulation-alters-perception-of-faces-scientists-find.html

Mmm The Cobra – Note: this exercise should not be done on a bed as a mattress will not provide enough support for the lower back. If getting down on the floor is too difficult repeat the Chair Neck and Upper Back Stretch from yesterday instead.

Lie face down on the floor. Bring the legs in close together and point the feet, so that the soles of the feet are towards the ceiling. Place the hands on the floor just below the armpits. Press the pelvis and hips strongly into the floor throughout to protect the lower back. Pull the shoulder blades back and down. Then on a slow in-breath, gently lift your head and look up. Lengthen the neck and curve it back gently without scrunching or wrinkling the skin at the back of the neck. If this is comfortable, continue to let the head be drawn upward so that upper back curves and the shoulders and chest lift off the ground. Hold for a few breaths, and then gently release back down. Bring the arms up to create a pillow for the forehead to rest on. Once or twice may be enough for this one.

— SET 296 —

WOW I have finally discovered what's wrong with my brain: On the left side there is nothing right, and on the right side there is nothing left. – Anonymous

3Rs What should every parent teach his or her children? Why? How should those lessons be taught? Are there things that you wish your parent's had taught you? Did you ever learn it? How or why not?

KISS 1. Say the following rapidly six times: "Black brings beloved."
2. Would you find a saguaro in a desert, a forest, or a jungle?
3. Chocolate is derived from the bean of what tree?

SOS How can you arrange the numbers 6-3-1 to create a number that can be divided evenly by seven? Tricky.

ICE You are a travel agent and you have been asked to nominate three places for the "Best Places in the Universe Contest". What places would you choose? Why?

TAB Nothing affects the brain more positively than a genuine belly laugh! Scientists agree that humor involves the whole brain, serves to balance and integrate the hormones and brain activity in both hemispheres of the brain, reduces emotional stress, gives one focus, and can even strengthen your immune system.

Mmm The Chicken Dance — Put on some music or sing the song if you know it. Start by placing your hands to create wings and flap your wings. Keeping your wings in place bend your knees, stick out your butt and wiggle. Then make your hands into chicken beaks. Open and close the hands—"Cluck, cluck, cluck!"

— SET 297 —

WOW Peace within makes beauty without. – English Proverb

3Rs What is too scary for you to ever try? Has this always been scary for you? What was the scariest thing you ever successfully did? How did you overcome your fear about it? How did you feel after you accomplished it?

KISS 1. Which musical instrument has more strings; the banjo or the guitar?
2. What is electrical resistance?
3. What was banned during Prohibition?

SOS A father paid $5 for each correct answer on a test, and the son pays $8 for each incorrect answer. The boy answered 26 questions, and no money was exchanged. How many correct and how many incorrect answers were given by the son?

ICE You are the person who puts fillings in donuts and you are trying to get fired. Create some wacky ideas for new fillings.

TAB "When researchers at UCLA compared the brains of meditators to non-meditators . . . non-meditators' brains are almost a decade younger by the time people reach their mid 50s."[175]

Mmm Seated Meditation: Underwater Meditation – In your mind, visualize a clear lake. Imagine yourself diving into the lake and swimming down to take a seat at the center of the bottom of the lake. The water is cool and crystal clear. You can see all the way up to the sunlight sparking on the surface of the lake. You can breathe underwater here, and the substance of this pure lake cleans and refreshes your lungs. Follow your breath. Whenever, you find your mind wandering breathe the thought out as air bubbles that float up to the surface of the lake and disappear.

— SET 298 —

WOW There is much pleasure to be gained from useless knowledge. – Bertrand Russell

3Rs Were you ever in plays, debate, or some kind of other dramatic performances at school or in the community? If so, describe your performance(s). How pleased were you with it/them, and why?

175 https://www.mindful.org/meditators-younger-brains/

KISS 1. What five letter word contains four personal pronouns in correct order?
2. How can you mathematically combine eight nines to equal 1125?
3. Which of the following is a Moslem place of worship: Cathedral, temple, mosque, or synagogue?

SOS What do all three of the following have in common: A doctor's office, a rattlesnake, the sign of Libra?

ICE List things with wrinkles.

TAB Contrary to popular opinion, there is no such thing as left-brain or right-brain learning. As demonstrated by a University of Utah study it is erroneous to imply that any learning occurs only on one side or the other. While some activities increase activity in particular areas of the brain, both sides of the brain are usually equally active and working together.[176]

Mmm Pushing Eight Horses – Throughout this exercise, keep the muscles of the hands and arms activated and move as if pushing them though a great force. Hold your hands out in front of you with the fingers together and the thumbs away to the side so one hand forms an "L" shape and the other forms a reverse "L". Maintaining the "L" shape, bring the hands to your sides. Take a solid stance with knees slightly bent. Keep the upper arms tucked in close to the body. Then as if resisting a great force, bend the elbows to bring the L-shaped hands up to the armpits. Touch the heels of your hands to the ribs. While keeping the thumbs up, push the arms out in front of you as if "pushing the weight of eight horses." Hold with arms extended for a breath or two. Then use your shoulders and arms to "pull the eight horses back," returning the hands first to their position by the armpits, and then down to your sides again. Repeat two times.

— SET 299 —

WOW I like nonsense; it wakes up the brain cells. Fantasy is a necessary ingredient in living; it's a way of looking at life through the wrong end of a telescope. Which is what I do, and that enables you to laugh at life's realities. – Dr. Seuss

3Rs If all of life's daily activities were Olympic sports, what would you be most likely to win a medal in? Why? How would you train for it?

KISS 1. Name five or more classical composers.
2. What are the three main layers of the earth?
3. Name the U.S. states that touch the Pacific Ocean?

176 http://www.apa.org/monitor/2013/11/right-brained.aspx

SOS Find a one word answer to the following so that the last two letters of each answer are also the first two letters of the next answer: Earth's path around the sun; Nation where Venice is found; Small harp-like instrument; Do or say again; Good-looking; Planet named for the goddess of love. Be creative!

ICE "If you twardle the merklo again, I'm going to dwankle up the yoppel." What does this nonsense sentence mean?

TAB Current research indicates that creativity involves strong and steady activity throughout the brain rather than a single specific "creativity area" of the brain.

Mmm Swords – Imagine you are a master at swordplay. Fend off a group of sword-wielding attackers with an imaginary sword. Remember they will be coming at you from all directions. You must block and thrust—high and low, right and left, to the front and behind. For extra challenge and benefit, switch your sword to the opposite hand.

—— SET 300 ——

WOW You've got to stand for something or you'll fall for anything. – Steve Bartkowski

3Rs List ten words to describe your day yesterday.

KISS 1. Which was invented first; the harpsichord or the piano?
2. List two animals that ruminate?
3. Which U.S. president never took a salary?

SOS A pail is tied to the outside of a boat. The pail hangs three yards above water level. The water rises two yards an hour. How long will it be before the water touches the pail?

ICE What if Cinderella's fairy godmother could give "The Three Bears" their wishes? What would the three bears wish for? Be creative.

TAB Be careful in making judgments about potential cognitive abilities. For example, F. W. Woolworth worked in a dry goods store at the age of 21, but was not allowed to wait on customers because "he didn't have enough sense." He later went on to create a multi-million dollar international corporation of discount stores.[177]

---

177 http://www.uky.edu/~eushe2/Pajares/OnFailingG.html

Mmm Clenched Fist Breathing – Stand in a shoulder-width stance with the arms hanging comfortably to your sides. Close the mouth and touch the tip of the tongue to the roof of your mouth as if you were about to say the letter "t." Make fists with your hands and turn them so that the thumbs point in toward your legs. Inhale deeply so that the belly expands, and at the same time relax the fists. Then as you exhale, pull the belly button in and squeeze the fists tight. Repeat 4 or 5 times.

— SET 301 —

WOW Obstacles don't have to stop you. If you run into a wall, don't turn around and give up. Figure out how to climb it, go through it or work around it. – Michael Jordan

3Rs Where do you feel most safe? Why? What do you consider the safest place in the world?

KISS 1. What do bullet, brace and bracket have in common?
2. What are some ways that metals are generally distinct from non-metals?
3. What oil tanker ran aground off the Alaskan Coast causing one of the worst oil spills in history?

SOS You are playing cards and three playing cards are placed face down on a table. For those three cards, the jack is immediately to the left of the queen. To the left of a spade is a diamond. A king is just to the left of a heart. A spade is to the right of a king. What is the placement of the cards on the table?

ICE List unusual things stored in a refrigerator.

TAB According to experiments at the University of Lübeck in Germany, to gain the benefit of sleeping to improve memory or learning, you must consciously believe that you will need the information in the future. Study participants were tested on their memory before and after ten hours of sleep. Only the ones who had been "warned" there would be a test in the morning showed improvement.[178]

Mmm Mindful Tracking: Media Consumption – For today consciously track how much time you spend to the nearest 15 minutes with various forms of media, such as internet surfing, TV, film, cell phone, social media, email, texting, etc. You can write it down or make a mental note and tally up at the end of the day. Any surprises?

---

178 http://www.newsweek.com/how-improve-your-memory-sleep-68745

— SET 302 —

WOW The most important things in your house are the people. – Anonymous

3Rs Which was more important to you when growing up, being good-looking or being smart? Why? How about now?

KISS 1. Which word means to place, lie or lay?

2. Who invented the telephone?

3. What is the only letter of the alphabet that is not used as the start of a country?

SOS If you were to paint two white lines dividing a road into three lanes and the cost is $100. What will it cost to paint lines dividing a road into six lanes?

ICE You find your house is now at the top of a tree. What are the challenges you now face?

TAB PET scans show that when you say people's names in their presence, you spark their brain's sense of worth and increase their interest in what you are saying.[179]

Mmm Word Meditation: Name of a Loved One –For this meditation, you will focus on the name of someone you love. This can be a romantic partner, a family member, or friend living or dead. Close your eyes. As you feel ready, repeat the name of your loved one aloud or silently in your head for one to five minutes.

— SET 303 —

WOW Humility is a strange thing; the minute you think you've got it, you've lost it. – E. D. Hulse

3Rs When was a time you took some good advice from someone? What was the advice, who gave it to you, and why was it good advice? What about a time someone gave you bad advice?

KISS 1. On a standard piano, which keys are longer; the black keys or the white keys?

2. What two words together make up the word smog?

3. What 19th Century "revolution" involved the transition from making things by hand to using complex machines?

SOS Sue eats an egg a day. She does not have any chickens at home, but she never buys, borrows, steals or receives eggs from someone else. Explain.

179 http://www.ncbi.nlm.nih.gov/pmc/articles/PMC1647299/

ICE You are a consultant who has been asked to recommend states that should be combined with other states. What states would you combine?

TAB Everyone can be extremely creative. Creativity is more an issue of whether we believe we are creative or not. Research shows that the brain definitely does create when we tell it to do something original or to "think outside the box."

Mmm Triangle Walk – Walk around the room filling the room with triangle pathways. Make large triangles and small triangles. High triangles and low triangles.

— SET 304 —

WOW Stand up for what is right, even if you're standing alone. – Anonymous

3Rs Where were you and what were you doing, when a national tragedy happened, such as the John F. Kennedy or Martin Luther King assassinations? How did you first hear about the event? What do you remember about your thoughts during the event? How did you feel?

KISS 1. What do "farther" and "further" measure?

2. What type of non-flying bird could be called an Emperor, a King, or a Fairy?

3. Name two of the three countries that are larger in area than the U.S.?

SOS The numbers of flowers in a garden doubles in size each day. In 28 days the flowers will cover the whole garden. In how many days will the garden be half-covered?

ICE List things that shine that would not need to be polished.

TAB The brain is designed to have empathy. A 2013 study reported in the *Journal of Neuroscience* found that although we have an "innate tendency" to be self-centered, a part of your brain (the *right supramarginal gyrus*) identifies that lack of empathy and "autocorrects."[180]

Mmm Walk as if: Life Stages – Take a few minutes to walk as if you were a person in the following life stages, and notice what changes. Walk as if you were: A toddler; Elderly; Middle-aged; A teenager; In grade-school; Pregnant.

— SET 305 —

WOW Take the attitude of a student. Never be too big to ask questions. Never know too much to learn. – Og Mandino

---

180 http://www.psychologytoday.com/blog/the-athletes-way/201310/the-neuroscience-empathy

3Rs What was the last thing you spent money on that you wish you hadn't? Why do you regret it?

KISS 1. Say this three times: One-one was a racehorse. Two-two was one too when One-one won one race. Two-two won one, too.
2. Hot liquid rock deep inside the Earth is called what?
3. Two 20th century U.S. presidents from different political parties had the same last name. What were their names?

SOS The following "witty words" contain either the letters "wit" or the sound "wit": 1) Carve wood; 2) Not outside; 3) Resign; 4) What a blacksmith might do to a horse (two words); 5) See and observe something.

ICE Compare a goblin and an elf.

TAB A German study in 2013 suggests that tongue twisters can be used to test for cognitive decline.[181]

Mmm Sun and Moon Embrace – Stand with your feet about hip-width apart. On an in-breath, raise the eyes skyward and reach the hands up above the head in a "V" shape, as if you are embracing the sky. Imagine that you hold the sun in your right hand and the moon in your left hand. On an exhale, bring the sun and moon together by touching your palms together and lowering the two hands to just in front of your heart. Follow your hands with your eyes. Hold the pose for 10-12 breaths. To release, turn the hands so that the finger tips point out away from your body, and then open your hands.

—— SET 306 ——

WOW Pride is at the bottom of all great mistakes. – John Ruskin

3Rs When do you feel undue pressure the most? How do you deal with that pressure? How could you make such situations easier?

KISS 1. Are lyrics a song's music or its words?
2. 16 12 2 3 = 99. What mathematical signs could you insert so that the total equals 99?
3. What is the oldest surviving college in North America?

SOS A lawyer in London has a brother in Paris who is a grocer. The grocer does not have a brother in London. How is this possible?

ICE If you were a sponge, what would be some of your favorite messes?

TAB Too much table salt causes electrolyte imbalances that temporarily slow down one's thought processes. Although some sodium is necessary for

---

181 https://www.ncbi.nlm.nih.gov/pubmed/24022211

the body, the American Dietetic Association advises no more than 2400 milligrams per day. But the problem is not just from salting your food at the table. According to the FDA, 75% of the sodium in one's diet is usually from packaged and restaurant foods.

Mmm Compass: Facing – If you do not have a compass and do not already know which way north is where you currently are, you can simply pick one direction to be north. Stand facing north. Turn southeast. Turn west. Turn northeast. Turn south. Turn southwest. Turn east. Turn northwest. Repeat.

— SET 307 —

WOW When you choose the behavior, you also choose the consequences. Choose carefully! – Dr. Phil Mc Graw

3Rs Who do you know in your family or another family (including you) that served in the military? Which military service was it; was it army, navy, air force, marines, or coast guard? What stories about this service do you remember? Do you do special activities on Memorial Day or Veteran's Day? If not, what do you do on that day?

KISS 1. Use the word "sit" and "set" in the same sentence.

2. If you have a problem with your feet, should you see a pediatrician, a pathologist, or a podiatrist?

3. What U.S. state has two separate land masses connected by the Mackinaw Bridge?

SOS In the following, take away the scrambled letters of a cold thing to find a hot thing, with the remaining letters in the correct order: CIFILICREE.

ICE "Can you qiv my rengle? I don't grevel for scuptors anymore." What does this nonsense sentence mean? Be Creative!

TAB Working memory is short-term memory that can be retained in your brain indefinitely with periodic repetition of the information. When the information is important enough to keep indefinitely the brain transforms information and associated experience into long-term memory. In order to get to long-term memory, the information must have **both** meaning and emotion.

Mmm Heart-Flow Breath – The oxygen brought into the lungs is pumped by the heart through the body to nourish and replenish all the cells of the body. As you breathe in, envision the breath going directly to the heart. As you exhale, see the breath flowing out from the heart. Continue in this way, for each in-breath say the word "heart" in your mind. For each out breath say the word "flowing." Do 10-12 breath cycles.

— SET 308 —

WOW This thing we call "failure" is not the falling down, but the staying down. – Mary Pickford

3Rs Describe a time that you "spoke your mind" about something, and why. Was that a good choice for you? For others?

KISS 1. Say the following quickly three times: "Nancy's noisy nose annoys an oyster."
2. What do you call plants that only last one year?
3. Known as the Father of Medicine, who gave his name to the doctor's oath?

SOS Happy Hostess invited some of her favorite scientists and inventors to a party and asked them to RSVP. Each reply relates to the person's claim to fame in some way. Whose RSVPs are the following: 1) Arrive at eight on the dot. Have to dash. Can't stop. 2) I'll let you know as my schedule evolves; 3) In theory, it should be relatively easy to come; 4) I am drooling at the thought. Shall I ring the bell or come right in?

ICE What would you do with a unicorn?

TAB Take a break from a problem that requires creativity. When we focus too long, the brain produces extra gamma waves, which can block it from finding a solution. Gamma waves are connected to narrow focused attention, when a creative solution requires us to think more broadly.[182]

Mmm Legs Up the Wall – This yoga pose can be very relaxing and according to *Yoga Journal* is good for headaches, de-stressing and calming the mind![183] The goal is to lie with your torso lying flat on the ground with your legs stretched up the wall as if the room had rotated and you are now "sitting" on the wall. Find a wall that is clear of furniture and art with at least 5 feet of clearance. Sit down a few inches from the wall. Lean back to brace yourself with your arms as you rotate your pelvis around so that your back comes towards the floor and the buttocks turn towards the wall. Gently swing both legs up against the wall and at the same time lower your upper body to lie down on the floor. Your body will form a capital letter "L"—with the

182 http://www.scientificamerican.com/article/mental-downtime/

183 https://www.yogajournal.com/poses/legs-up-the-wall-pose

legs going up the wall to form the vertical line and the torso on the floor pointing straight out away from the wall to form the horizontal line. If the back or neck hurt, use the blanket or towel to support the head or hips for more comfort. Rest and relax for five minutes or so.

— SET 309 —

WOW If you haven't got any charity in your heart, you have the worst kind of heart trouble. – Bob Hope

3Rs Have you ever "held your tongue" about something. Why didn't you speak up? Was that a good choice for you? For others?

KISS 1. What awards are given annually in the U.S. for outstanding achievement in theater?

2. True or false? Lightening can reach temperatures hotter than the surface of the sun.

3. What is the capital city of Greece?

SOS Why is a rainy day difficult for a mother kangaroo?

ICE Compare super glue and a stone wall.

TAB High blood pressure, radiation, microwaves, infections and head injury may interfere with the functioning of the blood brain barrier, and allow harmful substances into the brain that would otherwise be filtered out.[184]

Mmm Heart Health Meditation – This meditation is intended to help with blood pressure and heart health. It is included here because of the strong correlation between heart health and brain health. Close your eyes and bring your attention to your breath. Allow your breath to grow slower and deeper. As your breath changes, feel your heartbeat ease and slow down as well. It is as if time itself is in slow-motion. Now bring your attention to your hands and feet. Feel them getting warmer and warmer. You can play with images of heat to help, such as resting in front of a fire, holding a warm mug of your favorite hot drink, or whatever metaphor or image works for you. Successfully increasing the warmth of your hands and feet is correlated with dilating the blood vessels and enhancing the flow of blood through the body.[185]

---

184 http://faculty.washington.edu/chudler/neurok.html

185 Achterberg, Jeanne, Barbara Dossy and Leslie Kokmeir. (1994) *Ritual and Healing: Using Imagery for Health and Wellness.* New York: Bantam.

— SET 310 —

WOW Think left, think right, think low and think high. Oh the thinks you can think up if you only try. – Dr. Seuss

3Rs Who was your favorite teacher? Why? Who was your least favorite teacher? Why? From which teacher did you learn the most? Why?

KISS 1. "Is" and "are" are third person verbs. Which is plural and which is singular?

2. If three pieces of candy are worth two packages of gum, how many packages of gum are 24 pieces of candy worth?

3. What political party in the 19th Century was successfully led by Zachery Taylor? Hint it sounds like a hairpiece.

SOS Start with the word "Tears" and change one letter at a time to get to the word "Smile", making real words at each step. Tears ________________ _____Smile.

ICE List things that have attachments.

TAB Learned material can sometimes be moved to long-term memory more quickly using the material to create new lyrics for a familiar tune, such as "Mary Had a Little Lamb."

Mmm Rhythm Work: Verse and Chorus – Think of a song you know that has at least two verses and a chorus. Instead of singing the song, you will clap and snap out its rhythms. Clap for the verses, and snap for the chorus.

— SET 311 —

WOW A person who follows the crowd will never be followed by a crowd. – R. S. Donnell

3Rs What is something that you have surprisingly never done before? What has prevented you? Do you have any regrets about it?

KISS 1. Who is a "southpaw"?

2. What is the approximate distance in miles from the Earth to the Sun?

3. Guttenberg used movable type for the first time in history. What was the first book he printed?

SOS If you add a certain number to 3, the result is more than that number multiplied times 3. What is that number?

ICE What are things that should be discarded quickly?

TAB Neuro-scientists call a region in the far front of the brain the "rostro-caudal" or "rostral-caudal axis" of the frontal cortex. This area is responsible for higher levels of abstraction such as advanced reasoning, complex problem solving, application, analysis, assessment, evaluation, synthesis, imagination, logic, creativity, and mental flexibility.

Mmm Spool of Thread Meditation – This meditation can be helpful when your thoughts are scattered. Visualize your thoughts floating all around you as a blur of unwound thread. Now imagine that there is a spool inside your skull, and in your own time, begin to wrap the thread around the spool. As the thread winds around the spool, sense your mind becoming more and more focused and concentrated.

— SET 312 —

WOW A little nonsense, now and then, is relished by the wisest men. – Roald Dahl

3Rs What was/is your most common expression or saying?

KISS 1. The name of Tennessee Williams' Pulitzer-Prize winning play is "*A Streetcar Named*" what?

2. What is the scientific name for the windpipe?

3. What is the official language of Brazil?

SOS Decipher each of the following: you between me; noon good, japmadean. (Example: irighti = right between the eyes.)

ICE What would you find at the end of the rainbow?

TAB Your brain is especially good at remembering something that is silly or unusual. Therefore, it will help you remember things if you can somehow link each thing to something that is silly or unusual, e.g., , if a toothbrush is an item on your shopping list, picturing yourself brushing your hair with a toothbrush will help you remember.

Mmm Tongue "Workout" – See how many different ways you can move your tongue. Try to touch your tongue to your nose. To your chin. Can you curl your tongue? Fold it? What else can you come up with?

— SET 313 —

WOW Some cause happiness wherever they go; others whenever they go. – Oscar Wilde

3Rs Who was your first love? What was that person like? How old were you and what was the other person's name? What do you most remember about that person?

KISS 1. What do the following sequence abbreviations mean: nd; rd; st?
2. What plant's pistil forms a yellow mane like that of the animal in its name?
3. What massive timepiece helps keep time in London?

SOS Two children have cookies. Sue says, "If you give me one of your cookies, we have exactly the same number." Roger says, "If you give me one of your cookies, I will have twice as many cookies as you." How many cookies do Sue and Roger have?

ICE Design or think of new ways to store extra coat hangers.

TAB When we experience a sudden insight or flash of creative inspiration, there is a simultaneous synchronization of the two hemispheres of the brain.

Mmm Lightening Pose – This is a balance pose that strengthens the legs and core of the body. The first time you try this pose, it is advised that you have a stable chair behind you in case you lose your balance or need to rest until you build up strength. Start with feet close together, and be sure to keep the knees directly over the ankles throughout. Reach the arms up over your head in line with your torso. On an exhale, bend the knees, and keeping the back straight, lean forward as you push the buttock back and down. Your body now forms a zigzag bolt of lightning.

—— SET 314 ——

WOW Unless you try to do something beyond what you already mastered, you will never grow. – Ralph Waldo Emerson

3Rs What would other people be surprised to find out that you enjoy?

KISS 1. How can people without a common language communicate?
2. What was the name of the first cloned sheep?
3. Reykjavik is the capital of which country?

SOS What has hands but cannot clap?

ICE List as many uses of duct tape as you can.

TAB Research indicates that placing appropriate cues at the table can influence the brain concerning what, how much, and when to eat. For example, using red dessert plates can signal "stop" to the brain, and using smaller plates and tall narrow glasses rather than short wide glasses leads to people eating and drinking less while enjoying it more.

Mmm Mindful Tracking: Food Consumption – For today consciously track what you eat. Be specific. For example, "one cup of beef barley soup" rather than "soup." You can write it down or make a mental note and tally up at the end of the day. Any surprises?

— SET 315 —

WOW The person who does things that count doesn't usually stop to count them. – Anonymous

3Rs What is the most beautiful thing in the room you're in right now? What do you appreciate about it? What does that say about you?

KISS 1. List as many types (genre) of music as you can.

2. If you had chatterbox friends on the moon, why wouldn't you have to shush them?

3. Which word means a succession of rulers from the same family?

SOS Find a one word answer to the following so that the last two letters of each answer are also the first two letters of the next answer. Storage space above the house: A frozen drip: A citrus drink: Measurement of temperature: Spooky.

ICE Figure out some ways to make people more comfortable in seats on an airplane.

TAB A recent NPR report on a study in *Pediatrics* indicates thinking skills are better in elementary-aged children who engage in 70 minutes or more of active play (running around and playing on the playground) each day, compared to children who don't.[186]

Mmm Marionette – Imagine that you are a marionette and have strings tied to your knees, ankles, wrists, elbows, and the top of your head. Move as if you are being controlled by a puppeteer. How do you move, walk, sit, eat, and dance as a puppet?

— SET 316 —

WOW People in life who are the happiest don't have the best of everything; they make the best of everything they have. – Anonymous

3Rs Who was your first sweetheart? What was the attraction? Did you date? Was it a lasting relationship? Why or why not? As you think about such relationships, how did they contribute to your being the person you are today? If they did not make such a contribution to your life, why not?

---

186 http://www.npr.org/sections/health-shots/2014/09/29/352455278/more-active-play-equals-better-thinking-skills-for-kids

KISS 1. Which of the following words is a noun: require, requirement, or requiring?
2. Does the human body have more bones or more muscles?
3. Who flew the plane Spirit of St Louis?

SOS If five people can do five projects in five days, how many people that are equally capable and work equally hard can accomplish fifty projects in fifty days.

ICE What things are fragile?

TAB Perceptual filtering refers to the ability to forget what one doesn't need to remember. Purposeful forgetting is necessary to keep the brain from getting too cluttered with unimportant minutia that can interfere with purposeful remembering.

Mmm Doorframe Workout – Stand in the center of a stable doorframe. Put your hand out to the side on the door frame. Press you hand out against the doorframe and hold for a count of ten. Release. Then reach around behind you and grasp hold the door frame. Keeping your body straight, lean carefully forward to feel a gentle stretch along the back of the legs. Come back to center. Grab your hands around the opposite side of the door frame and lean back carefully to feel the stretch there.[187]

— SET 317 —

WOW Curiosity about life in all its aspects, I think, is still the secret of great creative people. – Leo Burnett

3Rs What do you spend too much of your "spare" time doing? Why is it a bad thing? What could you do to eliminate or reduce the time it takes?

KISS 1. What are aglets?
2. The Mojave prickly pear is a member of what plant family?
3. Which of the following is the shortest: Eiffel Tower, St. Louis Arch, or the Washington Monument?

SOS Jessie, Mackenzie, and Cloe are sisters. Cloe is three times older than Mackenzie, and in two years she will be twice the age of Jessie. Jessie is a year older than Mackenzie. What are the ages of the three sisters?

ICE The Hill's reverse Mother's and Father's Day. Explain why.

187 Rosas, Debbie and Carlos Rosas. (2004). The Nia Technique. New York: Broadway Books.

TAB In a 2014 *All Things Considered* radio program, neurobiologist Nina Kraus of Northwestern University describes how the brainwave "physically resembles the sound wave."[188]

Mmm Listening Meditation: Sounds in Your Environment – Settle into a comfortable relaxed position and close your eyes. Bring your attention to your breath for a few moments to quiet your mind. Then listen to whatever sounds surround you. Listen with curiosity and no judgment. What do you hear? Spend a few moments just listening to the orchestra of the present moment.

— SET 318 —

WOW Thinking is the hardest work there is, which is probably why so few engage in it. – Henry Ford

3Rs What is the best thing about getting older? What do you miss from when you were younger?

KISS 1. True or false? The barbershop quartet originated in barbershops.
2. What are the three physical states of matter?
3. Who was Amelia Earhart?

SOS The first letters of each word in the following descriptions are the same as the initials of the person being described. Name the famous person for each of the following: 1) Tinkerer Around Electricity; 2) Baseball Right-fielder; 3) Blonde Wit.

ICE What are some things you can shake?

TAB Even though the brain's weight is only three percent or less of your total body weight, it consumes 25% of all the oxygen you breath in, 25% of your blood glucose, 20% of the oxygenated blood that your heart pumps, and 20% of your body's total energy.[189]

Mmm Brain Breath Meditation: Briefly bring your attention to your breath for 2-3 breath cycles. Then for the next in-breath, close your mouth and breathe in sharply through the nose as if the breath were going directly to your brain in the center of your skull. On the out breath, open your mouth and breathe out through the mouth. Repeat for 10-12 breath cycles.

---

188 http://www.npr.org/blogs/ed/2014/09/10/343681493/this-is-your-brain-this-is-your-brain-on-music

189 http://www.scientificamerican.com/article/thinking-hard-calories/

— SET 319 —

WOW Opportunity is missed by most because it is dressed in overalls and looks like work. – Thomas Edison

3Rs What were some of your favorite clothes when you were young? What did you like about them? Were you more concerned with fashion or comfort then? How would you describe your current style of dressing? What does that say about you now? How do you choose the clothes you wear each day?

KISS 1. What are the adverbs in the following sentence: "The horse jumped extremely high."

2. A man bought a used car for $600, sold it for $800, bought it back for $1,000, and resold it for $1,200. Did the man make any profit?

3. Which two continents do not touch the Atlantic Ocean?

SOS What do all of the following have in common: Deck of cards, Jewelry store, Yankee Stadium?

ICE Create a sentence using the letters "L" "L" "I" "R" "F" at the beginning of each word.

TAB As noted previously, on average, people can only remember about seven (give or take two) pieces of information at a time. However, the size of the "piece" can be larger or smaller. Therefore chunking information into larger "pieces" enables you to remember more information at once. For example, you can remember the numbers 1 - 9 - 4 - 2 as one piece of information if you think of it as the year 1942.[190]

Mmm The Wind Moves the Lotus Leaf – Stand in a shoulder-width stance with your hands on your hips so that the fingertips are to the back. Close the mouth and touch the tip of the tongue to the roof of your mouth as if you were about to say the letter "t." As you slowly inhale, move the hands up and down, pressing and massaging the lower back and buttocks. Then on the exhale, make one clockwise circle with your hips. Repeat 4-6 times, alternating circling the hips clockwise and counterclockwise.

— SET 320 —

WOW You miss 100% of the shots you never take. – Wayne Gretsky

3Rs What is the angriest you have ever been? What happened that upset you, and how did you respond?

---

190 http://elearningindustry.com/3-chunking-strategies-that-every-instructional-designer-should-know

KISS 1. What does the Latin phrase *carpe diem* mean?
2. What eight-sided geometrical shape is often found on American street corners?
3. Read the following phrase: APEN NYSA VEDISAP EN NYE ARNED. Who said this?

SOS Joy was taking a bath at a friend's house. As she closed the big old wooden door it latched shut and could not be opened, but she decided to take her bath anyway. When the tub was full she went to shut the water off and found the faucet was broken, and the water could not be turned off. What should she do?

ICE Gloves are easily lost. What uses can you think of for a single glove?

TAB Unlike other parts of the body, if you add dye to a person's blood, it will not penetrate the brain. This is because the brain is protected by a semi-permeable "blood brain barrier" which filters out large and/or highly charged molecules.[191]

Mmm Force Field Meditation – Imagine that you have the ability to put up an invisible, protective force field around yourself. The force field will surround you like a semi-permeable bubble filtering out whatever you perceive as harmful while allowing in what is beneficial. Visualize your force field surrounding you and moving with you. Play with making it larger and smaller until it feels just right. See the way that negative thoughts, words and actions bounce right off of the force field.

— SET 321 —

WOW The highest reward for a person's toil is not what they get for it, but what they become by it. – John Ruskin

3Rs How do you like to celebrate your accomplishments? Describe a specific accomplishment you are particularly proud of and the way you celebrated it.

KISS 1. Which of the following composers was born first: Bach, Beethoven or Brahms?
2. Is the rhinoceros a carnivore or a herbivore?
3. In which building in England are the crown jewels on display?

SOS Each of following clues point to words with "bell": Peter Pan's fairy; Widely-flared pants; weightlifters' apparatus. What are those words?

ICE Three rooms of the house are full of old tables. Explain.

191 http://faculty.washington.edu/chudler/neurok.html

TAB Your brain's memory storage capacity is currently estimated to be about 2.5 petabytes (a million gigabytes). If your brain worked like a digital video recorder (it doesn't), 2.5 petabytes would be enough storage to hold three million hours of TV shows.[192]

Mmm Balancing an Object on the Hand – Find a small object with a flat narrow edge that can be safely dropped, such as a ruler, marker or small book. Now stand the object on the palm of your hand and try to balance it for as long as you can. The trick is to keep your eye on the top of the object. As it starts to tilt, gently move the hand in the direction it seems to want to fall.

— SET 322 —

WOW You never realize what a good memory you have until you try to forget something. – Franklin P. Jones

3Rs Which environmental problems today are the most important to you? What choices have you made that help the environment?

KISS 1. What is the correct spelling of the word pronounced "straight" when it means a narrow channel of water?
2. What is the difference between magma and lava?
3. What Scandinavian capital starts and ends with a vowel?

SOS What has a heart but is neither animal or human?

ICE List things that use batteries.

TAB A recent study used brain scans to monitor professional jazz musicians when they were playing a piece from memory "as written" and when they improvised based on the same piece. The findings indicate that areas associated consciously with monitoring, evaluating, and correcting behaviors were less active when improvising.[193]

Mmm Jazz Square Right Foot Leads – Stand with feet about hip-width apart. Lift the right foot and cross it over to step in front of the left foot (almost like you were going to step on your own toe). Pick up the left foot and step it directly back behind where it was. Now step the right foot out wide and to the right in line with the left foot. Bring the left foot alongside the right back to where you started. Repeat 8-10 times.

---

192 http://www.scientificamerican.com/article/what-is-the-mempry -capacity/

193 http://www.ncbi.nlm.nih.gov/pmc/articles/PMC2244806/

— SET 323 —

WOW You are never too old to set another goal or to dream a new dream. – C. S. Lewis

3Rs If you could travel to any time and place in history, when and where would you choose? Why?

KISS 1. What does the Latin phrase *e pluribus unum* mean? Hint: This phrase is on the Seal of the United States

2. Put a + or a - between each of these pairs of numbers to equal 88: 87 65 43 21.

3. What is the significance of Mecca?

SOS When will you first encounter a number word that contains both an "a" and "v" when you write the number word, not counting "and"?

ICE What qualities and actions would qualify a person for the world's worst waiter? Go wild with this one.

TAB Vitamin B1 (thiamin) shortage can lead to brain shrinkage and severe memory loss of recent events. B1 is available through eating beans, peas, grains, etc.

Mmm Jazz Square Left Foot Leads– Stand with feet about hip-width apart. Lift the left foot and cross it over to step in front of the right foot (almost like you were going to step on your own toe). Pick up the right foot and step it directly back behind where it was. Now step the left foot out wide and to the left in line with the right foot. Bring the right foot alongside the left back to where you started. Repeat 8-10 times.

— SET 324 —

WOW To acquire knowledge, one must study; but to acquire wisdom, one must observe. – Marilyn vos Savant

3Rs If you had the chance to talk to the person you were ten years ago, what would you talk about? What would you want that person to know?

KISS 1. How many "positions" are there for the arms and feet in ballet?

2. Human tongues can distinguish between four different types of tastes. What are they?

3. True or false? Baja California is part of the U.S.

SOS Which number is next in this series: 10, 4, 3, 11, 15, __?

ICE What are four reasons you might be turning the pages of a book 20 pages at a time?

TAB A speaker can assist the brains of the audience by moving around, using gestures in a natural manner related to the message, inserting relevant humor as appropriate, pausing now and then for relevant asides, modulating voice inflection, varying the pace, and keeping it brief.

Mmm Meditation: Invoking a Desired Quality – For this meditation, choose a valuable quality that you would like to embody more in your life, such as love, beauty, healing, or wisdom. Then, close your eyes and bring your awareness to your breath. As you inhale say or think "I am . . ." Then on the exhale say or think the quality you desire to increase. Repeat for at least 10 breath cycles.

—— SET 325 ——

WOW Know that you yourself are a miracle. – Norman Vincent Peale

3Rs Describe your first conscious memory. How old do you think you were? What sense (sight, sound, touch, etc.) is strongest in that memory?

KISS 1. Where does the apostrophe go in the following sentence: The chicken will sit on its egg?
2. True or false? Tortoises and turtles do not have teeth.
3. What does the word "suffrage" mean?

SOS What word can precede all of the following: sick, weed, and side?

ICE List things that people hide.

TAB Some scientists have calculated that the probability a person might forget his or her own name is about the same as that of getting hit by an asteroid: It could happen, but it's not very likely.[194]

Mmm Anchoring to the Self – Sit in a position of comfort with your back upright. As you are ready, think of a time and place that you felt free and safe to be fully yourself. Imagine yourself in that time and place and recall how you felt. Now say your name aloud and notice where the name resonates in your body. With a touch or gesture physically connect to that place in your body. Say your name again while you repeat the touch or gesture several times.

—— SET 326 ——

WOW Be kind; everyone you meet is fighting a hard battle. – John Watson

3Rs What quality of yours is most challenging for your friends and loved ones? Describe a time that quality affected one of your relationships.

---

194 http://www.supermemo.com/articles/myths.htm

KISS 1. What does the French phrase *Joie de Vivre* mean? Hint: Think happy!
2. Which real element discovered in 1898 is a threat for the fictional Superman?
3. Jerusalem is a holy city for which three major religions?

SOS Make as many words as you can create using the letters of your full name.

ICE Bradyn keeps fifty earthworms on his bedside table. Why?

TAB One theory for why we yawn is that yawning may cool the brain. Breathing through the nose is also believed to cool the brain.[195]

Mmm Yawning – Yawning is a great way to relax the body. Do several rounds of yawning. Use the whole body, stretch and open wide as if you just woke up. Or maybe you just escaped from a really boring lecture or conversation.

—— SET 327 ——

WOW Idleness is to the human mind like rust to iron. – Ezra Cornell

3Rs If you were an animal, what animal would you be? Why?

KISS 1. List three songs that each has an animal in its title.
2. What makes a black hole appear black?
3. Helsinki is the capital of what Scandinavian country?

SOS Take a luminous object, and add a letter of the alphabet (on the front or back) to get some joy. Example: A rubber wheel (tire) plus the letter N = All (N-Tire = Entire).

ICE Thinking creatively, what do the letters "BO" stand for?

TAB The healthy brain is active even when we are asleep. In fact, the brain patterns of a person at sleep are quite complex compared to a person in a coma. The brain activity of a comatose state is so slow that it can hardly be detected at all.

Mmm Hand Washing Meditation – The next time you wash your hands, bring as much mindfulness attention as you can to the experience. Fully sense the water as you start to run it. Sense the sensation of the water on your skin. Etc.

—— SET 328 ——

WOW I find the great thing in this world is not so much where we stand, as in what direction we are moving. – Oliver Wendell Holmes

3Rs When you were being "potty trained" as a child, what words were used?

---

195 http://faculty.washington.edu/chudler/yawning.html

KISS 1. What does the word "splay" mean?
2. Are most people more comfortable when the relative humidity is above 50% or below 50%?
3. From the 12th to the 19th century, what name was given to the Japanese warrior class?

SOS Using people's first names, fill-in the blanks to create the given meaning. 1) Let the water out: ______ the tub. 2) Cover the whole floor: Lay ______-wall carpeting. 3) Feed us until we aren't hungry: ______ up.

ICE In an imaginary kingdom, they have a very serious paper shortage. How many creative ways can you think of for conserving paper?

TAB John O'Keefe, May-Brit Moser and Edvard I Moser were awarded the 2014 Nobel Prize in Physiology or Medicine for their identifying the cells that function as a "GPS system" within the brain, allowing us to orient ourselves in space.

Mmm Compass: Marching Orders – Start facing north (real or imagined) and take the following marching orders: March north two steps; Turn south and march three steps; Turn southeast and march two steps; Turn west and march four steps; Turn northeast and march three steps. Repeat. Where are you?

— SET 329 —

WOW Organized people are just too lazy to look for things. – Anonymous

3Rs If you were a food, what food would you be? Why?

KISS 1. What does the German word *Wunderkind* mean? Hint: You'll be amazed.
2. What arachnid is given its name because it kills its mate?
3. What country has a flag like the Red Cross, but the colors are switched?

SOS There are two nine-letter words and one eight-letter word that start with the letters "TE" and end with the letters "TE" What are they?

ICE You are a toothbrush designer and want to create a unique toothbrush; what will be unique about it?

TAB A 2015 analysis of 32 studies of the effect of negative stereotypes about aging on the memory performance of older people, conducted by British researchers, found that exposure to such stereotypes caused older people to perform 20% worse on memory tests than older people who were not exposed to such negative stereotypes.[196]

196 https://www.ncbi.nlm.nih.gov/pmc/articles/PMC4360754/.

Mmm Compass: Marching Orders All Facing North –For this exercise stay facing the same direction throughout and take the following marching orders by stepping on an angle, sideways or backwards as necessary: East two steps; Southwest one step; Northeast two steps; West four steps; Southeast two steps; About-face to the south and repeat the marching orders.

— SET 330 —

WOW Praise can be your most valuable asset as long as you don't aim it at yourself. – O. A. Battista

3Rs If you were writing a book about yourself, what would the title of the book be? Why would you choose that title?

KISS 1. Name some famous choirs.

2. A fast-food restaurant had a ton of hamburger patties in stock, each weighing exactly one-quarter pound. How many hamburger patties does it have in stock?

3. What prime minister led Great Britain to victory in World War II, but lost the election at the end of the war?

SOS Find a one-word answer to the following so that the last two letters of each answer are also the first two letters of the next answer. Baghdad is its capital: Zodiac sign in February: Person who shows you to your seat: Mistake: Musical group that plays symphonies: Speeder's bane.

ICE Design a new wrapper for a candy bar.

TAB We remember better when we apply all five of our body senses—sight, smell, sound, taste, and touch—to imagine what we want to remember.

Mmm New Surroundings – Go for a walk in a new neighborhood or part of town. Use all of your senses. Look around you. Touch things. Notice sounds and how things smell. Notice how different or similar it feels.

— SET 331 —

WOW Age is something that doesn't matter, unless you are a cheese. – Billie Burke

3Rs What advice would you give to your fifteen-year-old self? Would that younger self take your advice?

KISS 1. Turn the noun "athlete" into an adjective.

2. What should you do first when helping someone who has been struck by lightning?

3. In what religion is the River Ganges considered sacred?

SOS A man had three children. For their allowance, he gave the first child $1 more than half of what he had in his pocket. The second child he gave $2 more than half what he had left in his pocket. The third child got $3 more than half of what was left. In the end, the man was left with $1. How much did the man start with? Hint: Work backwards.

ICE List seven common things kept in most wallets.

TAB After 30 years of age, the brain begins to lose a quarter of one percent of its mass each year, but the latest research is clear that cognitive decline with age is not inevitable. The hippocampus creates new neurons and continually fine-tunes neural connections up to the very end of life if one is healthy.[197]

Mmm Compassion Meditation: Elder Self –Close your eyes. Place your hands on your heart.. Invite an image of yourself in later years or at some point in the future. See your future self in front of you. Notice how your future self appears. How might age affect your body and emotions in the future? Smile to your older self. In your mind give that older self a hug, and send gentle, loving compassion to yourself in older age.

— SET 332 —

WOW Fulfillment is reaching your own expectations, not the expectations of others. – Walt Disney

3Rs Describe your most gratifying moment. What made it so special?

KISS 1. What does the Yiddish phrase *Mozel Tov* mean?

2. In the winter, is the water that gushes out of a geyser hot or cold?

3. Which two states share a border along the continental divide?

SOS Stan went to the rodeo. In the opening show there were only horses and rodeo clowns. Stan counted 34 legs and 22 eyes in the show. If none of the performers were injured, how many horses and how many clowns performed?

ICE Make up a really creative bumper sticker.

TAB While some research studies suggest that a glass of wine now and then is good for the brain, a 2012 study at Rutgers University indicates that even a glass or two of wine every day may kill too many brain cells; yes, alcohol does kill brain cells.[198]

---

197 http://www.ncbi.nlm.nih.gov/pmc/articles/PMC2596698/

198 http://www.personal.psu.edu/afr3/blogs/siowfa12/2012/10/is-a-glass-of-wine-per-day-good-for-you.html

Mmm Healing Ball – Imagine that there is a ball on the ground in front of you. Pick up the ball in both hands. Imagine that the ball contains healing power. Pat the ball, and play with it, making it larger and smaller until it feels just right. With both hands, take the ball all around your body. Touch the healing ball to your joints and anywhere you think your body needs healing. Don't forget to include your head and brain!

— SET 333 —

WOW Write in your heart that every day is the best day of the year. – Ralph Waldo Emerson

3Rs What occupation would you most hate to be in? Why?

KISS 1. In the song what did Yankee Doodle put in his hat and what did he call it?

2. Can magnets be made of steel or nickel?

3. What citizen endowed the most libraries in the U.S.?

SOS Using people's first names, fill-in the blanks to create the given meanings. 1) Get up from your seat: ______ up! 2) I genuinely care for that woman: _____ truly! 3) A woman's relationship to her brother's daughter: I am the aunt, and she is ______.

ICE Use the word "circle" as compound words or phrases. Example: Circle of Life.

TAB The latest national "Aging Survey " conducted by the National Council on Aging found preserving memory is the most important aging concern of 35% of older Americans.[199]

Mmm Ears – Imagine that your ears can change shape. Feel the ear growing tall and pointy. (If you are a *Star Trek* fan you can imagine you are a Vulcan.) Then let them grow even more into bunny or donkey ears. Feel the ears grow flat and wide like an elephant. Feel them grow long and floppy like a basset hound. Play with how you move your head and body with each new set of ears. Animal sounds are optional. ☺

— SET 334 —

WOW With time and patience the mulberry leaf becomes a silk gown. – Chinese Proverb

---

199 https://www.senioradvice.com/articles/what-matters-most-for-seniors-survey-results.

3Rs When you look back at pictures of yourself, what age are you most embarrassed about? What was your style at that time?

KISS 1. Name three words that have a silent "w".

2. What is the decimal for three hundredths?

3. What is the largest city in the world situated more than a mile above sea level?

SOS Fill in the blanks to create hyphenated words. 1) ______- thee-______ 2) ______ -o-______ 3) ______-me-______

ICE What if all roads were one-way?

TAB Celiac Disease can produce symptoms of memory loss and other neurological problems similar to Alzheimer's. Celiac disease is an allergy or intolerance for gluten found in certain grains like wheat.[200]

Mmm Victorious Breath – This breath technique is created by closing off the opening between the vocal cords and drawing the breath along the back of the throat, just like when you whisper. Before you begin, practice that sensation by speaking aloud first and then changing to a whisper. Notice what you do in the throat to create the whisper. For this exercise you will be breathing in and out through the nose with the throat closed like for a whisper. It will make a humming sort of hissing sound sometimes compared to the ocean and sometimes compared to Darth Vader. Gently constrict the throat as you practiced with the whisper. Gently and slowly inhale into the heart drawing the breath along the back of the throat and listening for that special sound. Then slowly and gently exhale. The sound will be slightly louder on the exhale than the inhale.

— SET 335 —

WOW Our greatest glory is not in never falling, but in rising every time we fall. – Confucius

3Rs Have you ever been involved in or seen a car accident? What was the situation? Did you learn anything from the experience?

KISS 1. What does the Yiddish word *Zaftig* mean?

2. Which planet in our solar system has the most moons?

3. Which branch of the U.S. government contains the Supreme Court?

---

200 Carper, Jean. *100 Simple Things You Can Do to Prevent Alzheimer's and Age-related Memory Loss.* NY: Little Brown, 2010. p. 61.

SOS Peter has a dangerous disease. The family decides Peter should have an operation, and they schedule one without telling him. The family takes Peter to a doctor who has never operated on a human before. When Peter resists going into the clinic, the family do not try to reason with him, they just use a restraint to force him to go in and get his surgery. Why did they not tell Peter, and who operates on him?

ICE Which is happier, a comma or a question mark? Why?

TAB Neurons have "limbs" that extend out from the cell body. The axon is the "limb" that takes information out from the cell body often to other neurons. Dendrites are branching "limbs" that carry information to the cell body.

Mmm Eagle Pose Hands – Bend the elbows and hold your arms in front of you with your hands pointing up. Lift one arm and place that elbow into the crook of the other elbow, so the arms form a "V." To whatever extent you can, reach the arms in towards one another (without dislodging the elbow lock). If possible, wrap the hand and wrist of the lower arm around the forearm of the top arm. Hold for 20-30 seconds. Then release and do the same on the other side.

— SET 336 —

WOW Toleration is the greatest gift of the mind; it requires the same effort of the brain that it takes to balance oneself on a bicycle. --Helen Keller

3Rs If you were a dog, what breed of dog would you be? Why?

KISS 1. For what kind of music is John Phillip Sousa known?

2. Why do people in the hot Arabian Peninsula prefer white horses to black horses? There is a scientifically valid reason.

3. What is the color of a U.S. Military General's stars?

SOS The first letters of each word in the following descriptions are the same as the initials of the person being described. Name the famous person for each of the following: 1) Brilliant Singer; 2) Writes Sonnets; 3) Iconic Broadway man.

ICE List petty annoyances that people experience.

TAB According to a new international study led by the Research Institute of the McGill University Health Centre, it may be possible to change the amount of information that the brain can store. The study identified a protein molecule that puts a brake on brain processing. When this protein is removed, brain function and memory recall improve.

Mmm The Opera Singer – Sit or stand with your back upright. Bring your hands in front of your heart and make two fists—one thumb up and one thumb down. Open the fists just enough for each hand to hook its fingers around the fingers of the other hand. Your fingers will wrap around each other inside of the joined fists. Let your thumbs rest on the top and bottom of the fists. Pull your elbows away from each other, creating tension in the hands without losing their interlocking grip. Hold for a few breaths. Then repeat with the opposite hand in front. Feel free to sing an aria if you like.

— SET 337 —

WOW You have to count on living every single day in a way you believe will make you feel good about your life—so that if it were over tomorrow, you'd be content with yourself. – Jane Seymour

3Rs Remember and think about your first ride on a carousel or other carnival ride.

KISS 1. What does "presumptuous" mean?
2. Name the type of bird whose "bill" can hold more than its belly can?
3. Four states share a border with Mexico. Name two.

SOS What do these have in common: A laptop computer, a flip phone, a weak poker hand?

ICE Your ship is sinking. What will you do?

TAB According to research by Gary Arendash of the University of South Florida, caffeine reduces amyloid, a substance that causes dementia in animal studies.[201]

Mmm Flying – Imagine that you are a bird and fly around the room. What type of bird are you and how do you fly? Does your bird soar, flap, flutter, zip? Try out different birds and different flight patterns.

— SET 338 —

WOW People are like stained glass windows; they sparkle and shine when the sun is out, but when the darkness sets in, their true beauty is revealed only if there is a light within. – Elizabeth Kubler Ross

3Rs What was your favorite comic book character as a child? What do you remember most about that character?

---

201 http://www.ncbi.nlm.nih.gov/pmc/articles/PMC3746074/

KISS 1. What does the Hebrew word *Shalom* mean?

2. If you were paid $6.00 per hour for the six seconds you took to close the door, how much pay would you receive for those six seconds?

3. Who is famous for saying "I will return"?

SOS Find a one word answer to the following so that the last two letters of each answer are also the first two letters of the next answer. Male or female: A test: Entertain with humor: Tranquil: Sewing implement: Rise off the ground.

ICE What are some ways to use a fireplace?

TAB Psychological research indicates that reflection on past experiences involves both the amygdala (involved in emotional reactions) and the hippocampus (involved in memory and learning).

Mmm Meditation: Guidance from Future Self – Close your eyes and bring your attention to your breath. After a few breaths, invite an image of yourself from some point in the future (at least five years older than you are now). Visualize this older self as if he or she were a separate person sitting in front of you right now. Notice how your future self appears in terms of dress, age, posture, etc. Look your future self in the eye and smile. Carry on a conversation with your future self in your mind for a while. Ask your future self what you could do now to improve the life of your future self. Imagine the response of your future self to that question.

— SET 339 —

WOW To know what you know and what you do not know, that is true knowledge. – Confucius

3Rs What would you like your "famous last words" to be?

KISS 1. In art, what does "perspective" mean?

2. What are some tips to stay safe during an earthquake?

3. What is the standard monetary currency in Mexico?

SOS Their are fore errers in this puzzle. Can you find all four of them?

ICE What if mosquitoes could talk? What would they say?

TAB Speed matters in retaining information. It is easier to remember a list of single syllable words than multiple syllable words.

Mmm Drink from the Back – This is a silly and challenging exercise sometimes used as a supposed hiccup remedy. Get a small glass of water. Rather than drinking out of the side closest to you. Try to drink out of the backside of the cup. Hint: you will have to tip your head over and support the cup on the upper lip rather than the lower one.

— SET 340 —

WOW A hunch is creativity trying to tell you something. – Frank Capra

3Rs Based on your past experiences, which person in the world (live or dead) do you think deserves most to be on the cover of a magazine? Why? Which magazine would you choose for that person to be on the cover?

KISS 1. Change the adjective "beautiful" into a verb.

2. Are bald eagles really bald?

3. What 1964 Republican presidential candidate had bumper stickers with "AUH2O"?

SOS If you counted all the days of the year starting with January 1 (not a leap year), Vicki's birthday would be between the 300th and 340th day. The sum of the digits of that number equals 9, and the number is divisible by 5. When is Vicki's birthday?

ICE Make a long and sensible sentence using only words beginning with the letter "S."

TAB A 2016 UCLA study suggests it is possible to boost your self-confidence by directly training the brain.[202]

Mmm Word Meditation: Chosen Word – For this meditation, choose a word that has meaning for you. It can be a word from your spiritual tradition, a name, a place, etc. Close your eyes. Bring your awareness to your breath. As you feel ready repeat the word you have chosen aloud or silently in your head for one to five minutes.

— SET 341 —

WOW Learn from the mistakes made by others. You won't live long enough to make them all yourself. – Eleanor Roosevelt

3Rs What is one thing you know more about than most any other person? What do you know the least about?

KISS 1. What does the Japanese word *Sayonara* mean?

2. Which is more than six pints, three quarts or one gallon?

3. What do the following have in common: Atlantis, Babylon, Pompeii, and Sodom?

---

202 https://www.sciencedaily.com/releases/2017/01/170103222701.htm

SOS John, Annette, Sherri, and Joel were all born in the same year. John is the oldest and Sherri is the youngest. When you write out the dates of their birthdays numerically, all of the digits 0-9 are used without repeating any digit. All of the digits in Sherri's birthday are prime numbers. One person's birthday has twice as many digits as the others, but when you add those digits together the total is less than adding the digits for any other birthday. The digits of Annette's birthday add up to John's birthday, and so do the digits of Sherri's birthday. All of the digits of Joel's birthday are divisible by 3. When is each of their birthdays?

ICE You are a sign maker and a new ordinance prohibits the use of the word "stop" on the stop sign. What words might you use instead of "stop".

TAB The myelin sheath is an insulating layer that usually surrounds the axon of a neuron and helps keep it functioning well. Without it, neurons lose their ability to fire and eventually die.

Mmm Mindful Cooking Meditation: Loving Effort – As you make one of your meals today, bring as much mindfulness as you can to filling the food you make with loving and nourishing intention. When you touch any food item, contemplate the kinds of nourishment it will provide for your body and the bodies of any others with whom you may share your meal. See the way that your efforts provide nourishment for body and brain. As you interact with the food imagine that each of your actions, from chopping to stirring, to pouring to serving, infuses the meal you are creating with love for yourself and others.

— SET 342 —

WOW The best way to get the last word is to apologize. – Anonymous

3Rs What good deed(s) do you usually do on a daily basis? What characterizes this behavior as a good deed? What motivates you to do it?

KISS 1. Name some shades of the following colors: Blue; Red; Yellow; and Green.

2. What is the "roar" we hear when we place a seashell next to our ear? It is *not* really the ocean.

3. What country are you probably in, if you are making purchases using rubles?

SOS In the following, take away the scrambled letters of a fast thing to find a slow thing with the remaining letters in the correct order: TBAUIRRTLTEB.

ICE You are king or queen of a very special imaginary kingdom. What interesting rules would you have in your kingdom?

TAB According to a study at Albert Einstein College of Medicine, 76% of seniors who danced regularly demonstrated less dementia compared with seniors who only read or did crosswords. [203]

Mmm Foxtrot Rhythm – The basic rhythm of the foxtrot is: *Slow, Slow. Quick-Quick. Slow.* Put on some music or make your own. Dance around the room doing the foxtrot rhythm with an imaginary dance partner.

—— SET 343 ——

WOW An effort made for the happiness of others lifts us above ourselves. – L. M. Child

3Rs If you could have changed one family rule when growing up, what would it have been? Why?

KISS 1. Which prefix means "less than normal": hypo or hyper?

2. What class of animals are frogs, salamanders, and toads?

3. The ________ won the battle of the Alamo, which is now located in __________.

SOS What do the following have in common: AVPC code, The Hershey Chocolate Company, A bird cage?

ICE Make a creative list of things that change color on their own. For example, a peeled apple is white and turns brown.

TAB Damage to the Myelin (which provides electrical insulation) in the brain and nervous system is connected to diseases such as multiple sclerosis.

Mmm The Wind Follows the Phoenix's Wings – Stand in a shoulder-width stance with the arms hanging comfortably to your sides. Close your mouth and touch the tip of your tongue to the roof of your mouth as if you were about to say the letter "t." As you exhale, bend forward at the waist and bend the knees slightly. Allow the hands to hang loosely in front of you. As you inhale, circle the left arm out to the side and as far overhead as you can. Follow the hand with your eyes and when you are at the top, rest the right hand on the left knee. Exhale and return to center before you repeat on the opposite side. Do a total of ten repetitions, counting each side as one.

---

203 New England Journal of Medicine reported on this; see http://examinedexistence.com/dancing-helps-the-brain-function-better/

— SET 344 —

WOW The groundwork of all happiness is health. – Leigh Hunt

3Rs What is the best compliment you ever received? Who said it to you? What made this compliment so special to you?

KISS 1. Who composed the Nutcracker?

2. Which two planets in our solar system have no moons? Hint: they are close to Earth.

3. What is the standard monetary currency in India?

SOS Start with the word "Mean" and change one letter at a time to get to the word "Kind", making real words at each step. Mean ____ ____ ____ ____ Kind

ICE You are in a contest to come up with the most interesting answer to the following question: What is the wiggliest thing in the world. To win the prize your answer must stand out from others by being original, engaging, or exotic in some way, e.g., snake in a patch of poison ivy. Brainstorm some ideas you might submit to the contest?

TAB You can't really fake a smile. When people are feeling miserable or frustrated their brain activity, timing, and behavior of little muscles around the eyes are different from genuine happiness.[204]

Mmm Face Massage – Starting at the jaw, gently massage the face with the fingers of both hands. Work up the cheeks then back down and inward to the chin. Rub the area above the upper lip and up and along the nose. Then gently stroke along the cheekbones, being especially tender under the eyes. Move up to the temples and then across the forehead and along the hairline.

— SET 345 —

WOW Reading furnishes the mind only with materials of knowledge; it is thinking that makes what we read ours. – John Locke

3Rs When traveling, do you like to listen to the radio, tapes, CDs, etc.? When you were growing up, did your family listen to the radio when traveling? If so, what are your memories and were there ever any disagreements about the choices made?

KISS 1. Name some characters in Shakespeare's plays that were based on real people.

---

204 http://www.livescience.com/20568-frustrated-smile-real-fak.html

2. How many pairs of ribs are there in the human body?

3. What British Parliamentary action required New World colonists to pay for an official stamp or seal, whenever they bought paper items?

SOS In what years did Christmas and New Year's fall in the same year?

ICE How can you stop chronic hiccups?

TAB Up to a point, the more challenging a book you are reading, the more likely it is that it will activate a new pathway in your brain. Furthermore, a recent study found that literary readers are better able to empathize with the emotions of others. The study attributes this finding to the practice readers get interpreting complex emotions and relationships in novels.[205]

Mmm Walk as if : Attitudes – Take a few minutes to walk as if you were a person with the following attitudes, and notice what changes. Walk as if you were: Insecure; Uptight; Egotistical; Immature; Flighty; Pained; Confident.

— SET 346 —

WOW Let us never negotiate out of fear, but let us never fear to negotiate. – John F. Kennedy

3Rs Recall from memory things that are out of place in your bedroom. Then go check to see how many things you remembered. Do you often have a messy bedroom or do you tend to keep things extremely tidy? What expectations did you have to live up to for caring for personal and family spaces when you were growing up?

KISS 1. How many letters are silent in the word "knight"?

2. Express the decimal .75 as a proper fraction?

3. The way of life that includes people's language, customs and beliefs is called what?

SOS What year is the same upside down and backwards?

ICE List as many words as you can that have "ring" in them.

TAB Midnight snacking is probably bad for the brain. A recent study found that "snacking" during normal sleeping times caused mice to do less well on memory tests even if they still got their normal amount of sleep.[206]

Mmm Skull Shining Breath – Sit in a position of comfort with your back upright. Place your hands on your belly. On your next in-breath, breathe

---

205 *Better Homes and Gardens*, June 2014, p. 184.

206 http://www.smithsonianmag.com/ist/?next=/science-nature/midnight-snacking-bad-your-brain-180954295/

in slowly. Then exhale strongly through the nose by consciously pulling the diaphragm in sharply to force the air out. Release to let the inhale come naturally. On the exhale you should feel the belly contract beneath the hands. If you do not feel the belly move, you can push the hands into the belly to help stimulate the necessary sensation of contracting. Imagine that each strong exhale seeps up around the skull cleansing and brightening it. Repeat 8-10 times. If at any time you feel light-headed, stop and return to a normal breath.

— SET 347 —

WOW No mud, no lotus. – Thich Nhat Hanh

3Rs Did you name any of your animals or things (e.g., car, boat, toy) when you were growing up? What were they?

KISS 1. Name some Rodgers and Hammerstein musicals.

2. What two-word term describes frozen carbon dioxide?

3. What country are you probably in, if you are making purchases using shekels?

SOS Tim can't seem to keep a job. The following reasons for losing each job are hints to where he worked or what job he had: 1) I took this job to add spice to my life, but found that I didn't really have the thyme. 2) I liked this job until they put the squeeze on. I got canned because I couldn't concentrate. 3) I enjoyed being in the forest, but I couldn't hack it and I got the axe. 4) This job was noteworthy, but I just couldn't work in harmony with my colleagues.

ICE The answer is excellent; thinking creatively, what is the question?

TAB Some memory loss serves a psychological function. For example, *repression* is an unconscious act the brain uses to protect the person's well-being and prevent emotional paralysis by getting rid of memories pertaining to unpleasant experiences or trauma.

Mmm Mud to Lotus Meditation – This meditation uses the image of mud-to-lotus. In much of Asia the lotus is a significant symbol of transformation because although it rises out of the mud, the lotus flower emerges pure and beautiful. And as the quote above indicates, the mud is necessary for the lotus to grow. Consider what mud you have in your life (anger, grief, suffering, regrets, irritations, etc.) that you would like to transform into a lotus. Close your eyes and see that the mud at the bottom of the pond is thick and murky. Then notice a bump in the mud, and see it gradually become a stem growing up out of the mud. Follow the stem up to the surface where it blooms into a beautiful flower. Enjoy the beauty of the flower for awhile. Then express your gratitude to the lotus and to the mud it has transformed.

— SET 348 —

WOW If I cannot do great things, I can do small things in a great way. – Martin Luther King Jr.

3Rs After you have saved your family and friends, what one item would you save if your house caught on fire? Why would you choose that?

KISS 1. What does the word "rendezvous" mean?

2. Estimate the sum of 14,021and 709 to the nearest hundred.

3. Who is America named after?

SOS Tim still can't seem to keep a job. The following reasons for losing each job are hints to where he worked or what job he had: 1) The recruiter reeled me in, but I just couldn't live on that net income; 2) This job was stimulating, but kept me up nights and got to be a grind. 3) I thought I had this job down stone-cold, but my relationship with the boss was rocky; 4) I was all fired up about this job, but then it went up in smoke.

ICE Mr. and Mrs. Plunkett have lost their car in a massive parking lot at the stadium. How can they find their car?

TAB 24 hours must pass to determine if previously learned information is in long-term memory.[207]

Mmm Flamingo Stance –. Stand hip-width on both feet so that you feel solid. Then as you feel ready, lift one foot off the ground to stand like a flamingo. It is better to be stable with the foot closer to the ground than to lift so high that you cannot keep your balance for long. Count to see how long you can comfortably stay balanced in that position. Repeat on the other foot. How did the two sides compare?

— SET 349 —

WOW Once you say you're going to settle for second, that's what happens to you in life, I find. – John F. Kennedy

3Rs Would you leave America never to return again for one million dollars? Why or why not? If you had to leave, what place would you choose to live instead?

---

207 http://arc.duke.edu/documents/Learning%20and%20Memory%20handout.pdf

KISS 1. What are the first names of Haydn, Liszt and Schubert?

2. What is the medical name for the breast bone?

3. Several nations use the word "dollar" for their national currency. Name some of them.

SOS Polly's street address is between 240 and 250. All the digits of the address are even, and two digits are the same. What is the number of Polly's address?

ICE List things that return.

TAB Some studies suggest that Alzheimer's may be connected to infections such as cold sores, gastric ulcers, Lyme disease, pneumonia and the flu. Researchers theorize that infections lead to increased beta amloid, which kills neurons in the brain.[208]

Mmm You Walk Funny – Intentionally do a funny walk. Walk around with that walk. Then try a different one.

— SET 350 —

WOW Reprove a friend in secret, but praise him before others. – Leonardo da Vinci

3Rs What one item that your parents owned would you most like to have inherited? Describe it. Why would you have liked to have it?

KISS 1. Name some characteristics of Gothic architecture.

2. True or false? Swallows chew their food.

3. The Declaration of Independence states the following: "We hold these truths to be self-evident . . . ." What is the first truth?

SOS The first letter of each word in the following descriptions are also the same as the initials as the person described. 1) Betrayed America; 2) Artist Romantic; 3) Made Television's Mary; 4) The Trio Slapstick (a group).

ICE You have a scratch on your face. What is the story?

TAB In addition to the skull, the brain is protected by three layers of meninges which limit the movement of the brain within the skull to protect the blood vessels of the brain. Meningitis is an infection in these layers that can be fatal.

Mmm Meditation: Color Bathing – Imagine that you are seated at the edge of a deep and beautiful pool of water. The color of the water of the pool is constantly changing. Spend awhile just visualizing the many colors the water can be. Notice how each color makes you feel. When you are ready, let the color of the water stabilize into one color that pleases you and dive

208 http://epirev.oxfordjournals.org/content/early/2013/01/23/epirev.mxs007.full

in. Swim and bathe in the color. Allow the color to wash over and penetrate through every pore of your entire body.

— SET 351 —

WOW A person who knows nothing is closer to the truth than a person whose mind is filled with falsehoods and errors. – Thomas Jefferson

3Rs Which was/is your favorite cartoon character? Why? How often did you watch cartoons when you were young?

KISS 1. What prefix means under and could be put in front of "way" and "marine"?

2. Divide the number of degrees in a semi-circle by the number of degrees in a triangle. What is the answer?

3. American colonists who agreed to work for four-to-seven years on the farms of those who paid for their journey to the New World were called what?

SOS What do these initials stand for: 1) Tired fairy tale – S. B.; 2) Colorful song – Y. R. of T.; 3) Revolutionary musical: L. M.

ICE Imagine that you are creating a band with some friends. Brainstorm some good names for your band.

TAB Neurobiologist Lawrence C. Katz identifies three key ingredients for making an activity more brain-enhancing: 1) Use senses in a unique way, such as adding scent or doing something with eyes closed; 2) Engage attention with things that stand out as unusual, arousing, playful or meaningful; 3) Break routines in significant ways to stimulate novelty.[209]

Mmm The Blind Flamingo Stance –Do the Flamingo Stance again: Start in a solid stance and as you feel ready, lift one foot off the ground to stand like a flamingo. This time, however, close your eyes. Count to see how long you can comfortably stay balanced in that position with eyes closed. Repeat on the other foot. How did you do compared with your eyes open?

— SET 352 —

WOW Better to bend than to break. – Scottish Proverb

3Rs What experience, if any have you had outside of the United States or interacting with people who are from other cultures?

---

209 Katz, Lawrence C. and Manning Rubin. (1999) *Keep Your Brain Alive*. New York: Workman.

KISS 1. What do you call the introduction of a play or speech?
2. The renal artery supplies blood to which organs?
3. In what country do you always pay by the pound? Think: Pounds sterling.

SOS Use the same three letters to fill in the blanks to create legitimate words from the following: ___dom, ___ect, ___ler, ___ ves.

ICE List things that can involve a roll?

TAB A 2013 study by researchers at Montclair State University in New Jersey found that if you clench your right hand, it activates the left frontal lobe of the brain where memories are stored. If you clench your left hand, it activates the right frontal lobe of the brain where memories are retrieved. People who squeezed with their right and then their left hand remembered 15% more words from a list.[210]

Mmm Wrist and Finger Workout – Put arms out in front of you. Wave hands up and down at the wrist. Circle the wrists, first in one direction, then in the other. Pull the fingers one-at-a-time into the palm to make a fist. Nod the fists up and down and side-to-side. Circle the wrists again in each direction again with the fingers in fists. Release the fingers one-at-a-time and shake out the hands and wrists.

— SET 353 —

WOW Life is not measured by the number of breaths we take, but by the moments that take our breath away. – Vicki Corona

3Rs Not including food, clothing, or shelter, what would be the hardest ten things you would not want to give up for 30 days? What would make it hard to give up?

KISS 1. What instrument did Louis Armstrong play?
2. True or false? Flamingos have pink feathers because they eat shrimp?
3. A shelter made of tanned hides fastened to a framework of poles is called what?

SOS Marie has a desk calendar made up of long blocks with the months and two smaller, numbered blocks that can be rotated for the dates. What number appears on each small block so that Marie can use one or both of them to represent the date.

ICE If you were hired to create a new costume for the devil, what would you design?

210 http://healthland.time.com/2013/04/29/grasping-memory-with-both-hands/

TAB According to the Foundation for Critical Thinking "Experience may be the best teacher, but biased experience supports bias, distorted experience supports distortion, self-deluded experience supports self-delusion. We, therefore, must not think of our experience as sacred in any way but, instead, as one important dimension of thought that must, like all others, be critically analyzed and assessed."[211]

Mmm Bellows Breathing – Lie on your back, and place your hands on your belly. Start with a few rounds of Skull Shining Breath: exhale strongly through the nose by consciously pulling the diaphragm in sharply to force the air out explosively. Release to let the inhale come naturally. On the exhale you should feel the belly contract beneath the hands. When you are ready, break the strong exhale into 3-5 smaller quick bursts. Repeat 8-10 times. If at any time you feel light-headed, stop and return to a normal breath.

— SET 354 —

WOW Struggles in life are like fertilizer; they stink but they help us grow. – Anonymous

3Rs What words of wisdom would you like to pass down to future generations? How did you gain this wisdom that you want to share?

KISS 1. Which is two words: haystack or hayfever?

2. How were the Hawaiian Islands formed?

3. What is a Euro?

SOS List as many words as you can with at least 5 letters that do not contain the letters a, e, i, o, u? (Hint: Use the letter Y).

ICE Complete the following statements with something completely new: A hug is like a ____; A laugh is like a _____; A tear is like a ____. Be original!

TAB How you feel affects how you learn. Bad emotions interfere with learning; good emotions create excitement about and love for learning, and result in effective learning.

Mmm Mindful Tracking: Emotions – For today consciously track your emotions. Be conscious to identify even very subtle and transitory emotions. For example, in the course of a conversation, one might feel confused, slightly irritated and then relieved in a very short period of time. Since emotions

---

211 http://www.criticalthinking.org/pages/critical-thinking-distinguishing-between-inert-information-activated-ignorance-activated-knowledge/488

are so fleeting, it is suggested that you write down notes for this one and tally up at the end of the day. Were you surprised by what you observed?

— SET 355 —

WOW To have a great idea, have a lot of them. – Thomas Edison

3Rs If you were running for political office, what would you prioritize in your campaign? What would your opponent say about you?

KISS 1. Who is the most famous classical composer of the western world, even though he began to go deaf at age 28, known for writing nine extraordinary symphonies?

2. If you only have nickels and dimes, how many of each do you need to equal $1.35?

3. Who was the first woman to serve on the US Supreme Court?

SOS Take a word for vim and vigor (Pep) and add a letter of the alphabet (on the front or back) to get a brand of soda. Example: A rubber wheel (tire) plus the letter N = All (N-Tire = Entire).

ICE Name some sources of happiness!

TAB Researchers from The University of Texas Health Science Center at Houston and the University of California, San Diego used brain imaging to identify the areas of the prefrontal cortex associated with self-control and "braking" ability in relation to certain behaviors. They then demonstrated that harmless electrical stimulation of these areas can boost self-control by amplifying the brain's "brakes."[212]

Mmm Figure-Eights – Create as many different ways as you can to draw figure-eights with your body. Consider how you can use all the major joints. Play with speed, angle, and direction. For example, you can make a figure-eight from the shoulder at different angles: with arms hanging at your side, with arms out to the side, with arms over head or with arms out in front.

— SET 356 —

WOW Without winter, there can be no spring. Without mistakes, there can be no learning. Without doubts there can be no faith. Without fears, there can be no courage. My mistakes, my fears and my doubts are my path to wisdom, faith and courage. – Anonymous

212 http://www.medicalnewsmediasource.com/study-shows-that-electrical-stimulation-can-boost-the-brains-brakes-forbes/

3Rs If you were to act on a whim, what would you do? Why do you consider that a whim?

KISS 1. What is a ballad?
2. What do the initials ICU stand for in a hospital?
3. What cemetery has over 240,000 military service members buried there?

SOS Daisy, Lucy, Belle, and Rex are purebred dogs. Their breeds are Miniature Poodle, Cocker Spaniel, German Shepherd, and St. Bernard. Belle is smaller than both the Cocker Spaniel and Rex. The St. Bernard is younger than Daisy. Lucy is the oldest and friends with the Cocker Spaniel. What breed is each dog?

ICE Make as long and sensible a sentence as you can using only words beginning with the letter "O."

TAB Recent research at the Harvard Medical School suggests that the same protein that stimulates brain growth via exercise could potentially be bottled and given to patients experiencing cognitive decline, including those in the beginning stages of Alzheimer's and Parkinson's. [213]

Mmm Visualization Meditation: Winter – Metaphorically, winter is a time of resting and containment: buried under snow and burrowed in to keep warm. This meditation can reflect on the season or can be used to acknowledge or invite calm and patience in some phase or aspect of your life. As you are ready, visualize yourself or some area of your life as a small burrowing animal. Notice how the days are shorter, light grows paler and air gets colder. Yawn and travel down inside your earthen home where you have a warm bed of dried grasses. Nestle down for a cozy, long winter's sleep. Let your body slow down to hibernate while above, the earth is blanketed in snow and ice.

— SET 357 —

WOW Art is the only way to run away without leaving home. – Twyla Tharp

3Rs What were some of your favorite TV or radio programs during your childhood? What did you like about them? With whom did you watch/listen to them? Describe the plot of a favorite episode.

KISS 1. Find the nouns in the saying "His bark is worse than his bite."
2. Is a zebra black with white stripes, or white with black stripes?
3. Where is the Forbidden City?

213 http://harvardmagazine.com/2013/10/an-exercise-pill-for-the-brain

SOS A brown house, a blue house, a white house, and a green house are all in a row. The green house is not first. The white house and the brown house are on either side of the blue house. The brown house is next to both the green house and the blue house. What order are the houses in?

ICE How can you make someone move (as in walk or drive away)?

TAB The University of Pennsylvania School of Medicine conducted a study on older people with existing memory problems. The participants had better blood flow to the brain and improved cognitive functions after two month of practicing meditation for twelve minutes a day.[214]

Mmm Visualization Meditation: Resting in a Natural Environment – Visualize yourself out in nature in a place that you find restful and enjoyable. You can visualize an actual place that you have been to before, a real place that you long to visit, or an imaginary place. In your imagination explore this new environment around you. What season is it? Is it flat or mountainous? Is there water nearby? What plants and animals are around? Rest here awhile.

— SET 358 —

WOW The test of a first-rate intelligence is the ability to hold two opposed ideas in mind at the same time and still retain the ability to function. – F. Scott Fitzgerald

3Rs What was the happiest/most exciting time in your life? What made it so?

KISS 1. What Shakespeare play contains the line "To be or not to be"

2. How many weeks are in a century?

3. What national landmark in Washington, DC includes 14 museums?

SOS Delores has 9 bills and 1 coin in her pocket. She has two times as many tens as one-dollar bills. The coin is not a penny, nickel, dime, or half-dollar. How much money does Delores have in her pocket, and what is the breakdown of denominations?

ICE What are some things that come in a bunch?

TAB Omega-3 fatty acids are concentrated in the brain and crucial for effective brain functioning. They are found in certain fish/seafood (halibut, herring, mackerel, salmon, sardines, trout, tuna, halibut, algae, krill), nuts and non-hydrogenated nut butters (almonds, cashews, Brazil nuts, filberts,

---

214 See http://mcleanmeditation.com/meditation-research.html

hazelnuts, peanuts, walnuts, tahini), and seeds (flax seeds, sesame seeds, sunflower seeds).[215]

Mmm Change your bedtime ritual in some way today.

— SET 359 —

WOW If you tell the truth, you don't have to remember anything. – Mark Twain

3Rs Describe what "homecoming" was like at your school. What did you like and dislike about it? Why?

KISS 1. Name some dance styles.
2. What part of the body is affected by glaucoma?
3. Tehran is the capital of what country?

SOS What do the following have in common: A light switch, a wall calendar, a coin?

ICE If you had to choose a verb for a last name, what would your name be?

TAB Young children who are fluent in more than one language are less likely to develop Alzheimer's later in life.[216]

Mmm Supersonic Hearing – Imagine that you have super sensitive hearing. Close your eyes and move your head and body to tune into the sounds around you. Imagine that you can hear sounds that others cannot hear, tune into those sounds, too.

— SET 360 —

WOW We should not let our success go to our heads, or our failures go to our hearts. – Anonymous

3Rs Think of gardens you have known. Which one was your favorite? Where did you see it? What made it so special? Do you like doing gardening?

KISS 1. Place a single letter in front of each of the following words to form three new words: Randy; Adios; Axmen.
2. Where could you go to celebrate New Year's Eve in the summer?
3. Where does the U.S. Congress meet and conduct business?

SOS What English word has all of the vowels a, e, i, o, and u in it in alphabetical order?

ICE If God asked you to redecorate heaven, what would be your color scheme?

---

215 For example, see http://www.ncbi.nlm.nih.gov/pmc/articles/PMC3738731/

216 http://www.theguardian.com/science/2011/feb/18/bilingual-alzhairmers-brain-power-multitasking

TAB Gratitude increases the level of serotonin in your brain, and that fuels your sense of well-being and your ability to remember.

Mmm Staff Pose – Sit on the floor with legs extended out in front of you with toes up. If this is uncomfortable, use a few folded blankets or towels to sit on. Feet are together and spine is long. Press the back of the legs against the floor gently, and extend the heels away from you, keeping the toes up. Place the hands or fingertips on the ground alongside the hips and press down lightly to invite the spine to lift up from the pelvis. Keep the face forward and the chin level. Sense a lengthening out the top of the head and out the soles of the feet. Hold for 20-30 seconds, and then release.

— SET 361 —

WOW We must become the change we seek in the world. – Mahatma Gandhi

3Rs Do you have a hometown? If not, what place do you consider your home? What is your that town like and why do you consider it to be your home?

KISS 1. What does the Shakespeare quote "Et tu, Brute?" from *Julius Caesar* mean?

2. How many minutes are there in a week?

3. What is the 16th word of the "Pledge of Allegiance"?

SOS Billy, Luis, Irene, Marci and Scott are all on the same baseball team. They play first base, pitcher, shortstop, catcher, and right field. They all made a different number of hits in the last game, but everyone had at least one hit. No one had more hits than the shortstop, and she was tired after getting her fifth and final hit. Billy is positioned furthest from home plate, and he had exactly twice as many hits as the pitcher. Shane had more hits than all the other infielders except for Irene. Luis wears a mask when he plays. How many hits did each player get?

ICE What are some things that have spots on them?

TAB Recent studies have concluded that excessive viewing of television and use of smartphones and computers by children can adversely affect their ability to pay attention when they become adults.[217]

Mmm Bee Breathing – According to *Yoga Journal*, bee breathing helps one to relax and reduce anxiety.[218] Sit in a position of comfort with your back upright. Close your lips gently but firmly, and take your next inhale through

217 http://www.nature.com/articles/srep21129#ref-link-section-8/

218 https://www.yogajournal.com/practice/buzz-away-the-buzzing-mind

the nose. As you exhale, make a humming sound like a bee. Let the hum continue through the entire out-breath. Stop and inhale through the nose when you need to, then go back to your bee buzz again for the exhale. Repeat for 10 breath cycles or longer.

— SET 362 —

WOW You do not have to be good. You do not have to walk on your knees for a hundred miles through the desert, repenting. You only have to let the soft animal of your body love what it loves. – Mary Oliver

3Rs Based on your own experience, what do you consider to be "good manners"? Think of a time or situation where you did not show good manners. What do you consider the most important aspects of good manners?

KISS 1. Colors that are opposite one another on the color wheel are called what?
2. What shellfish produces a pearl?
3. How many provinces and territories are in Canada?

SOS The following descriptions can be rephrased to create rhyming word pairs (Example: chubby feline = fat cat). 1) Paris ballet; 2) A lively bird; 3) Wet highway exit;

ICE Name things that are caught.

TAB Recent studies indicate that the flavonols in hot cocoa boost the blood flow to your brain and other organs, thin the blood to reduce one's blood pressure as much as a low-dose aspirin, and can reverse age-related memory decline in healthy older adults.[219]

Mmm Wave the Flag – Get a bandana, loose scarf, flag or other small piece of light-weight fabric. Wave the fabric in the air as if you are trying to get someone's attention. Wave first with one hand, then the other, then both hands. Wave high. Wave low. Wave all around you. See if you can catch and keep a breeze so the fabric billows. Swirl the fabric in the air. Toss it up and catch it as it floats down. Feel free to add music and make it a dance.

— SET 363 —

WOW If a voice inside you says, "I cannot paint," then by all means, paint, and that voice will be silenced. – Vincent Van Gogh

219 https://www.washingonpost.com/national/health-science/compound-in-chocolate-found-to-reverse-age-related-memory-loss-study-finds/201410/26/cee91aac-5bcb-11e4-bd61-346aee66ba29_story.html

3Rs Describe some important relationships with family friends, cousins, or other relatives of a similar age to you. How did these relationships shape your behaviors, beliefs and attitudes?

KISS 1. Which of the following pairs of words cannot be combined to make a contraction: I would; I did; I can?

2. Which of the following conduct electricity: copper, plastic or wood?

3. What is the official language of Quebec, Canada?

SOS What device in an orchestra is not blown, bowed, plucked or struck?

ICE List as many compounds or known phrases using the word "brain" as possible.

TAB In 2013, European researchers reported that they were able to grow miniature human brains from stem cells. The research team formally acknowledged that they had not created a full-scale, fully functioning human brain, and that doing so is a long way off.[220]

Mmm Remote Control Meditation – This meditation is intended to reduce worry and fear. Sit in a position of comfort with your back upright. You are going to imagine that you can watch your life like a movie and control it with your "remote control". As you are ready, begin to play a scene from your life of a situation that causes you anxiety or worry. Whenever you want to, use your remote to change the movie. Turn the volume up or down. Adjust the color, focus, or frame. Fast-forward or rewind. Imagine that you can change the content of the scene, making different decisions about how you speak, act, and respond.[221]

— SET 364 —

WOW Age is a question of mind over matter. If you don't mind, it doesn't matter. – Satchel Paige

3Rs What is your favorite sport? Why? Was it always your favorite sport?

KISS 1. What famous composer had the first name "Wolfgang"?

2. Divide 40 by ½ and add 5. (Hint: Invert)

3. Which landmark holds records of the three branches of the U.S. government?

---

220 http://www.bbc.com/new/health-23863544

221 Achterberg, Jeanne, Barbara Dossy and Leslie Kokmeir. (1994) *Ritual and Healing: Using Imagery for Health and Wellness.* New York: Bantam.

SOS What same word can come before "nut," "fly," and "cup" to form them into compound words?

ICE Create some bad business names. For example, Drippy's Plumbing.

TAB According to scientific evidence, neurons last a lifetime; they are some of the oldest cells in the body.

Mmm Charleston Dance Step – Begin with both feet together and arms at your sides. You can turn your hands up at the wrist flapper-style if you want. Start by stepping back on your right foot. Kick your left foot back behind you. Step forward with the left foot. Kick forward with the right foot. Repeat with music and add arms movements if you wish.

SET 365

WOW Feeling gratitude and not expressing it is like wrapping a present and not giving it. – William Arthur Ward

3Rs What favorite items of clothing have you had? Why? Where did you get them?

KISS 1. Name some artists associated with Impressionism.
2. What colors are the five Olympic rings, and why were they chosen?
3. In what city do you find the following: Louvre; Left Bank; Latin Quarter; Bastille?

SOS The following descriptions can be rephrased to create rhyming word pairs (example: chubby feline = fat cat). 1) Rain of petals; 2) The White House; 3) Noisy cumulus; 4) Obstacle for a tortoise.

ICE The authors are tired. Please make a list of other prompts to use for the next edition.

TAB Several studies suggest that chewing gum may accelerate and/or recover the process of working memory and also improve one's arousal level[222]

Mmm Blessings Meditation – Take the time to visualize the various things in your life right now that you appreciate or that are a blessing for you. When you finish, express your gratitude for all these wonderful parts of your life in whatever ways feels good to you.

---

222 https://www.ncbi.nlm.nih.gov/pubmed/18403120

Books and Websites to Help Improve Brain Health

Books

Annibali, Joseph A. (2015). *Reclaim Your Brain*. New York: Penguin Random House.

Carper, Jean. (2012). *100 Simple Things You Can Do to Prevent Alzheimer's and Age-Related Memory*. New York: Little, Brown and Company.

Gelb, Michael J., and Kelly Howell. (2012). *Brain Power*. Novato,CA: New World Library.

Goldberg, Elkhonon. (2013). *The SharpBrains Guide to Brain Fitness*. San Francisco: Sharpbrains, Inc.

Hagerty, Barbara B. (2016). *Life Reimagined*. New York: Penguin.

Kiraly, Stephen J. (2014). *Your Healthy Brain, 2nd ed. Vancouver, BC Canada:* West Coast Reproductions.

Lotto, B. (2017). Deviate: The Science of Seeing Differently. London: Weidenfeld & Nicolson.

Medina, John J. (2008). *Brain Rules.* Seattle, WA: Pear Press.

Mehta, Mira. (1998). *How to Use Yoga*. Berkley, Ca :Rodmell.

Michelon, Pascale. (2011). *Max Your Memory*. New York: DX Publishing.

Nhat Hanh, Thich. (2009). *The Blooming of a Lotus*. (Revised). Boston: Beacon Press.

Perlmutter. David, & Carol Colman. (2005). *The Better Brain Book*. New York: Penguin.

Rosas, Debbie and Carlos Rosas. (2004). *The Nia Technique.* New York: Broadway Books.

Small, Gary, & Gigi Vorgan. (2015). *2 Weeks to a Younger Brain*. Boca Raton, FL: Humanix Books.

Swanson, D. (2001). *Hmm? The Most Interesting Book You'll Ever Read about Memory*. New York: Scholastic.

Tan, Zaldy S. (2006). *Age-Proof Your Mind*. New York: Time Warner Books.

Unger, Karen V. (2015). *Brain Health for Life***.** Portland, OR: Inkwater Press.

Wayne, (2012). Peter M. with Mark L Fuerst. *The Harvard Medical School Guide to Tai Chi*. Boston: Shambala.

Websites

https://www.nianow.com/about-nia

http://www.yougajournal.com

http://www.aarp.org/health/brain-health/info

http://www.alz.org/we_can_help_brain_health_maintain_your_brain.asp

http://www.aplaceformom.com/blog/10ways-to-keep-the-mind-sharp/

http://www.beautiful-minds.com/four-dimensions-of-brain-health/brain-health-tips

http://www.brainpower.org/maximize-brain-power.html

http://www.brainrules.net/about-brain-rules

https://health.clevelandclinic.org/2015/07/6-ways-to-maintain-your-brain-health-infographic/

http://www.mayoclinic.org/healthy-lifestyle/healthy-aging/in-depth/memory-loss/art-20046518

http://www.sparkpeople.com/resource/wellness_articles.asp?id=1613&page=2

http://www.signchido.com/art-of-moving-prayer/

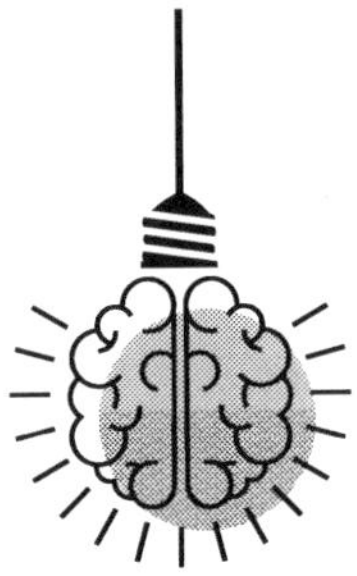

POSSIBLE SOLUTIONS FOR KISS, SOS AND ICE ITEMS WITHIN EACH SET

SET 1	KISS	1. Neat, funny, smart, etc. 2. George Washington Carver 3. Lincoln, Jefferson, Franklin Roosevelt, Washington.
	SOS	"I am a liar."
	ICE	Backhand, handcuff, handbag, handshake, handsome, etc.
SET 2	KISS	1. Meg, Jo, Beth, Amy, Marmee, Laurie, etc.; 2. Glenn, Armstrong, Aldrin, etc.; 3. Connecticut, Delaware, Georgia, Maryland, Massachusetts, New Hampshire, New Jersey, New York, North Carolina, Pennsylvania, Rhode Island, South Carolina, and Virginia.
	SOS	Paradox ("pair of docs"); Turned inside out.
	ICE	Antennae, radio transmitter, fake eyebrows, etc.
SET 3	KISS	1. "Twinkle, Twinkle Little Star"; 2. Measles, mumps; polio, smallpox, etc.; 3. Alabama & Wyoming.
	SOS	Carrot and karat.
	ICE	"Gee, is it February again?"; "Do you like cherry pie?"; "Are you a Whig?"; etc.
SET 4	KISS	1. N – Turn on the fan, V- Do not fan the fire, Adj. – Lay them out fan pattern, etc.; 2. Currants, grapes, pineapples, raspberries, watermelons, etc.; 3. Apple.
	SOS	Spider—number sequence of legs.
	ICE	Clichés, wrapping paper roll, bowl, etc.
SET 5	KISS	1. A. A. Milne; 2. Celsius: Boiling water is 100°C and 212° F; 3. Egypt, Kenya, Nigeria, Tanzania, South Africa, etc.
	SOS	Wombat; batter; and combat or battle.
	ICE	Seat your pet snake at the table; Put your head on table and don't move; Drop your plate on floor; etc.

SET 6	**KISS**	1. Mount Rushmore Memorial (completed) and Crazy Horse Memorial (not completed as of 2017); 2. =7, 11, 13, etc.; 3. Jefferson, Lincoln, T. Roosevelt, Washington.
	SOS	Your name.
	ICE	Your feet wouldn't hurt; You'd save money on shoes; It would be easier to fall head over heels; People would look you in the belly button; etc.
SET 7	**KISS**	1. Gnat, gnome, knight, pneumonia, etc.; 2. A, B, AB, O; 3. Columbus, Magellan, Lewis & Clark, etc.
	SOS	Birth order: Junior – August 1; Kev-June 1; Walter – July 1; Mike – May 1; Arnold & Harold (twins) – April 1.
	ICE	Will probably call you late at night; If no one pays attention; Dreams of fire hydrants; Me sweat; etc.
SET 8	**KISS**	1. Percussion; 2. Redwood and spruce; 3. 100-2 for each state.
	SOS	A sundial has smallest number of parts. An hourglass filled with grains of sand has largest number.
	ICE	Since Saturday, silly Sally sold sixty-seven stupendous suede shoes; Simple Simon saw seventy-seven sentimental swans singing slow, sweet songs; etc.
SET 9	**KISS**	1. Bassoon, flute, oboe, piccolo, saxophone, etc.; 2. 0°C and 32° F; 3. Alkaline battery, incandescent light bulb, motion picture, phonograph, etc.
	SOS	1 hour.
	ICE	He saw an alien; He bumped into Elvis Presley; He's being audited by the IRS, etc.
SET 10	**KISS**	1. Q; 2. Equator; 3. Germany.
	SOS	A zipper.
	ICE	"I took the wrong diet pill, and . . ."; That is how tall I felt after being really embarrassed; I got mistaken for a foot-long hotdog, and then . . . "; etc.
SET 11	**KISS**	1. Paul Bunyan; 2. Middle ear; 3. Washington, John Adams, Jefferson, Madison, Monroe, John Quincy Adams.
	SOS	A shoe.
	ICE	"Please do not use my bedspread as a hankie"; "My home owner's insurance "snot" going to cover this"; "Gesundheit"; etc.
SET 12	**KISS**	1. Michelangelo; 2. Snake, lizard, toad, etc.; 3. The Netherlands.
	SOS	There is no smoke since it is an electric train.
	ICE	"Tick" is first in the alphabet; Tock has the final say; Ticks cause diseases; Who has ever heard of a "tock"?; "Tock" radio can get people riled up; etc.

SET 13	KISS	1. Answers will vary; 2. Iron; 3. New York, Los Angeles, and Chicago in that order.
	SOS	Doing the laundry.
	ICE	Brains, campfire, eyes, flashy clothes, fluorescent bulbs, lamps, etc.
SET 14	KISS	1. Ben Franklin; 2. 11, the last two pieces are cut at the same time; 3. Florida, St. Augustine (1565).
	SOS	Candy = lemon.
	ICE	Snow falling; a cotton ball fight; the house after the grandkids leave; etc.
SET 15	KISS	1. Leonardo da Vinci; 2. Brain, heart, kidney, liver, pancreas, etc.; Colorado and Wyoming.
	SOS	All are slang for money.
	ICE	They both have a point; both can hurt you; etc.
SET 16	KISS	1. Deer, moose, Mrs., Geese, Octopuses, oxen, teeth; 2. True; 3. Agnew, Bush, Ford, Gore, Mondale.
	SOS	Gallery; Largely; Regally.
	ICE	No calendars; No census; No speed limits; Money denominations indistinguishable; etc.
SET 17	KISS	1. Alice Walker, Ernest Hemmingway; 2. Ant; 3. Algonquin, Apache, Arapaho, Blackfeet, Cherokee, Chickasaw, Chippewa, Choctaw, Fox, Iowa, Kansas, Kickapoo, Kiowa, Mohawk, Navajo, Ottawa, Pottawatomie, Quapaw, Seminole, Shawnee, Sioux, Winnebago, Wyandot, etc.
	SOS	Lenora ate fish and ice cream. Melissa ate salad and apple pie. David ate chicken and chocolate cake. William ate steak and cheesecake.
	ICE	New world; Best abode; Greatest show on earth; etc.
SET 18	KISS	1. Mozart, Beethoven, Grieg, Handel, Haydn, Schubert, etc.; 2. Stethoscope; 3. East-to-West Interstates end in even numbers; North-to-South Interstates end with odd numbers.
	SOS	Liz and Sue.
	ICE	"When the spacecraft hits the asteroid belt, check the monitor for signs of life"; "When the liquid hits the boiling point, check the radiator for signs of distress"; etc.
SET 19	KISS	1. Squeak, mosque, unquote, etc.; 2. Pulley, lever, inclined plane, wheel and axle, screw, wedge; 3. Gave women the right to vote.
	SOS	H has only straight-lines, and goes in the first group; D and Q are curved and go in the second group.
	ICE	Cut with dental floss or string; Use hands; Use a screw driver; Eat your part first; Pull off pieces by layers; etc.

SET 20	**KISS**	1. *Comedy of Errors*, *Hamlet*, *Henry VIII*, *King Lear*, *Macbeth*, *Merry Wives of Windsor*, *Midsummer Night's Dream*, *Much Ado about Nothing*, *Romeo and Juliet*; etc.; 2. Mongoose; 3. China.
	SOS	Answers will vary. Example: lying; dried; plump; and trial.
	ICE	Doughnut; belly button; Chinese money; skull; etc.
SET 21	**KISS**	1. Most of his comedies end with at least one marriage; 2. [1) The sun heats the water which evaporates. 2) The water vapor forms clouds. 3) The water vapor cools, condenses, and falls as rain or snow.]; 3. The flag must be hoisted to the peak for an instant before being lowered to half-mast.
	SOS	Uphold, upheaval, upholster, etc., where "p" is at the end of one syllable and "h" begins next syllable.
	ICE	Don't bite off more (than one head at a time.); He who laughs last (doesn't get the joke.); A bird in the hand (may lay an egg there.); The more things change (the more stress I feel.); etc.
SET 22	**KISS**	1. Dwarf, dwell, dwindle; 2. Mercury, Venus, Earth, Mars, Jupiter, Saturn, Uranus, Neptune. (Pluto was demoted from planet status!); 3. Pyramids.
	SOS	Elephant – mouse.
	ICE	Your outfit would be "back in style"; your children would be embarrassed; etc.
SET 23	**KISS**	1. October, *The Hunt for Red October;* 2. The liver's main job is to filter and detoxify the blood coming from the digestive tract, before passing it to the rest of the body; 3. China, India, Indonesia, Korea, Mongolia, Vietnam, etc.
	SOS	Ara makes the words "bearable", "guarantee", and "caravan".
	ICE	Your house has a side door instead of a front door; The carpenter accidentally nailed your front door shut; You are homeless and live in the great outdoors; Your house has no walls; etc.
SET 24	**KISS**	1. Cubism; 2. A fierce marsupial from "down under" in Australia; 3. Arizona.
	SOS	99+9/9.
	ICE	Possible answers: The early bird (has to wait for those who come late); A penny saved (often gets hoarded); The Grass is always (needing to be mowed); It's always darkest (when you get lost at night).
SET 25	**KISS**	1. 8 – Noun, verb, adjective, adverb, pronoun, interjection, preposition, conjunction; 2. Ants, bees, wasps, etc.; 3. Belgium, Greece, Italy, Norway, Poland, etc.
	SOS	He is completely bald.
	ICE	"I Gave Him My Number"; "OMG, LOL"; "She's Just the O-N-E"; etc.

SET 26	KISS	1. Alex Haley / Walt Whitman / Lorraine Hansberry; 2. 999+999=1,998; 3. Margaret Thatcher.
	SOS	Take the first letter and place it at the end of the word; spell the word backwards and it will be the same word as you originally had spelled frontwards.
	ICE	No one would know if you were a twin; Crimes would be more difficult to solve; You wouldn't need mirrors; etc.
SET 27	KISS	1. Beethoven was a music composer & the others are artists; 2. Our eyes; 3. "Four score and seven years ago our forefathers brought forth on this continent a new nation, conceived in liberty and dedicated to the proposition that all men are created equal."
	SOS	Boy – Bay – May – Man.
	ICE	"You might want to ask my fairy godmother for a breath mint"; etc.
SET 28	KISS	1. Dad, deed, mom, pep, radar, etc.; 2. They cannot see in total darkness; they do see better than humans in semi-darkness; 3. Lake Superior.
	SOS	Tennessee, fluency, literacy, consistency, prophesy.
	ICE	Throw water on them; Shout "The British are coming";Set off the smoke alarm; etc.
SET 29	KISS	1. James Baldwin, W.E.B. Dubois, Langston Hughes, Zora Neale Hurston, etc.; 2. Nitrogen (about 78%) and Oxygen (about 21%); 3. Patrick Henry.
	SOS	Your mother.
	ICE	"The navigator gave bad directions"; "The flight attendant got sick"; "We ran out of fuel"; etc.
SET 30	KISS	1. Eeyore, Tigger, Roo, Owl, Kanga, etc.; 2. Nothing, because there is no air to carry sounds; 3. West Virginia.
	SOS	Turkish; Swiss; Italian; and Japanese.
	ICE	This book; My body; Boomerang; etc.
SET 31	KISS	1. Answered, replied, screamed, shouted, suggested, etc.; 2. It's an optical illusion. Generally our vision reflects a blending of what each eye sees. As you move your finger closer the image from each eye is separated. 3. Canada.
	SOS	1. Sitting duck; 2. Babysitter; 3. Sitar; 3. Sitting Bull; 3. Sit-in.
	ICE	You've joined the secret service; you lost your voice; etc.
SET 32	KISS	1. Andy Warhol; 2. Vipers are poisonous and constrictors are not. 3. South Carolina, Mississippi, Florida, Alabama, Georgia, Louisiana, Texas, Virginia, Arkansas, North Carolina, Tennessee.
	SOS	Steve sells appliances on the west corner. Victoria sells candy on the south corner. Roxanne sells shoes on the north corner. Ali sells fruit on the east corner.
	ICE	ANNAlyze, BOBcat, CRYSTALize, EDucate, etc.

SET 33	**KISS**	1. "Happy Birthday"; 2. Ostrich; 3. Acadia National Park in Maine.
	SOS	Hershey; Kit Kat; Baby Ruth; Mounds.
	ICE	Stay on the plane; Jump without it—parachutes are for wimps; Make it into some pants; Give it to a friend; Grab hold of someone whose chute is working; etc.
SET 34	**KISS**	1. Quick, brown, lazy; 2. Haircut; 3. Freed all people held as slaves in Confederate states. It also allowed black soldiers to serve in the Union army. Freedom for <u>all</u> people held as slaves in the U.S did not come until the ratification of the 13th Amendment.
	SOS	Mirror: Organ: Annually: Lye: Yellow.
	ICE	Drink tea; hire someone to hold your cup, wait to have coffee at work, etc.
SET 35	**KISS**	1. Writing a dictionary; 2. Bowling, boxing, golf, tennis, weightlifting, etc.; 3. Alaska.
	SOS	S (so)—do, re, mi, fa, so, la, ti, do.
	ICE	Back, elbow, Gumby, the road, etc.
SET 36	**KISS**	1. Elizabeth Barrett Browning, EmilyDickenson, Adrienne Rich, Sylvia Plath, May Sarton, etc.; 2. Oxygen, fuel, ignition (heat); 3. Italy.
	SOS	Example: Area, Bib, Chronic, Test, Window, yummy, etc. We couldn't think of any for J, Q, V, and Z; can you?
	ICE	The invisible man, my own funeral, air, wind, faith, fairies, etc.
SET 37	**KISS**	1. Apostrophe, asterisk, backslash, brackets (angle, square or curly), colon, comma, dash, ellipsis points, exclamation point, forward slash, hyphen, parentheses, period, question mark, quotation marks, semi-colon, and single quotation marks; 2. Mercury; 3. Present-day Arkansas, Iowa, Kansas, Missouri, Nebraska, and Oklahoma were entirely included in the purchase. Most of North and South Dakota were included, and parts of Colorado, Minnesota, Montana, New Mexico, Texas, and Wyoming.
	SOS	Two quarters and one nickel; two of them are not a nickel.
	ICE	Belly button, middle child; middle of the night, Middlesex in England, etc.
SET 38	**KISS**	1. He created written Cherokee, even though he did not read in any other language; 2. $E=MC^2$; 3. Vatican City.
	SOS	Roll of toilet paper or roll of paper towel.
	ICE	"Did I leave the oven on?"; "Does this chute match my shoes?"; etc.
SET 39	**KISS**	1. Bach; 2. The ribs; 3. The Cherokee, Chickasaw, Choctaw, Muscogee, and Seminole, also known as the Five Civilized Tribes. Thousands of people died of exposure, disease and starvation en route.
	SOS	9 left; the others died.
	ICE	Could change size, color, shape, use, break into parts, add to it, etc.

SET 40	KISS	1. Japanese; 2. As a type of whale, the orca is a mammal; 3. Lanterns.
	SOS	I ought naught to owe for I ate nothing.
	ICE	Put your ring in an ice cube tray of water and freeze it; Pull up a piece of carpet in the corner; Tape it to the underside of a drawer; Weave it into a tapestry hung on your wall; etc.
SET 41	KISS	1. Cheshire; 2. Caves; 3. Abraham Lincoln.
	SOS	One hour; it is a wind-up clock.
	ICE	Do an ink spots painting; cast shadows; make origami; cover a hole in the wall; etc.
SET 42	KISS	1. The Limbo; 2. X; 3. British Library.
	SOS	A touchdown.
	ICE	You lost courage to run away; You left the stove on at home; etc.
SET 43	KISS	1. Misspell; 2. White blood cells; 3. Guatemala is in Central America.
	SOS	Get off the merry-go-round.
	ICE	Spiderman climbing the building; a loose elephant; skywriting; you, of course; etc.
SET 44	KISS	1. John Steinbeck's *Grapes of Wrath*; 2. Wandering Albatross (wingspan of up to 3.5 meters or 11 ft. 6 inches); 3. Lewis and Clark, Mark Anthony and Cleopatra, and Juan Peron and Evita.
	SOS	Thrifty; curiosity; variety.
	ICE	An array of hands holding one another; A beautiful sphere where the surfaces are different but equal; a circle of barbed wire; etc.
SET 45	KISS	1. Tchaikovsky; 2. Red, orange, yellow, green, blue, indigo, violet; 3. Provinces and territories.
	SOS	"e".
	ICE	Create a ballet company; Add a music room to the house with full orchestra; Indoor basketball court in the basement; etc.
SET 46	KISS	1. Hawaii, ski, spaghetti, etc.; 2. Milky Way; 3. Levi Strauss, makers of Levis, Dockers, Denizen, etc.
	SOS	Possible answers: Barber, beautician, a gossip, etc.
	ICE	Roof's leaking; The kids are dressing up with turbans for Halloween; She's having a garage sale; They are moving and she's using them to pack dishes; etc.
SET 47	KISS	1. *Romeo and Juliet*; 2. Leg; 3. France.
	SOS	The two apples that I took.
	ICE	Pay the $100; Place a post on your land three inches from his fence to hook your fence onto; Leave the opening just as it is and do not let children or pets roam your yard; Purchase your neighbor's house and hook on before reselling it; etc.

SET 48	**KISS**	1. Bow; 2. Praying mantis; 3. Ireland.
	SOS	You are the driver, what color are your eyes?
	ICE	Dry cleaning, your paycheck, a psychologist; etc.
SET 49	**KISS**	1. Don't, we've, you'll, etc.; 2. Cirrus, cirrocumulus, cirrostratus, cumulus, nimbus, stratocumulus, stratus, etc.; 3. Arizona, California, New Mexico, Texas, Utah, and parts of Colorado, Kansas, Oklahoma, and Wyoming.
	SOS	A map.
	ICE	Pay the person at the gate to watch it; hide it in a bathroom stall with "out of order" sign; get a wheelchair for it; etc.
SET 50	**KISS**	1. 17 syllables total, 5 – 7 – 5; 2. Pi is the ratio of a circle's circumference to its diameter, which is 3.14 when rounded to the nearest hundredth; 3. South Africa.
	SOS	The doctor hits the newborn baby so it cries and can then use its lungs.
	ICE	Sing To Our Pizza; Stop to open padlock; Send to obvious person; etc.
SET 51	**KISS**	1. A conductor; 2. Disc; 3. Arizona, Alaska, and Hawaii.
	SOS	1. Willa Mary; 2. Arthur; 3. Andy.
	ICE	Valiant Valerie vows victory very vociferously; Vibrant violet velvet vests violate vision; etc.
SET 52	**KISS**	1. Is, has, have, was, etc.; 2. The jaguar. Most other cats go for the throat; 3. President Theodore Roosevelt because he kept a bear from being killed.
	SOS	No; it still seems to be a mystery whether sharks ever sleep, so why take a chance.
	ICE	Never leave home; Use a conveyor belt; Walk on your hands; Put bread sacks over your shoes; etc.
SET 53	**KISS**	1. Two lines in poetry with the same meter that usually rhyme at the end; 2. Zinc; 3. Brazil, Chile, Peru, Venezuela, etc.;
	SOS	Armchair, grandfather clock, etc.
	ICE	Answers will vary. Can change others' thoughts and actions positively through mind control; Can walk through walls; Can make bosses give raises or promotions; etc.
SET 54	**KISS**	1. Rembrandt; 2. Isaac Newton; 3. Mandarin Chinese.
	SOS	False teeth.
	ICE	Paint an un-removable identifying ink mark on each; Give each distinctive clothes and forbid them from borrowing each other's clothes; send one to live with relatives; teach them to say their names whenever they enter the room; etc.

SET 55	**KISS**	1. "ly"; 2. The cranium; 3. The Ural Mountains.
	SOS	A dead centipede.
	ICE	A box of candy; A check to pay off the mortgage; A notice that you won the sweepstakes, etc.
SET 56	**KISS**	1. Miles Davis; Dizzy Gillespie; Charlie Parker; Sarah Vaughn, etc.; 2. Salt; 3. Longitude lines run north and south, and latitude lines run east and west.
	SOS	(1) Side – downside, inside, outside sidewalk; (2) Sign – sign language, neon sign, sign-off, stop sign; (3) Horse –workhorse, racehorse, horseradish, horsepower.
	ICE	"You think you're so hot"; "You look dog tired"; "Haven't I seen you around the grill?"; "Lets' play ball. You be the bat and I'll be the ball." etc.
SET 57	**KISS**	1. Brass, Strings, Percussion, Woodwinds; 2. Helium; 3. St. Andrews.
	SOS	July; the months are listed in alphabetical order.
	ICE	Run a mile on the potatoes because they provide more support; Put on waterproof diving gear to swim through the syrup without your body touching it; Refuse to do either no matter what the personal cost to you; etc.
SET 58	**KISS**	1. Pronouns; 2. 10; 3. Indonesia.
	SOS	The serious offense is voting twice in one day; it is a fraud.
	ICE	"I don't know how to tie it"; "I used my tie as a tourniquet to save someone on my way over"; etc.
SET 59	**KISS**	1. Curious George; 2. 32; 3. India.
	SOS	Mom – Mod – Mad – Dad.
	ICE	The stars; wind; love; another person's inner being; the center of the earth; the past; etc.
SET 60	**KISS**	1. Cymbals, kettle drums, tambourine, triangle, etc.' 2. Cricket—number of chirps in 15 seconds plus 39; 3. Australia; Mexico has the world's second largest barrier reef.
	SOS	Tree-T = Treaty.
	ICE	Drag over cookie dough to make a design; Make into a mobile; Sell as an antique; Use as a noise maker; etc.
SET 61	**KISS**	1. Listing items, between city and state, between day and year, when a pause is called for, etc.; 2. The *wrong* answer is a squirrel. It can run 12 mph, but bears can run 30 mph; 3. Prohibition of alcohol.
	SOS	Don't groan—a walker.
	ICE	"We're drilling for oil"; Stick up your hand if you think this latest gossip I heard yesterday is true; "Wonder what we'll find down there"; etc.

SET 62	**KISS**	1. *Pride and Prejudice*, *Sense and Sensibility*, *Emma*, etc.; 2. Mars—a day on Mars is 24 hours and 37 minutes, while a day on earth is 24 hours; 3. Augustus Caesar.
	SOS	Side, Wide, Wade, Wale, Walk.
	ICE	Cover it with clear plastic wrap; Do not drive your vehicle; Install an automatic wiper with sensor that detects dirt; Place it inside the back window; etc.
SET 63	**KISS**	1. Renaissance, 1400-1600. Baroque, 1600-1760. Classical, 1730-1820. Romantic, 1815-1910. 20th Century, 1900-2000; 2. Soles of the feet; 3. Peru's La Rinconada has an elevation of 16,732 feet.
	SOS	12 – the 2nd of each month. Did you groan? Okay, if you wanted to do the math that's 31,536,000 sec/year in a non-leap year.
	ICE	"Which of us will make the first move?"; "We are from different worlds. Can't we learn from each other?"; "Where is the rest of your family?"; "Darling, you look delicious!" "I'm told I have very bad taste"; etc.
SET 64	**KISS**	1. "Cried" – Exclaimed, screamed, wept, sobbed, etc. "Grumpy" – Cranky, peevish, irritable, etc. "Great" – absolute, awesome, distinguished, eminent, fantastic, first-rate, impressive, magnificent, sumptuous, wonderful, large, etc. 2. Trees that shed their leaves annually. 3. The Civil War, which began in 1861.
	SOS	Brown had a black tie; Black had a green tie; Green had a brown tie.
	ICE	Be polite; Offer money; Say you have five kids in the car; Say you have ice cream melting; etc.
SET 65	**KISS**	1. "American Cousin"; 2. Sedimentary, igneous, and metamorphic; 3. The Amazon and the Nile. Official title is disputed; different opinions as to how the measurement should be calculated.
	SOS	Abbreviation, condensation, hippopotamus, Pennsylvania, undercoating, etc.
	ICE	Homework, make work; workaholic, work of art, yard work, etc.
SET 66	**KISS**	1. Duet = 2, solo =1, trio = 3; 2. 144 square feet are needed--since there are nine square feet in one square yard, you would need to order 16 square yards; 3. (1) Freedom of speech, press, religion and petition; (2) Right to keep and bear arms; (3) Conditions for quarters of soldiers; (4) Right of search and seizure regulated; (5) Provisions concerning prosecution; (6) Right to a speedy trial, witnesses, etc.; (7) Right to trial by jury; (8) Protection from excessive bail and cruel punishment; (9) Rule of construction of the Constitution; and (10) Rights of the states under the Constitution.
	SOS	A hand.
	ICE	Cook up taffy to place in the hole; Sit on the hole in your raincoat when the storm occurs; Open your umbrella and place the handle down through the hole; borrow needed materials from neighbor; etc.

SET 67	**KISS**	1. Before a list of items, introduction to a long quotation, after a salutation in a business letter, etc.; 2. The humerus bone, which is near the largest unprotected nerve in the human body, and so it hurts a lot when you hit it; 3. Campbell.
	SOS	ACB.
	ICE	Have a prom where everyone gets a date; Have a Best True Compliment contest; etc.
SET 68	**KISS**	1. *Mein Kampf* by Adolph Hitler; 2. Eucalyptus tree; 3. Death Valley, CA.
	SOS	Aspen – pizza; Bradyn – cheeseburgers; Hannah – chicken; and Jack – hot dogs.
	ICE	*The Purple Prose Book*; *Recipes for the Bold at Heart*; *The Grapest Story Ever Told;* etc.
SET 69	**KISS**	1. David, Moses, Pieta, etc.; 2. False; 3. Ellis Island.
	SOS	(1) house; (2) school; (3) shoe.
	ICE	It keeps them from rusting; she has them ready whenever she serves a frozen dessert; She ran out of room in the utensil drawer; The spoons are made of ice; etc.
SET 70	**KISS**	1. The; 2. Electronic; 3. Egypt.
	SOS	Answers will vary. Example: Crest, frown, great, hover.
	ICE	The three bears; Three strikes; Trios; Triplets; Wise men at Christmas; etc.
SET 71	**KISS**	1. Cinderella; 2. Bubonic and Pneumonic Plague spread by fleas on rats; 3. The stock market crash in 1929 that led to the Great Depression.
	SOS	You are adding the legs of four cows (16 legs), two birds (4 legs) and one spider (8 legs) to get a total of 28 legs.
	ICE	Bring, ringing, ringworm, sharing, swearing, etc.
SET 72	**KISS**	1. 4; 2. Growing plants; 3. Actually, 116 years.
	SOS	Drop.
	ICE	Dust rag, mouse sleeping bag, hole plug, stuff a pillow, etc.
SET 73	**KISS**	1. Stationery—remember envelope when thinking whether this word should end with "ary" or "ery"; 2. Condensation; 3. China and India
	SOS	The numeral 8; take away the top half or the bottom half, and a zero will remain.
	ICE	Give her an umbrella; Put her in the ice box; Send Dorothy back to Kansas early with your frequent flier miles; etc.

SET 74	**KISS**	1. Allan a-Dale, Friar Tuck, Mush, Sebald, Maid Marian, Will Scarlett; 2.350 ft. fence; 3. Germany.
	SOS	Pain; main; drain.
	ICE	Computer keyboard, price tags, radio dials, road signs, swimming pools, prize ribbons; etc.
SET 75	**KISS**	1. Soprano, alto, tenor, bass; 2. Kinds of joints; 3. Arctic, Atlantic, Indian, and Pacific; the Pacific Ocean is the largest.
	SOS	There isn't such a thing as a mommy bull. Are you groaning again?
	ICE	Freezer in the trunk for groceries and frozen treats; periscope to see over vehicles ahead; a passenger mute button; etc.
SET 76	**KISS**	1. Aye & eye, flea & flee, pair & pear, etc.; 2. They are hatched there—insect lays egg in the apple blossom and at some point later the worm hatches in the heart of the apple; 3. The White House.
	SOS	(1) bean; (2) horn; (3) potato.
	ICE	Pillows, mud, cookie dough, gummy bears, etc.
SET 77	**KISS**	1. They were all famous writers who were blind; 2. H_2O; 3. New Zealand.
	SOS	OHIO.
	ICE	Blend, mend, tight end, the end, pretend, end of an era, etc.
SET 78	**KISS**	1. Athens; 2. Blue stars are the hottest; 3. The Himalayas.
	SOS	February, since it has the least amount of days.
	ICE	"How do you like my new hat?"; "What do you think of the answers the authors have provided so far?"; "What comes after 'ridicule' in the dictionary?"; etc.
SET 79	**KISS**	1. Examples: anti, dis, fore, inter, mid, mis, non, pre, pro, re, semi, sub, under, etc.; 2. Carry oxygen to all parts of the body; 3. Mao Zedong; also spelled Mao Tse Tung.
	SOS	Did you say June? Jackson has to be the third child.
	ICE	Who made a mess on the statue in the park?; What bird brings mail?; What do you want for dinner?; etc.
SET 80	**KISS**	1. There were 13 people at the Last Supper; 2. Dog, fox, horse, and man; 3. Gobi Desert.
	SOS	Build three pens and put three puppies in each; then build a fourth pen around the other three pens.
	ICE	On a dare; She had a date with the rooster over there; The grass looked greener on the other side; She was looking for her chicks; She was on a lark adventure; etc.

SET 81	**KISS**	1. 88; 2. Igneous; 3. A census.
	SOS	Bryan.
	ICE	Cake and frosting, snaps, tapes, two friends, Velcro, etc.
SET 82	**KISS**	1. Newspaper, sidewalk, pancake, etc.; 2. Tip travels faster than speed of sound (noise); 3. Hirohito.
	SOS	11 is the maximum possible; how many did you get?
	ICE	To get over insomnia; To get into the *Guinness Book of Records*; To get bored; etc.
SET 83	**KISS**	1. They are all literary devices; 2. 300; 3. Austria.
	SOS	Chris was digging a hole to plant a tree.
	ICE	Equal sign in math, identical twins, rights, pieces of candy, etc.
SET 84	**KISS**	1. Moderately fast, joyful and lively; 2. Clara Barton; 3. Mahatma Gandhi; Gandhi was a leader in the movement to free India from British colonial rule through non-violent civil disobedience. His work continues to inspire non-violent activism around the world.
	SOS	C, for Cupid, one of Santa's reindeer.
	ICE	Inauguration of the first female U.S. president; Rose Bowl; etc.
SET 85	**KISS**	1. Five (as-tro-nom-i-cal); 2. Cheetah; 3. Russia.
	SOS	The man was a professional blind hanger for window blinds.
	ICE	When did you retrofit the Universe, or did it enter the fifth-dimension by merit?; When did you drop the paperweight, or did it shatter the glass by earthquake?"; etc.
SET 86	**KISS**	1. Alliteration, specifically consonance; 2. Answers will vary. Examples: carbon, gene, molecule, stars, tungsten; 3. Washington, Jackson, Van Buren, Taylor, Fillmore, Lincoln, Andrew Johnson, Cleveland, and Truman.
	SOS	Possible: The mother is a goat with her kids; They were camping with appropriate equipment; etc.
	ICE	A cake baked in a measuring cup; Jelly stored in a hollow log; Clean the springs of a bed; A new wardrobe for the turkey; etc.
SET 87	**KISS**	1. Two violins, a viola, and a cello; 2. Uniform Resource Locator; 3. Christopher Columbus' flagship.
	SOS	All of the men were married.
	ICE	"What is your name?"; "What did you use for shortening for the cake?"; "What did the matador say to the senorita?"; "Was he an "ole" man or "young" man?"; etc.

SET 88	**KISS**	1. Kindergarten (German); 2. Answers will vary, Examples: badminton, hockey, horse racing, running, sailing, skiing, etc.; 3. Italy.
	SOS	Al swims for the Dolphins. Pam plays basketball for the Tigers. Bob plays soccer for the Sharks, and Sue runs track for the Road Runners.
	ICE	Be a "night owl"; Own your own ear plugs; Have a driver's license; Degree in psychology; Crowd control skills; etc.
SET 89	**KISS**	1. Assonance; William Wordsworth; 2. Stones; 3. Susan B. Anthony and Sacagawea
	SOS	She was reading Braille.
	ICE	A broken chair, gelatin, nose, worms, etc.
SET 90	**KISS**	1. Franz Joseph Haydn; 2. A six-sided figure; 3. Alaska.
	SOS	A notable surgeon had no table and therefore was not able to operate.
	ICE	Snap, fingers, hand, shake, French fries; Snap, crackle, leaves, break ups, lonely; etc.
SET 91	**KISS**	1. Earnestly, efficiently, quickly, quietly, etc.; 2. Bowling, golf, tennis, football; 3. Prisoner of War.
	SOS	Wild – Mild – Mile – Tile – Tale – Tame.
	ICE	Hide; Listen and keep your mouth shut; Show up and ask questions; Quit; Call in sick; Pretend you have laryngitis; etc.
SET 92	**KISS**	1. John Bartlett, author of *Familiar Quotations*; 2. 12 years; 3. Cultivation of land, wheel, Pyramids.
	SOS	Pajamas, Aspirin: Indigo: Gopher: Erase: Severe: Retire.
	ICE	Never go out at night; When you see a shoe, run; Walk in line; Save the queen at all costs; etc.
SET 93	**KISS**	1. Play or sing strong and loud; 2. Nail rusting; 3. Pacific.
	SOS	Lea, because the higher the elevation the lower the boiling point.
	ICE	A flying arrow; A boat floating with the current; A bright ray of light; A cloud; etc.
SET 94	**KISS**	1. Come, give, moved, sang, told, etc.; 2. The Big Bang is the prevailing scientific theory explaining the origins of the universe. It suggests that at the beginning of the universe all space was contained in a single point that exploded (BANG!). And the universe has been expanding ever since. As we hope your mind is! ☺; 3. July.
	SOS	Probably, because a panther, a mountain lion and a puma are all different names for the same animal.
	ICE	Make them glow in the dark; Perm the feathers, Do a Mohawk, etc.

SET 95	KISS	1. *Gone With the Wind*; 2. No; 3. Japan.
	SOS	Put a predator in the tank with them.
	ICE	Coins, houses, mattress, pancakes, your lid, etc.
SET 96	KISS	1. Germany; 2. A caterpillar has 4000 muscles, a human has 792; 3. Gross National Product.
	SOS	She had an automatic transmission.
	ICE	Busy as a (mosquito); Stubborn as a (spoiled child); Arrogant as (politician); etc.
SET 97	KISS	1. WOW! (interjection) The (article) brown (adjective) dog (noun) jumped (verb) quickly (adverb) over (preposition) my (pronoun), fence (noun) and (conjunction) gate (noun); 2. Diamond, ruby, sapphire, opal, amethyst, etc.; 3. Lye.
	SOS	Mike had wished for "a hundred bucks."
	ICE	California – Dreaming in the Sun; Texas, You're always Home in the Lone Star State; etc.
SET 98	KISS	1. "It was the best of times; it was the worst of times; 2. 24; 3. Denver, CO.
	SOS	Yes, fold your arms before you pick up each end of the rope and then pull your arms apart.
	ICE	Jennifer had surgery; Jennifer was dreaming that she was waking up and that the Lone Ranger was there to save her; Jennifer was actually married to the Masked Marvel; etc.
SET 99	KISS	1. Sister Rosetta Tharpe; 2. Yes, the tags were originally used as a health measure to let people know it was a used mattress; 3. Dynamite.
	SOS	Grape: Permafrost: Sty: Typhoon: Onset: Etcetera.
	ICE	*Entering the Stream of Life*; *I Had to Write a Book and This is It*; *At the Top of the Mountain: Now What?*; *It Wasn't Me; An Ordinary Life*; etc.
SET 100	KISS	1. Example: N – He took a fancy to her. V- I fancy her, too. Adj. – She wore fancy coats.; 2. Piranha; 3. Indonesia.
	SOS	Fresh: Shame: Mean: Annex: Except.
	ICE	They were playing badminton; In a popular golf tournament, Tim hit his golf ball too near Bob, which put him in a position to earn a birdie; Tim and Bob were playing a computer game with cheering crowd sound effects called "Little Birdie; etc.
SET 101	KISS	1. Anne Frank; 2. Carbon dioxide; 3. Military Police.
	SOS	"It" – This is an "oldie".
	ICE	Black-out, blueberry, orange grove, Red River, etc.

SET 102	**KISS**	1. Three; 2. Void of matter, including air, as in outer space; 3. The Vatican.
	SOS	They all have heels.
	ICE	Canned or frozen foods, letters, people, professions, displays, photos, etc.
SET 103	**KISS**	1. She has no one to mow her lawn; 2. It can lead to antibiotics-resistant bacteria; 3. About 70%.
	SOS	Three; one pig, one cow and one horse.
	ICE	Two talking mouths in a circle with the phrase "Chatfield, MN, the Center of Friendly Conversation" around it; etc.
SET 104	**KISS**	1. Pearl Buck; 2. Flounder; 3. George Gallup.
	SOS	Seas, sees, seize.
	ICE	Come in second because "I hate being a 'loser'"; Come in last four times but win every fifth contest because "I am an official winner"; Refuse to participate "Because I never want to lose"; etc.
SET 105	**KISS**	1. An eighth note counts as one beat; 2. Small; 3. Missouri and Tennessee.
	SOS	21.
	ICE	Great cast! Can't wait for the reviews!
SET 106	**KISS**	1. Communication, communicator; 2. Remainder; 3. Answer will vary depending on the state and point in time.
	SOS	The wagon.
	ICE	Container for dirty clothes; Make a ghost; Doll's table cloth; etc.
SET 107	**KISS**	1. Iris; 2. False; if one is eating a balanced diet and getting enough calories, it doesn't matter if food temperature is hot or cold; 3. In addition to being famous, they all went deaf or hard of hearing.
	SOS	Sleeplessness.
	ICE	Don't want to eat certain icky food; It's your turn to give a speech and you are unprepared; You are acting in a play; etc.
SET 108	**KISS**	1. A ballet movement in which the dancer bends at the knees with back straight; 2. Wild rice is not rice, it is marsh grass seed; 3. Lichtenstein, Luxemburg, Monaco, Vatican, etc.
	SOS	(8888-888)/8 = 1000.
	ICE	Possible answer: Braid her hair, cut off the braid, tie it to something in the room, and climb down; Throw her mattress down on the ground and jump down on the mattress; Call fire department; etc.
SET 109	**KISS**	1. Moccasin; 2. Hydrogen; 3. The Japanese attacked Pearl Harbor on December 7, 1941.
	SOS	Push the cork into the bottle and shake the coin out.
	ICE	Your mind, your body, elastic, rubber bands, fishing stories, the truth, etc.

SET 110	**KISS**	1. A metaphor; it does not use "like" or "as"; 2. Cheese . . . we mean basalt; 3. About 2800 miles.
	SOS	Answers will vary. Examples: con, confident, dent, dental, find, etc.
	ICE	You catch more flies with (a baseball glove); (All work and no play) is just plain mean; Fools rush in (whenever there's a sale); Slow and steady (annoys the driver behind you); etc.
SET 111	**KISS**	1. France (in the Court of Louis XIV); 2. Ultraviolet; 3. Two—Andrew Johnson and Bill Clinton were impeached by the U.S. House of Representatives, but acquitted by the Senate. Richard Nixon resigned before he could be impeached.
	SOS	A square cover could fall in if it is inserted into the hole diagonally, but a round manhole cover cannot fall through its circular opening. In addition, round covers do not need to be rotated or precisely aligned when placing them on the opening, and a round manhole cover can be easily rolled and moved along the street or ground.
	ICE	Ideas, because they are not limited by facts and happen when awake; Knowledge, because knowledge can be verified and shared while ideas and dreams can be contested; Dreams, because they can take us beyond the limits of the everyday world; etc.
SET 112	**KISS**	1. Principal; 2. False; 3. France.
	SOS	Pickle-O = Piccolo.
	ICE	An arm and a leg, Anthony and Cleopatra, bacon and eggs, Bert and Ernie, Beauty and the Beast, the Smothers brothers, etc.
SET 113	**KISS**	1. A simile; it uses "like" or "as"; 2. Limestone; 3. United States.
	SOS	Answers will vary. Examples: axe, elation, lax, relax, tear, etc.
	ICE	Chairs, clothes, hide-a-bed, paper, slice of bread, etc.
SET 114	**KISS**	1. Brazil; 2. Any problems? 139 is not divisible by 9; 3. Liberia, an African nation founded by ex-American slaves, which adopted its current flag in 1847.
	SOS	One hour 20 minutes and 80 minutes are the same duration.
	ICE	It's your symbol. Things to consider: What shape, color, animals or object do you see as powerful?
SET 115	**KISS**	1. "Pig"; 2. Closed; 3. Massachusetts, North Carolina and South Carolina.
	SOS	Snail, deer, horse.
	ICE	Young at Heart; Those Were the Days; Tired and Retired, etc.
SET 116	**KISS**	1. Antithesis; 2. A horse, Secretariat; 3. Grover Cleveland.
	SOS	The time and date is 12:34, 5/6/78.
	ICE	Surprise birthday party; Internal affairs investigation; Use of anti-aging cream; etc.

SET 117	**KISS**	1. Kiln; 2. Yes, when head wind is greater than the maximum air speed.; 3. No, he signed the Declaration of Independence.
	SOS	40 – 12 = 28.
	ICE	It's not over 'til (I win.); People who live in glass houses (should keep their clothes on.); A rolling stone (can squish you.) You can't judge a book (by how much it costs.); etc.
SET 118	**KISS**	1. Front of the ship, weapon, knot, lowering one's head in worship, Japanese expression of respect for another, bending under weight, tool to play a string instrument, etc.; 2. Isaac Newton; 3. New Mexico.
	SOS	Answers will vary. Example: three, ruled, bunny, meant.
	ICE	Duct tape hanging on a string inside the door; Fine people who make noise; Require everyone to take off their shoes at entry; etc.
SET 119	**KISS**	1. Personification; 2. basketball, baseball, basketball, football; 3. Italy, Mexico, Japan.
	SOS	They said "Hi Jean" (hygiene).
	ICE	Fly, to save airplane fares; Invisible, because I'm nosy; Neither, because I'd feel out of place; etc.
SET 120	**KISS**	1. 1800s; 2. Zoologists; 3. Hawaii, Arizona, and Kentucky.
	SOS	Mt. Everest has always been the tallest mountain in the world, even before it was discovered.
	ICE	Cutting in line; long-winded stories; people thinking they "know better"; unsolicited advice; etc.
SET 121	**KISS**	1. Examples: saw; did; 2. It boils at a higher temperature; 3. Answers will vary. Example: Countries, Geography, Map, Sociology, Timeline.
	SOS	One; you have birthdays, but only one birth day.
	ICE	Jam on celery; Banana on steaks; Peanut butter on cereal; etc.
SET 122	**KISS**	1. Gertrude Stein / Rudyard Kipling / F. Scott Fitzgerald; 2. Lines that never meet or cross each other, like railroad Tracks; 3. Arlington National Cemetery in Arlington, Virginia.
	SOS	(1) Market; (2) Cut; (3) Light.
	ICE	"How old are you?"; "How many train cars did you have to wait for?"; etc.
SET 123	**KISS**	1. She was a documentary photographer; 2. The **hyoid bone** in the throat, which has as its only purpose to support/anchor the tongue; 3. United Kingdom.
	SOS	(1) Russian; (2) German; (3) Dutch; (4) Hungarian.
	ICE	Many bugs buzz over Jackson's friend Quinn while he plays with boxes; etc.

SET 124	KISS	1. Desert; 2. A snail; 3. J. Edger Hoover.
	SOS	Pup – Pug – Dug – Dog.
	ICE	"Leave a message if I won the lottery"; "You have the wrong number"; "Greetings from outer space"; etc.
SET 125	KISS	1. Oedipus; 2. Carbon; 3. Kansas; North Dakota.
	SOS	Gangster, hamster, monster, plaster, register, roaster, rooster, etc.
	ICE	1 square X 2 = 1 rectangle; 2 geniuses X 3 tornados = 6 brainstorms; 3 cats + 2 mice = 0 mice; 2 pieces of candy ÷ 3 children = a fight; etc.
SET 126	KISS	1. Landscapes; 2. Common denominator, Geometry, Multiplication, Subtraction, Tabulate, etc.; 3. Turkey.
	SOS	There are no two exactly alike.
	ICE	Contact paper; A rug; A gift bag; String; Staples; etc.
SET 127	KISS	1. Anyway; 2. Food—most people can survive for a month or more without food. However, sleep- deprived last only 10 days before they will die; 3. The Great Wall of China.
	SOS	House numbers.
	ICE	Noun – because nouns get to play in every sentence, but sometimes the adjectives get left out; Noun – because "fun" is a noun. Adjective – because adjectives are "flashy" and "adaptable"; etc.
SET 128	KISS	1. The use of humorous exaggeration to ridicule or criticize human stupidity and vices; 2. Flea; 3. Delaware, Pennsylvania, Texas.
	SOS	Examples: dream; spent; pecan; waist; etc.
	ICE	Cell phone, toilet paper, photos, myself, etc.
SET 129	KISS	1. It emphasized individual craftsmanship in reaction to the industrialization of design; 2. Generally, things contract when they are cold, making them more brittle; 3. Driving while intoxicated.
	SOS	Four years ago.
	ICE	A bee, because folks would get the point; An ant, as long as I was the queen with all those workers spoiling me; etc.
SET 130	KISS	1. **Subservient** – Inferior or less / **Rescind** – Cancel or repeal / **Contiguous** – Connected or adjoining; 2. Turn the second fraction upside down and multiply it times the first fraction, then reduce; for example, 2/3 ÷ 1/3 = 2/3 X 3/1 = 6/3 = 2; 3. Arizona.
	SOS	Successfully; unsuccessfully.
	ICE	A grumpy red and yellow fuzz ball that illustrates boredom; A special name for an inexperienced bungee jumper; etc.

SET 131	**KISS**	1. Aphrodite, Apollo, Ares, Artemis, Athena, Demeter, Hades, Hera, Zeus. etc.; 2. The Heimlich Maneuver; 3. "We the people . . ."
	SOS	Six small and four large peaches.
	ICE	A tree farm owner to the police; Santa Claus, after coming down the chimney and finding that this year they don't have any Christmas trees for his gifts; etc.
SET 132	**KISS**	1. Amish, Shakers, etc.; 2. Blue stars are the hottest; 3. House of Commons.
	SOS	You drove in reverse.
	ICE	Tricky trigonometry triggers teen test takers to trepidation; etc.
SET 133	**KISS**	1. Carnation, Illumination, Resignation, Indignation; 2. Jade; 3. London, Rome, Paris, San Francisco.
	SOS	Hannah-trucker; Bradyn-engineer; Aspen-accountant; Jackson-teacher.
	ICE	Use juice to trap insects; Do a Marlon Brando impression from the *Godfather* movie; Use to illustrate the color orange for preschoolers; Use them to fertilize your grounds; etc.
SET 134	**KISS**	1. He lies and cries wolf as a joke too many times, so when the wolf really comes, no one believes him; 2. False; Lasers focus light waves; 3. The toothbrush.
	SOS	Cold, hot, light.
	ICE	Stunt double speaking to the designer of the volcano movie set; Pele to the bellhop at her vacation resort; Athlete to the coach of the Volcano's team; etc.
SET 135	**KISS**	1. Late 19th-early 20th century—French phrase *Nouveau Riche* means "Newly rich"; 2. Hearing, sight; 3. Germany.
	SOS	French; Scotch; Swedish; English.
	ICE	Toothpick for a dragon; picture hanger; make jewelry; etc.
SET 136	**KISS**	1. Catalog, Catnip, Category, and Catcher; 2. Five pairs of legs; 3. Antarctica.
	SOS	Made mashed potatoes or potato salad.
	ICE	A burned marshmallow; Black and white jelly beans; Oreo cookies; etc.
SET 137	**KISS**	1. Slow and steady wins the race; 2. A bridge is exposed to wind and cold air above, below and on either side, but the road is insulated by the earth, so it only loses heat from the top; 3. They were all famous walls.
	SOS	A sponge.
	ICE	Make people carry wastebaskets at all time; Get rid of fast food restaurants; etc.
SET 138	**KISS**	1. Antoni Gaudi, Thomas Jefferson, Christopher Wren, and Frank Lloyd Wright; 2. Zero—any number times zero is zero; 3. Zambia, Zimbabwe.
	SOS	Act makes the words "exact", "enact", and "react".
	ICE	Alisha – Always let Ida share her apples; Renie – Run every night into eternity; etc.

SET 139	**KISS**	1. Bellhop; *For Whom the Bell Tolls*; Queen Isabella; 2. Femur; 3. All competed in Olympic Games.
	SOS	Daylight savings time in all states that observe Daylight savings time.
	ICE	Sell tickets to see the haunted house; Tell the sellers you are allergic to ghosts; Donate it to the historical society; Charge the ghosts rent; etc.
SET 140	**KISS**	1. Travel and communication; 2. Five; 3. Chicago, London, New York City, Paris.
	SOS	Three; one apple tree, one cherry tree, and one peach tree.
	ICE	Make a large pin cushion; Sell house; Make a food trail leading outside; Have your spouse do it; etc.
SET 141	**KISS**	1. Grant Wood; 2. The liquid mercury expands and rises as it gets warmer, and it contracts and drops as it cools down; 3. Canada.
	SOS	Monday.
	ICE	Noah's 40 days and 40 nights of rain during the flood; The back forty; The big 4-0 (birthday); etc.
SET 142	**KISS**	1. Pittsburgh—people forget the "h" at the end; 2. The Moon passes between the Earth and the Sun, blocking all or part of our view of the sun; 3. Mayflower.
	SOS	Paul Revere – "The British are coming!"
	ICE	"Duh"; "Puke," "The Song I Wrote Because My Ex Did Me Wrong And I Don't Know What to Do, Because My Car Won't Start"; etc.
SET 143	**KISS**	1. Love and beauty; 2. Facial communication, keeping sweat out of your eyes, and they provide shade; 3. Reno. It's true; check the map.
	SOS	Blades; keys.
	ICE	Xs & Os; Dog and Cat; etc.
SET 144	**KISS**	1. Neoclassical; 2. Box Turtle – 100+ years; Chimpanzee – 20 years; cow – 15 years; 3. England, France, Spain.
	SOS	(1) startling; (2) starting; (3) staring; (4) string; (5) sting; (6) sing; (7) sin; (8) in; (9) I.
	ICE	Have them say the alphabet backwards; Have a quiet contest; etc.
SET 145	**KISS**	1. My house is your house; 2. Iron is an element, while steel is an alloy of iron with carbon and other elements. Among other things, steel is stronger and less brittle than iron, making it a more stable building material; 3. England, Scotland, Wales, and Northern Ireland.
	SOS	Outside back.
	ICE	Keep vacuum cleaner sales up; As magic fairy dust; Make fine sand paper out of it; To sell furniture polish; To write in; etc.

SET 146	**KISS**	1. War; 2. 50%; 3. The value to you of what is needed or wanted that you will have to do without because you chose something else.
	SOS	Smile: Lean: Andes: Estimate: Tentacles.
	ICE	Root beer; Peanut butter & jelly; etc.
SET 147	**KISS**	1. Using only one color; 2. The stirrup, in the ear; 3. Okay.
	SOS	Bread, not toast; of course you can also toast bagels, baguettes, and even tortillas in a toaster.
	ICE	Morning Glory; Eat Quick; Yucky Bran, etc.
SET 148	**KISS**	1. Brain; 2. Grafting; 3. Italy.
	SOS	That was a sample number.
	ICE	Horror movie scene; mouse; surprise party; etc.
SET 149	**KISS**	1. The sea; 2. Rock vein of ore in a mine; 3. Spoiled meat.
	SOS	Denise placed first.
	ICE	Principle, because you have to be brave to stand up for it; Principal, because he or she can choose principles or not; etc.
SET 150	**KISS**	1. A mural or mural technique painted on wet plaster; 2. Colds are caused by viruses that do not respond to antibiotics; 3. Thomas Jefferson.
	SOS	**Grown**; **defe**at; **koala**; **mark**; **porcupine**; **jazz**; **quiet**; **yucca**; extra; **violin**; **bash**ful, **tur**tle.
	ICE	Eyebrows, mountains, moonbeams, clouds, etc.
SET 151	**KISS**	1. "The"; next most often is "of" and third most often is "and"; 2. Backstroke, rowing, tug of war; 3. The U.S. Constitution.
	SOS	Let some air out of the tires.
	ICE	"Ever happen to you?"; "I'm so very sorry Mr. President, here is my napkin"; "Congress should pass a law about these cups"; etc.
SET 152	**KISS**	1. The king of the gods; 2. Raptors; such as eagles, falcons and hawks that can see eight times better than humans; 3. Pop-up toaster (1919), lie detector (1921), TV (1923).
	SOS	1) Julia Child; 2) Pablo Picasso; 3) Marcel Marceau.
	ICE	Lizard-shaped taco called the harp taco; I munched on my taco as the lizard ran back and forth over the harp strings; Lizards like to eat tacos while harp music is playing; The band named the Lizards has a harp, and they are also taco lovers; etc.
SET 153	**KISS**	1. A painting technique which uses small dots of color to create an image; 2. Most plastics are made from petrochemicals, which include oil, natural gas, coal, or renewable sources such as corn or sugar cane; 3. Arabia, Italy, and France.
	SOS	Drawing an "I" over the bottom line of an "L" gives you a four, which means L+I=4.
	ICE	And the Emmy goes to . . .

SET 154	**KISS**	1. Rotaregirfer (Cool!); 2. Reduce using 19 for 4/5; and 17 for 5/6; 3. Buddhism, Christianity, Hinduism, Islam, Judaism, Paganism (or Indigenous Traditional Faiths)
	SOS	The word "ton".
	ICE	A good, long book; camera; extra oxygen; a cat; a fishing pole; etc.
SET 155	**KISS**	1. Athens was named for Athena, and she gave them the olive tree; 2. Human; 3. Alaska.
	SOS	Pencil sharpening.
	ICE	Trunk of a car; On the torch of the Statue of Liberty; the International Space Station; etc.
SET 156	**KISS**	1. Corinthian; Doric are the plainest, Ionic are scrolled, and Corinthian are fluted with both leaves and scrolls; 2. Elephant; 3. Lincoln; President Ford was not elected.
	SOS	He juggled the gold coins all the way across the bridge.
	ICE	Cold snap, fingers, jeans, gingersnap cookies, "pans" spelled backwards, etc.
SET 157	**KISS**	1. "Tree"; 2. $; 3. Examples: Siddhartha/Buddha, Maya, Prajapati, Tara, Ananda, Dalai lama, etc.
	SOS	Jack-of-all-trades; Jack-be-nimble; Jackknife; Jack Frost.
	ICE	Move away; Invest in better curtains; Ask them why they did it, since those bushes stood on your land; Share your disappointment and concern with them; Forgive them; Build a fence; Take them to court; etc.
SET 158	**KISS**	1. In autobiography the author writes about her/his own life, and in a biography the author writes about someone else; 2. The equator; 3. Washington.
	SOS	The future.
	ICE	Leave it; Try to sell it; Give it to someone you don't like; Throw it in the dumpster; Check on its appraised value; etc.
SET 159	**KISS**	1. It was the theatre where Shakespeare and his theatre troop originally performed most of Shakespeare's plays; 2. 60-100 beats per minute; 3. Answers may vary. Examples: Jesus, Peter, Paul, Virgin Mary, Mary Magdalene, John the Baptist, etc.
	SOS	Remove "Raccoon" and you have ORANGE.
	ICE	Porcupine meat balls; A ball of barbed wire; Me before I've had my coffee in the morning; etc.
SET 160	**KISS**	1. First word in a sentence, the pronoun "I", the first word and all other major words in a book or article title, proper names, etc.; 2. False; 3. Chicago.
	SOS	Your breath.
	ICE	Is a good thing; Buy an air conditioner; There'd sure be a lot of manure; Think and think some more.

SET 161	**KISS**	1. Gods and goddesses from Norse mythology, Odin was the ruler of the gods, Thor was god of thunder and battle, Loki was the trickster god of mischief, Freyja was goddess of love and fertility, and Hel was goddess of the underworld; 2. Sleet; 3. Seven.
	SOS	Stairs.
	ICE	Ice tray, fireplace, under the rug, light socket, etc.
SET 162	**KISS**	1. A poetic meter, or rhythm, made up of 5 two-syllable "feet" in which the second syllable is stressed and the first syllable is unstressed; 2. A pair of dice contains a total of 42 dots; 3. Answers may vary—Examples: Rama, Sita, Hanuman, Brahma, Krishna, etc.
	SOS	Birthday candles.
	ICE	Bake more things with peanut butter; Easily get gum and glue out of fabric and bugs off windshields; Eliminate odors and squeaks; Leather cleaner; Bait for mousetraps; use as door stops, etc.
SET 163	**KISS**	1. I, me, you, your, their, myself, herself, yourself, ourselves, themselves, etc.; 2. Below 120/80; 3.Istanbul, Turkey.
	SOS	Roller skates.
	ICE	"We wouldn't have to fix the broken garbage disposal"; "My uncle is a vet"; "You would finally have a friend"; "You won't need an alarm clock"; "We can keep up with the Jones' barking dog" etc.
SET 164	**KISS**	1. Biography, fable, memoir, myth, novel, play, poem, short story, etc.; 2. Pads of paws, nose and tongue; 3. Mohamed, Ali, Rumi, Maryam, etc.
	SOS	desert – rain.
	ICE	Knock it around the edge and try again to open it; Get a big wrench to give you leverage in opening it; Take a hammer and knock a hole in the cover; Ask someone stronger; etc.
SET 165	**KISS**	1. A contrived ending—It comes from the ancient Greek theatre conventions of using a machine to bring in an actor playing a god or goddess at the end of the play to resolve the plot in an excessively easy manner; 2. One million years; 3. Arizona, Colorado, New Mexico, and Utah.
	SOS	(1) ha; (2) pe; (3) co.
	ICE	Sponge Bob Square Pants; City square; Square frame; You're a square; Tool square; Square root; Square dance; etc.
SET 166	**KISS**	1. Eat your heart out!; 2. When the Moon is on the far side of the Earth, opposite the Sun, the Moon passes through the shadow of the Earth; 3. Hawaii.
	SOS	These nine words are all contained within the word "therein" when read left-to-right.
	ICE	Lying under a tree in solitude; Clear water in a still pool; etc.

SET 167	KISS	1. In the Trojan War, the Greeks built the horse as a fake gift for the Trojans. In the night after the Trojans brought the horse inside the city wall, two Greek soldiers hidden inside the horse were able to let the Greek army in to defeat them; 2. In the neck; 3. Abraham, Sarah, David, Moses, Ruth, Esther, Elijah, etc.
	SOS	Place a large sheet of paper over the threshold under a closed door with the brothers on opposite sides of the door standing on the paper.
	ICE	Turn back; Stop and wait for them to pass; Step over them; Bring your pet aardvark along; etc.
SET 168	KISS	1. "Silent Night"; 2. False, it is a live marine animal; 3. Ohio.
	SOS	They are all different words when spelled backwards – diaper, drawer, and spools.
	ICE	Get paid to nap/go to the beach; A lost friend returns; Your favorite celebrity proposes to you; etc.
SET 169	KISS	1. Lie; 2. An instrument that registers earthquake activity; 3. Members of the labor union for workers in transportation industries, the name reflects that originally these people drove teams of horses.
	SOS	None; they were blackbirds. However, there were four and twenty blackbirds in the nursery rhyme.
	ICE	Bed bugs in the clothes; A genuine Van Gogh painting for ten dollars; etc.
SET 170	KISS	1. Limerick, sonnet, haiku, villanelle, ode, elegy, blank verse, etc.; 2. A quadrillion; 3. Wyoming.
	SOS	Toenail.
	ICE	Stick Your Nose Up, MA; Too Hot, AZ; No Vacancy, NE; etc.
SET 171	KISS	1. Ceramics or pottery, glass blowing, macramé, metal work, weaving, wood working etc.; 2. When a person is exposed to cold and the body's core temperature drops below the level needed for normal body functioning. Mild hypothermia leads to mental confusion; severe hypothermia can be fatal; 3. The straight sections are usable as airstrips in times of war or other emergencies.
	SOS	Many eggs are laid on ledges rather than a nest, and this shape makes them roll in a tight circle which can keep them from falling off the ledge.
	ICE	Flower secrets; Silence; The willow weeping; The buzz on the bees; Time passing; etc.
SET 172	KISS	1. See, sea, sequential, siesta, etc.; 2. Giraffe; 3. The period after World War II when political tensions were high between Eastern Block (the Soviet Union and its Warsaw Pact allies) and Western Bloc (The U.S. and its NATO allies).
	SOS	Saturday.
	ICE	An elephant without a trunk; A monkey gymnast; A new fad diet; etc.

SET 173	**KISS**	1. Aeschylus, Aristotle, Euripides, Homer, Pindar, Plato, Sappho, Sophocles, etc.; 2. Yeast; 3. Siberia in Russia.
	SOS	The oil to pack them in is more expensive per ounce than the fish per volume.
	ICE	Crossed out; Teepee; Two crossed sticks; Signature of someone who doesn't know how to write; etc.
SET 174	**KISS**	1. Japan; 2. X-rays; 3. U.S.; Italy, France, United Kingdom, Russia, etc.
	SOS	Hula: Latin: Inch: Chintz: Tzar: Artist: Star.
	ICE	He was in trouble; he was a gunslinger in the Wild West; it was the only seat available; etc.
SET 175	**KISS**	1. Metro; 2. Cardio-Pulmonary Resuscitation; 3. Minnesota.
	SOS	Chicken (egg and chicken).
	ICE	Brillo®, Jello®, Kleenex®, etc.
SET 176	**KISS**	1. Characters, times, setting, plot, etc.; 2. Kodiak, or Alaskan Brown Bear; Nine.
	SOS	All of them are types of candy.
	ICE	Vote for the Polka Dot Party; Make Pancake Day a national holiday; Start a "Total Forgiveness for Politicians" campaign; etc.
SET 177	**KISS**	1. *Aida, Carmen, Die Fledermaus, La bohème, Madama Butterfly, Marriage of Figaro, Tosca*, etc.; 2. H2O water; 3. They were labor organizers and civil rights activists who advocated for the rights of migrant workers and started what would become the United Farm Workers labor union.
	SOS	Contact lenses, eyeglasses, optometrist, ophthalmologist, etc.
	ICE	Underwear through the Ages; Teetotalers Propaganda; Things That Go Bump in the Night; etc.
SET 178	**KISS**	1. What was, isn't what is / What was, was / What is, is; 2. A decimal point; 3. Arizona.
	SOS	U-Knight =unite.
	ICE	Pick your teeth, prick holes in something, Pick a lock, etc.
SET 179	**KISS**	1. The one less traveled; 2. The mosquito, because it carries and transmits deadly diseases such as malaria and yellow fever. Statistically: Humans are #2; 3. Ella Baker, James Farmer, Martin Luther King, John Lewis, Rosa Parks, Malcolm X, etc.
	SOS	He is playing baseball.
	ICE	Well Worn Sneakers contest, winner receives an odor eater; Worst Chicken Clucking Contest, winner receives a wet hen statuette; Ugly Baby Beauty Pageant, winner receives a covered stroller; etc.

SET 180	**KISS**	1. Frida Kahlo, Rembrandt, Van Gogh, etc. / Rembrandt–62; Van Gogh–40; 2. Green; 3. Chicago.
	SOS	The authors are guessing it is a hot air balloon! What is your guess?
	ICE	Wait 'til it rains; Car wash; Give her a washtub for her birthday; Get the fire truck to hose her off; etc.
SET 181	**KISS**	1. The teacher says, "The principal is a fool." "The teacher," says the principal, "is a fool."; 2. Peanut oil; 3. Presidents Carter, George H. Bush, Clinton, George W. Bush, Obama, and Trump were all living at this writing, so none of them are currently buried on U.S. soil.
	SOS	A good buy or a goodbye.
	ICE	Soup; Sand; Water in a glass; etc.
SET 182	**KISS**	1. Victor Hugo, Charlotte Bronte, Mary Shelley, Edgar Allen Poe, John Keats, etc.; 2. Sunlight reflecting off the surface of the moon; 3. In front of the Lincoln Memorial in Washington, D.C. as part of the 1963 March on Washington.
	SOS	Your sister; you have the same parents and get half of your genes from each, while you and your mom each only have half of the same genes!
	ICE	Bat, cat, cow, dog, pig, rat, etc.
SET 183	**KISS**	1. Triangle; 2. An emetic is a medicine or potion that makes you vomit, which you should take if you've consumed certain poisons or other harmful substances; 3. Venezuela; these falls are 15 times higher than the Niagara Falls.
	SOS	Anyone see the bee?
	ICE	Heat the floor of his pen; Use fire crackers; etc.
SET 184	**KISS**	1. "Its" has an apostrophe only when it is a contraction; 2. Examples: Anemone, crocus, daffodil, Dutch iris, onion, tulip, etc.; 3. George III.
	SOS	You are absolutely right.
	ICE	Surprise party; You forgot that you sold your house; The cleaning crew is running late; You mixed up the dates of your dinner party; your house is on fire; etc.
SET 185	**KISS**	1. Schoolmaster; 2. True; 3. New Hampshire.
	SOS	You are a cutie, I am one too!
	ICE	Chatter; Laughter; Nothing; switch the light on and fill the room with light; Open the windows and fill the room with fresh air; etc.
SET 186	**KISS**	1. The leading female singer; in Italian, it is literally the "first lady"; 2. Jugular vein; 3. Lame duck.
	SOS	A pair of birds, etc.
	ICE	What time is the duel scheduled?; When should I take a nap?; When do you think the world will end? When are you making my fondest wish a reality?; etc.

SET 187	**KISS**	1. Should be "among," not "between"; 2. Sire, dam, colt, and filly; another name for the father and mother are stallion and mare; 3. King Charles I, William Penn, King George II, Queen Elizabeth I, since she was known as the "Virgin Queen"
	SOS	On calendars; two days are put together at the end of the month when the month ends on a Sunday.
	ICE	Committees; Time on a broken clock; etc.
SET 188	**KISS**	1. Lincoln; 2. The glass is sorted, ground up, melted and formed into new products; 3. Switzerland.
	SOS	Moses; he broke the tablets on which they were written.
	ICE	A cane; a stick; a drone; a slinky; etc.
SET 189	**KISS**	1. The lead singer sings a line and then other singers sing a line to respond to or complete the thought of the first line; 2. 6, 19, and 25; 3. Akhenaton, Cleopatra, Nefertiti, Psusennes, Ptolemy, Ramses, Tutankhamen (Tut), etc.
	SOS	Bowling.
	ICE	Someone planted a nickel; A practical joke; A wealthy person paid to have the trees decorated with bills; etc.
SET 190	**KISS**	1. Onomatopoeia; 2. Black eye; 3. Opened in 1869, it connects the Mediterranean and Red Seas.
	SOS	Hand – Band – Bond – Fond – Food – Foot.
	ICE	Costs too much; Hard on eyes; Kids get addicted; Too many reruns; etc.
SET 191	**KISS**	1. It was written without the letter "e"; 2. Squirrel family (Sciuridae in Latin); 3. Woodrow Wilson.
	SOS	Horsepower.
	ICE	"Is my brain working?"; "You can think of the rest on your own, can't you?"; etc.
SET 192	**KISS**	1. The volume levels different parts of a piece are to be played, i.e. forte, pianissimo, etc.; 2. Dew; 3. Mesopotamia (in the Middle East), Egypt, India, and China.
	SOS	July 2.
	ICE	Moonbeam; Saturday night smile; Tree; etc.
SET 193	**KISS**	1. Luminary, featherweight, low (as in low-fat); bright, easy, gentle, ignite, pale, etc.; 2. Hot air in the balloon has a lower density (is lighter) than the air around the balloon, and so it rises; 3. The Washington Monument.
	SOS	Rose.
	ICE	Its brain, extra arm, marbles, ray gun, replacement eyes and teeth, moon glasses, etc.

SET 194	**KISS**	1. Study of how people interpret the world around them; 2. Example: If you see lightning, and are able to count to ten before you hear the thunder, you know that the storm is about two miles away; 3. Jesse Owens.
	SOS	All are used to start a race.
	ICE	Life is hard sometimes like uncooked spaghetti; They both take time to yield results; Their both better when you spice them up; etc.
SET 195	**KISS**	1. Good Luck!; 2. King Cobra; 3. Carson City, Jefferson City, and Oklahoma City.
	SOS	Crabapple.
	ICE	Bubble-gum; Saffron; Zucchini; Nutmeg from Zanzibar; etc.
SET 196	**KISS**	1. Father-in-law's; 2. An educated guess or assumption that is tested in science to see whether it is true or not; 3. Wampum.
	SOS	Do it during daylight.
	ICE	Clues, gum, money, spider, spy phone, etc.
SET 197	**KISS**	1. They are all characters in *The Legend of Sleepy Hollow*; 2. 24; 3. They were destroyed and buried when the volcano Mount Vesuvius erupted.
	SOS	The cup had only instant coffee in it and the water had not yet been added.
	ICE	"I could use 50 bucks"; "That's the way the cracker crumbles"; "Beware of vicious dog—woof!"; etc.
SET 198	**KISS**	1. Frank Lloyd Wright; 2. Chromosomes (in most cells); 3. They are all capitals of states starting with the letter "M".
	SOS	Half way, because after that the dog is running out of the woods.
	ICE	Balloon, ball, broom, domino, feather, cup, pencil, etc.
SET 199	**KISS**	1. Sisters-in-law; 2. Skunk; 3. Arabia, Italy, and Japan.
	SOS	The masked man is professional hockey player serving as goal tender for his team, and is wearing a pair of ice skates on his feet.
	ICE	How does the Merry go?; What kind of cake pan do you need?; How shall we sing it?; etc.
SET 200	**KISS**	1. A preface introduces a book; 2. Electricity, lightening is a highly visible form of energy transfer, in other words an electric current; 3. Australia.
	SOS	Woman's intuition; Good after noon; Just in time.
	ICE	"My mother wouldn't let me"; "My homework is haunted"; "My dog ate my homework"; etc.

SET 201	**KISS**	1. Octave; 2. The Earth's tilt shifts gradually throughout the year. The solstices mark the shortest and longest days of the year as first one pole and then the other move closer to the sun; 3. Franklin D. Roosevelt (1933-45).
	SOS	Neither; the first day of the 21st century was January 1, 2001. The beginning of a century will start with the year "one," not the year "zero."
	ICE	Cicadas; "We're locked in!" Who cares, nobody will recognize me in that photo wearing that get-up; Paparazzi!; etc.
SET 202	**KISS**	1. 9632; 2. Blood pressure. Hope you didn't feel any "pressure" trying to answer this; 3. Pencil with an attached eraser, 1858; ball point pen, 1888.
	SOS	Johnny was born and always lived in the southern hemisphere. Seasons are reversed in the northern and southern hemisphere.
	ICE	Both can be slow; Both require fuel; Can both stop and start; Hard exterior; etc.
SET 203	**KISS**	1. Fox; 2. The locust; 3. Answers will vary.
	SOS	1. Ulysses S. Grant; 2. Charles Schultz; 3. Harpo Marx.
	ICE	Muffin tin, half of an egg carton, layout of an array of nuclear reactors, a plastic building block, etc.
SET 204	**KISS**	1. Spain, Italy, Poland; 2. Blizzard, dust storm, flood, hurricane, ice storm, tornado, thunder storm, wildfire; 3. Unarmed.
	SOS	It must be dead.
	ICE	Balloons, cotton balls, frosting, marshmallows, etc.
SET 205	**KISS**	1. Yak; 2. 74 mile per hour; 3. Europe.
	SOS	Examples: 1. Man-of-war; 2) Mother-in-law; 3) Jack-in-the-box.
	ICE	Compost, Mr. Potato Heads, potato salad, a battery, etc.
SET 206	**KISS**	1. *Moby Dick*; 2. Tsetse fly (as a carrier of a parasite); 3. Denmark.
	SOS	East.
	ICE	Baked Alaska in Alaska; Rocks in Little Rock, AR; Strawberries in Strawberry Point, IA; etc.
SET 207	**KISS**	1. A sharp takes a note one-half step higher; a flat takes a note one-half step lower; 2. Pig; 3. France, Germany, Germany.
	SOS	The two defendants were Siamese twins. It would be wrong to punish an innocent man.
	ICE	Spoon; Yo-yo, Baton; Bat hitting a ball; Lollipop; etc.
SET 208	**KISS**	1. Cysts, gypsy, hymns, lymph, lynch, myrrh, nymph, pygmy, synch, etc.; 2. Cream; that is why it rises to the top; 3. Valencia.
	SOS	1. Penicillin; 2. Appendages; 3. Aspen; 4. The Pentagon.
	ICE	Insulted the queen; Cut down your neighbor's hedge; Toilet papered someone's house; etc.

SET 209	**KISS**	1. Sherlock Holmes; 2. The ratio of mass to volume, or in simpler terms, how tightly packed the molecules are in space; 3. Lewis and Clark.
	SOS	Stand back-to-back.
	ICE	Doors, extender bars, love handles, CB talkers, etc.
SET 210	**KISS**	1. Red, yellow, blue; 2. All are ways of scoring in games; 3. Germany, Japan.
	SOS	At -40 degrees Celsius, the temperature is the same as -40 degrees Fahrenheit.
	ICE	There was a water balloon fight; Pipes are leaking; Hose was left on; Your walk in pool dried up; etc.
SET 211	**KISS**	1. To jump; 2. Arctic; 3. Madison, Monroe, Polk, Buchanan, Garfield, Carter.
	SOS	"Cousin" because the others refer to a specific gender.
	ICE	Have llamas in your back yard; Have a noisy car; Open up a zoo; Change their locks; Haunt their house; etc.
SET 212	**KISS**	1. *Little House on the Prairie*' 2. Water—ice floats in water; 3. Salary.
	SOS	100; work backwards.
	ICE	Scream; Fib; Fix it; Blame someone else; etc.
SET 213	**KISS**	1. Keystone; 2. VII; 3. Pennsylvania.
	SOS	Unite; untie.
	ICE	Toilet paper on your shoe; You won the lottery; Your fly is down; etc.
SET 214	**KISS**	1. I say, "Let's eat, Grandma."; 2. Sinuses; 3. Baseball; 1883; football, 1892.
	SOS	Kennedy was elected at age 43; Vice President Theodore Roosevelt, who was not elected president, was 42 years of age when sworn in after the assassination of McKinley.
	ICE	Spackle the wall; Fix a squeaky door; Create a cheese-head mascot; Moon in a painting; etc.
SET 215	**KISS**	1. He reversed last two numerals of "1948," year book was published; 2. Soybeans; 3. Vatican City.
	SOS	Galaxy: Xylophone: Neat; Atoll: Llama.
	ICE	As jewelry; hang a Christmas ornament; take out a sliver; as a paper clip; attach insects on a specimen board; etc.
SET 216	**KISS**	1. Piano; original name "pianoforte", which is Italian for soft-low; 2. Mercury; 3. Known as "the father of the American cartoon," he created the elephant and popularized the donkey as the symbols of the U.S.'s two current primary political parties.
	SOS	$45; $5 for each letter to spell the item.
	ICE	You are failing the test; You are passing gas; Your cell phone is ringing; etc.

SET 217	KISS	1. Did you have to resort to Pig Latin?; 2. December and June, usually around the 21st of the month; 3. Mothers Against Drunk Driving.
	SOS	Heartbeats.
	ICE	Everything, if you are in a soundproof room; dog whistles; snow falling; your own snoring; etc.
SET 218	KISS	1. Atlas; 2. $A=\pi r^2$; 3. Oslo, Norway.
	SOS	Fill the three-gallon pail with water and pour it into the five-gallon container. Do it again until the five-gallon pail is full, which leaves the needed one gallon in the three-gallon container.
	ICE	Eat crackers; Read an instruction book you don't like; Count stars; Call a boring friend; Drink some herbal tea; etc.
SET 219	KISS	1. All of the colors; 2. abbreviations for Internet domains: commercial, education, organization; 3. Priesthood.
	SOS	UCLA.
	ICE	"The picnickers are here. Dinner is served."; "Beware of the ant trap near the radish dish"; "Sugar in Aisle 6"; etc.
SET 220	KISS	1. "Capital" is a city, and "Capitol" is the legislative building; therefore, Washington, DC is the Capital of the U.S.; 2. Shifting of tectonic plates, volcanic activity; 3. Columbus, Cleveland, and Cincinnati.
	SOS	Normal, some fingers are on each hand.
	ICE	A sports team; A billion items at the dollar store; 1000 rides to the International Space Station; etc.
SET 221	KISS	1. Troubadour; 2. Zero (0) — 88-64-24=0; 3. Cashmere.
	SOS	He asked the patient to take off his shoes.
	ICE	They make good coat hooks; They have sweet dispositions to make up for their looks; They have cute ears; They have nice accents; etc.
SET 222	KISS	1. German and Latin; 2. Vanilla; 3. Sahara.
	SOS	22, 23, 24, 25.
	ICE	Reality show called "So You Think You Can Be Mayor"; Comedy cooking show called "Burn the Buns"; etc.
SET 223	KISS	1. Be sure to buy <u>fine</u> sandpaper : I feel <u>fine</u> : She bought <u>fine</u> clothes : etc.; 2. Eight swans and seven elephants; 3. Arkansas.
	SOS	Chris collects model airplanes that he makes; Jennifer collects old coins.
	ICE	Bull Run, in the long-run, rerun, roadrunner, runaround, runaway, runner-up, runway, etc.
SET 224	KISS	1. Five; 2. James Watson; 3. Henry Ford.
	SOS	Charcoal; used when you barbeque.
	ICE	A seed; An ant; Salt; Coin; etc.

SET 225	KISS	1. Base (bass), pitch, slide, score, tie' 2. If the weight of the water displaced is less than the weight of the object, the object will sink; otherwise the object will float, with the weight of the water displaced equal to the weight of the object; 3. Peru.
	SOS	He was standing on the bottom rung.
	ICE	Odd socks and bookends; Oddballs and dead ends; Clothes pins; Last chapters of novels; etc.
SET 226	KISS	1. Pheasant; 2. Smallpox; 3. The sinking of the Titanic.
	SOS	IOTUVWXY.
	ICE	Roof; Taking the blame for a friend; Hands when you cough; etc.
SET 227	KISS	1. Becky Thatcher; 2. Earthworm; 3. Hershey, Pennsylvania.
	SOS	The letter "r".
	ICE	Count flies in a research lab; Dust antique cars in an auto museum; Make duck calls, Rub someone's back; etc.
SET 228	KISS	1. Chord; 2. A spiral shape called a double helix; it looks like a spiraling ladder; 3. Lake Ontario and Lake Erie.
	SOS	Dianne's bags were empty.
	ICE	They both can cause a stir; They both can be healthy; They both can be on television; etc.
SET 229	KISS	1. Succession, sequence, command, etc.; 2. Subtraction and division; 3. "The Star Spangled Banner" (by Francis Scott Key in 1814, during the bombing of Fort McHenry)
	SOS	Three.
	ICE	Two goose bumps on your forehead; Straws in a drink; pig's nose; etc.
SET 230	KISS	1. World War II; 2. Deteriorated lead paint chips or dust from older housing; 3. West side.
	SOS	Catapult, catastrophe, cataract.
	ICE	"I already paid my dues"; "I only lie to my friends"; "The length of my nose should be ignored"; "I don't know how I ended up in a liars club"; etc.
SET 231	KISS	1. Metronome; 2. All are; 3. William Henry Harrison, Zachary Taylor, Abraham Lincoln, James A. Garfield, William McKinley, Warren G. Harding, Franklin D. Roosevelt, and John F. Kennedy.
	SOS	First Tuesday in July.
	ICE	"I packed you a nice lunch"; "Your teacher is really Mary Poppins"; etc.
SET 232	KISS	1. Larynx; 2. Neutrons and protons; 3. The Alamo.
	SOS	Water.
	ICE	Lost the other for each pair; Want to be different; Designated school "Mismatch Day"; It was dark when I got dressed; etc.

SET 233	**KISS**	1. The letter "A"; 2. Equinox is when the sun is directly over the equator, so that the day and the night are equal in both hemispheres. It happens twice a year around the 21st of March and September; 3. Oahu.
	SOS	Mountain.
	ICE	Covers, a deal, hair, a heist, pull off the road, someone's leg, things from the fridge, etc.
SET 234	**KISS**	1. A prelude or overture; 2. The liver (three-to-four pounds); 3. White.
	SOS	Write, Wright, right.
	ICE	Full of stuff; Have aisles; Carefully designed displays; Specimens are prominent; Can be overwhelming; Items are labeled; Colorful; etc.
SET 235	**KISS**	1. Examples: over, under, beside, in, off, on, of, up, with, toward, etc.; 2. False, they jump; 3. India.
	SOS	Eye; it could also possibly be "sea".
	ICE	Rock climbing wall; Mural portraits of my guests; Live orchestra on call; etc
SET 236	**KISS**	1. Leo Tolstoy / John Bunyan / Geoffrey Chaucer; 2. Square; the bases are equidistant and are set at right angles; 3. Gavel.
	SOS	Stars.
	ICE	A period because you generally put it after the fact; A semi-colon because it makes more complex sentences; etc.
SET 237	**KISS**	1. Rap; 2. Wednesday; 3. Egyptian.
	SOS	Few – fewer.
	ICE	Cell phone for use on the moon; Umbrella with holes in it; Two heels on a single shoe, etc.
SET 238	**KISS**	1. The prefix "poly" means many or much; therefore, "polyrhythm" refers to the use of two or more conflicting rhythms at the same time in a piece of music; 2. Apricot pits; 3. Japan.
	SOS	Place "eci" within each to obtain precise, special, and species.
	ICE	A comedian on TV; A little boy trying to eat by himself for the first time; A woodpecker trying to peck on a steel building; They are each in hilarious Halloween costumes; etc.
SET 239	**KISS**	1. Robert Lewis Stevenson's *Treasure Island*; 2. The pistil; 3. Interstate.
	SOS	Nine; the sisters all had the same brother, which makes seven, and then add the parents.
	ICE	It can be a matter of luck; You take a chance; Things can get competitive; You want to win; You have to move to succeed; You can try hard and still come in second; etc.

SET 240	KISS	1. Voice(s); 2. A series of giant waves caused by the displacement of water; 3. Osaka.
	SOS	Eight.
	ICE	The envelope, pedal to the metal, children in school, buggy, doors, swing, dead car off highway, etc.
SET 241	KISS	1. Underprivileged; 2. Vibrate; 3. Virginia.
	SOS	Answers will vary; as an example, four of the children could each have arrived in a separate car (16 wheels), two could have ridden their bikes (four wheels), and one could have walked to school (Zero wheels).
	ICE	The authors say that at this point their minds are blank; etc.
SET 242	KISS	1. Fighting windmills; 2. Prism; 3. Clara Barton.
	SOS	1. Spine; 2. Alpine; 3. Pineapple.
	ICE	Hard boil him; take him home with you; tear down all the walls in the kingdom; line the wall with mattresses; put him in your Easter basket; etc.
SET 243	KISS	1. Palette; 2. Peanut; it is considered a legume because it grows in the ground; 3. Mexico (Pyramid of the Sun).
	SOS	1. Agatha Christie, 2. Cecil B. DeMille; 3. Paul Revere 4. Isadora Duncan.
	ICE	Put plastic around it so it doesn't break; Mix colors within each crayon, etc.
SET 244	KISS	1. Answers will vary—supposedly there are 79 of them; 2. Electrons; 3. Peru.
	SOS	Shakespeare never saw an actress, because in those days there were none in England; only men and boys played acting roles in the time of Shakespeare.
	ICE	Have no thorns; Make it have more petals; Make it live longer; etc.
SET 245	KISS	1. Three; 2. They are all math terms; 3. Arizona.
	SOS	Bell; box; fire.
	ICE	Taped to the bottom of a wastebasket; At a friend's house; etc.
SET 246	KISS	1. Octave; 2. Incisors, canines, bicuspids, and molars; 3. Ethan Allen.
	SOS	The three people are a son, his father, and his grandfather.
	ICE	Road kill, litter, sign post, eating place, dirty diaper, quarter, hitchhiker, etc.
SET 247	KISS	1. Ge – ra - ni – um; 2. Four; 3. The Eiffel Tower in Paris, which was built for the Exposition of 1889.
	SOS	Coffee break; Wind breaker; Commercial break.
	ICE	Your skin; Roads; Things in the night; Pregnant women; etc.

SET 248	**KISS**	1. Bob Cratchett; 2. In a chemical compound, through a chemical reaction the atoms of two or more different elements have been bound together to form a new substance. A mixture consists of two or more different elements and/or compounds physically intermingled but not chemically bound together; 3. Yellowstone, established in 1872.
	SOS	The parrot was deaf.
	ICE	People's teeth might decay; The price of jelly beans would go down; Would need more workers to plow the roads; The song "Purple Rain" would be too literal; etc.
SET 249	**KISS**	1. Piccolo; 2. Acid rain; 3. The South Vietnamese.
	SOS	$11,010.
	ICE	Jane Austen and Madonna discussing courtship; Daniel Boone and Beethoven sharing about their respective life's work; P.T. Barnum and Cecil B. Demille discussing showmanship; etc.
SET 250	**KISS**	1. Immediate, mediate, meaning, permeable, etc.; 2. Zero; 3. The United States.
	SOS	Scythe.
	ICE	The astronaut's children who were expecting a present; An ad for a new Mars candy bar; Mission Control when the astronaut arrived without the rocket; Martian's mother when they unpack at the Venus resort; etc.
SET 251	**KISS**	1. Beauty; 2. Enamel and dentin; 3. Windsor.
	SOS	General.
	ICE	The mail carrier is jealously in love with you; Someone put gum in the mailbox; Dropped out of the mail truck and blew away; Mail plane crashed; etc.
SET 252	**KISS**	1. Japan; 2. They do not retract; 3. Bismarck, North Dakota.
	SOS	An unopened parachute.
	ICE	The kids; Water; Food; Pans; Spices; Soap; Candles; Animals; Rags; Rope; Medicine; etc.
SET 253	**KISS**	1. Incorrectly; 2. Gold; 3. The Andes, along the west coast of South America, this mountain range also boasts some of the highest peaks in the world.
	SOS	Sue sculptures ice, and of course ice melts.
	ICE	Don't take a shower, so no one wants to stand near you in line; Shop at 4 a.m.; Tell people there is a quicker line at the end; Cross your eyes at the cashier; etc.
SET 254	**KISS**	1. He has to slay the monster Grendel and Grendel's mother, too; 2. The gravitational pull of the Moon (and Sun) on the water; 3. Honolulu.
	SOS	Heel, heal, he'll.
	ICE	"How full does this elevator get before it collapses?"; How angry does this monster get before it spits?; etc.

SET 255	**KISS**	1. In a piece of music; it is a musical technique where notes in a chord are played or sung one after the other (either going up or down) in sequence rather than simultaneously; 2. Black on Yellow—Note: school buses and road signs; 3. Indian Ocean.
	SOS	A coffin.
	ICE	To whistle; Boil water; Send a note; Roll out pie crust; etc.
SET 256	**KISS**	1. Et cetera; 2. Rodents; 3. Must: (1) have been born in the U.S., (2) be at least 35 years of age, (3) currently be a U.S. citizen, (4) have resided in the U.S. for at least 14 years, and (5) be elected.
	SOS	The letter "e".
	ICE	A baby bowling ball; A globe bank; A rotten orange; A round paper weight; A round rock; A baseball; etc.
SET 257	**KISS**	1. They were probably sour anyway."; 2. True; 3. Elizabeth Blackwell.
	SOS	One word.
	ICE	A cup, paper clip, and sponge can make a cup holder for your car, with removable sponge to wipe up any spills; etc.
SET 258	**KISS**	1. ". . . Far away from the cold night air," from *My Fair Lady*; 2. 12; 3. Hemispheres.
	SOS	S-cape = Escape.
	ICE	What can we say, they're your friends and family?
SET 259	**KISS**	1. Bass, bat, desert, record, wound, etc.; 2. Almost any part of the body. Did you say "colon"? Remember, we were looking for the *wrong* answer; 3. Spice—valuable at that time.
	SOS	A pound of gold is always worth more than half a pound of gold.
	ICE	They are both "on call"; They both have volume; You don't want either one to interrupt your vacation; etc.
SET 260	**KISS**	1. They do not rhyme; the "o" is pronounced differently in each word; 2. True; 3. Turkey.
	SOS	The President is still the President. If the President happened to also be dead, the next in line of succession would be the President Pro Tempore of the Senate.
	ICE	Caskets, hatchets, hurtful feelings, secrets, seeds, treasures, dog bones; etc.
SET 261	**KISS**	1. Washington, John Adams, Jefferson, Madison, Monroe, John Quincy Adams; 2. False; 3. A coup.
	SOS	A coin.
	ICE	Nothing would get done because everyone would be describing things; The verbs would revolt; Nouns would live very pampered lives; etc.

SET 262	**KISS**	1. Examples: able, ed, en , er, es, est, ful, ing, less, ly, ment, tion, y, etc.; 2. Patterns of stars in the sky; 3. Libel is printed/Slander is oral.
	SOS	They are all animals and they are also all the name of dances.
	ICE	They make connections; They can collapse; They don't want to be all wet; etc.
SET 263	**KISS**	1. A container which some people pour wine into before serving; 2. Third degree; 3. Utah.
	SOS	1. Funny bunny; 2. Boar store, 3. Mall ball.
	ICE	The editor didn't like it; Computer malfunction; Couldn't spell it right; It was lousy; Someone stole the idea; etc.
SET 264	**KISS**	1. Leonardo da Vinci; 2. They have bills and lay eggs; 3. Benjamin Franklin.
	SOS	Trees grow at their tops.
	ICE	Sleepwalkers; Spooks; People without flashlights; etc.
SET 265	**KISS**	1. Awesome, fantastic, great, wonderful, etc.; 2. The nucleus; 3. World's largest of its category, mountain, ocean, waterfall by height
	SOS	One way to do this is fire, fine, mine, mint.
	ICE	Electronics, paper plates, drapes, Witches of the West from Oz, etc.
SET 266	**KISS**	1. Usually, the person in a graduating academic class who has earned the highest grade average or ranking; 2. 21; 3. Farmer.
	SOS	July, August, September, October, November – JASON.
	ICE	Full of hot air; Important; Long winded; etc.
SET 267	**KISS**	1. C; 2. Did you find this challenging?; 3. The Mexican War.
	SOS	Heroine—he , her, hero, heroine.
	ICE	Balloons; Musical instruments; Hot food; Whistles; Hands; Enemy bridges; air mattresses; Tires; etc.
SET 268	**KISS**	1. How long did it take?; 2. Four; 3. Madagascar.
	SOS	Worm; it is the only word in the group that is not a palindrome (makes another word when spelled backwards).
	ICE	Hey, it's your party! You choose!
SET 269	**KISS**	1. Thesaurus; 2. Tectonic plates; 3. Iroquois.
	SOS	Dry – Day – Pay – Pat – Pet – Wet.
	ICE	Both begin with the letter "P"; Both are soft; Both get filled; You're not supposed to play with them, but . . .; etc.
SET 270	**KISS**	1. Greece; 2. An object's speed. "Honest, Officer, I was going the speed limit!"; 3. Colorado River.
	SOS	They all have degrees.
	ICE	Mata Hari; Thomas Jefferson; Al Capone; Martin Luther King; Joan of Arc; etc.

SET 271	KISS	1. When they are used as a name or at the beginning of a sentence; 2. Cool the burn, often by holding under cool (not cold) water; 3. Paper.
	SOS	None; unlisted numbers will not be in the phone book.
	ICE	They have rank; Work together; Need to follow the rules; Both might have jokers; Card suits are like uniforms; Often encounter cheaters; etc.
SET 272	KISS	1. Exaggeration; 2. Silk worms-mulberry leaves, pandas-bamboo, koalas-eucalyptus leaves; 3. West Virginia fought for the Union side.
	SOS	Throw in the towel; Just in time; I am beside myself; H2O.
	ICE	A flushed face, heated rock, water when you add gelatin or drink mix, newspaper, etc.
SET 273	KISS	1. Left—the right hand is usually used to play the treble clef; 2. 36 pairs; spiders have eight legs, while bees and flies both have six legs and there are two shoes in a pair; 3. True.
	SOS	52.
	ICE	"Try again"; "You will win a fortune . . . cookie"; "Much luck will come your way if you leave a BIG tip"; etc.
SET 274	KISS	1. Commas and periods; 2. =0; 3. Renaissance.
	SOS	The jewels were found in a poison ivy patch, so only when one of the men broke out with poison ivy did they know which one of them was guilty.
	ICE	Kids' hair; Things from the trash; A child's doll house; Nothing—Why bother?; Buy a ready-made nest; Steal another bird's; etc.
SET 275	KISS	1. Cupid, Washington, Antarctica; 2. Intestines; 3. Colorado.
	SOS	The same weight because all the materials are taken from the earth.
	ICE	Kindness – it reaches the soul; Understanding – Love and kindness can be misunderstood; etc.
SET 276	KISS	1. Julie Andrews; 2. Triceratops; 3. Begins a new term.
	SOS	Tim stands under a container of water and lights the match beneath it.
	ICE	What did Dela wear to the ball?; How aii you today?; Go the Io way.; I ran a good race.; Does Tennes see very well?; etc.
SET 277	KISS	1. Black Beauty, Coca-Cola®, Dunkin Doughnuts®, Krispy Kreme®, Park Place, etc.; 2. Photosynthesis; 3. China.
	SOS	Snake: Key: Eyelash: Shower: Erupt: Ptarmigan: Angel.
	ICE	Shut off a pipe; Keep someone quiet; Give the little Dutch Boy a break; Fishing weight; etc.
SET 278	KISS	1. Homer. 2. Northern Lights; 3. Baghdad.
	SOS	Example: I; do; met; shot; timed; desist; methods; moistest; Methodist; Methodists.
	ICE	Colds, bedspread, mayonnaise, spread-eagle, seeds, etc.

SET 279	**KISS**	1. Music produced by instruments without electrical enhancement; 2. Two; 3. Russia.
	SOS	The opposite numbers on a die always add up to seven.
	ICE	Uses all the same letters, although the "s" is used twice; Can be dry; Can be colorful; Too much is unhealthy; etc.
SET 280	**KISS**	1. Truck, gasoline, a line of something (like people waiting); 2. Hummingbirds and ostriches 3. Olympia, Greece.
	SOS	The score before any game starts is always zero to zero.
	ICE	Pick it up, smile and keep walking; Take the other shoe off also so you are more balanced; Throw it at the groom; Act like you were bowing to the altar; etc.
SET 281	**KISS**	1. Spine; 2. False—hail forms when precipitation is blown up and down from warm low to freezing high altitudes; 3. Filibuster.
	SOS	"Inkstand".
	ICE	Shipwrecks, pogo sticks, rainbows; etc.
SET 282	**KISS**	1. Supercalifragilisticexpialidocious; 2. =0; 3. Hitler.
	SOS	Windows.
	ICE	Backpacks, your lips, sweaters, zip line, Ziploc bag, etc.
SET 283	**KISS**	1. Boom; Voices; Thunder; etc.; 2. Four; 3. Brazil—India is by far the world's leading grower of bananas and plantains but most of them are consumed internally and not exported.
	SOS	The woman was a minister or a justice of the peace.
	ICE	National anthem; Parade; Worship Service; As a citizen on an important issue; Judge enters the courtroom; Wedding day; etc.
SET 284	**KISS**	1. Enjoy!; 2. Horns are made of bone and they are permanent, while antlers are made of the same material as fingernails (keratin) and will fall off and re-grow; 3. The host country.
	SOS	Cut the pie into four quarters with two cuts; then pile four quarters of pie one on top of one other, and make a cut through the center.
	ICE	Watering can; Your breath; A bag of dirt; Sunrise; etc.
SET 285	**KISS**	1. Painter; 2. They are all plants from which drugs are derived; 3. Mississippi.
	SOS	1. *Much Ado About Nothing*; 2. *Star Spangled Banner*; 3. *Star Wars*.
	ICE	Square jack-o-lantern; Street light; Carrots under ground; etc.
SET 286	**KISS**	1. Common errors include: comma errors, apostrophe errors, sentence fragments, lack of subject/verb Agreement, misplaced modifiers, pronoun errors, etc.; 2. Leeward; 3. True.
	SOS	She works in a library, and people are taking books.
	ICE	Christmas trees; Ambulances; Car turn signals; Traffic lights; Song by American rap artist Kanye West titled "Flashing Lights"; etc.

SET 287	**KISS**	1. Enjoy!; 2. Femur or thighbone; 3. Red.
	SOS	1. Buzz Aldrin; 2. Francis of Assisi; 3. Carol Burnett.
	ICE	Rhinocergator – two-ton, scaly animal with a nose horn and sharp teeth that lies in wait in the mud to charge you; Tigaroo – striped and toothy pouched animal that growls and boxes; etc.
SET 288	**KISS**	1. A flute; 2. True; 3. West.
	SOS	Portugal; Iceland, Sweden.
	ICE	Charge them rent; Sic the cat on them; Beg them not to reveal your secrets; etc.
SET 289	**KISS**	1. Sing, Work, Play, Think, etc.; 2. Erosion; 3. 300 B.C.
	SOS	When you add two hours to eleven o'clock.
	ICE	Could rescue up to eight people at a time – good; Arms could get tangled up – bad; etc.
SET 290	**KISS**	1. How is your tongue?; 2. In this case, it does not matter which you do first; 3. Greenland.
	SOS	Water.
	ICE	The toilet and how it works; A drive through at a fast-food restaurant; Niagara Falls; etc.
SET 291	**KISS**	1. Mona Lisa; 2. Fingerprints; 3. Caesar.
	SOS	To the right. The hand that you use does not matter.
	ICE	His garden had a piano plant; His garden was shaped like a piano; He had a dog named "Piano"; He used a broken piano as a planter; etc.
SET 292	**KISS**	1. A dash connects thoughts and a hyphen connects parts of words or makes compound words.; 2. Peas; 3. $10.00 bill.
	SOS	Eleven; the count does not start until the first strike.
	ICE	Glue, paint, shower, water, hairspray, etc.
SET 293	**KISS**	1. Twist your tongue?; 2. Chlorophyll; 3. Guatemala (Guatemala City) and Panama (Panama City).
	SOS	1. Mean bean; 2. Fish Dish; 3. Mouse Spouse.
	ICE	A mural of a hockey game between the starfish and the pickle; Use a starfish shaped pickle to play hockey; Starfish could use the puck as a table to eat its pickle; etc.
SET 294	**KISS**	1. Crescendo; 2. Comets; 3. Marco Polo.
	SOS	Spain; Italy; Ecuador.
	ICE	Helicopter; Trampoline; Put glue on your hands so they will stick to the pole and allow you to climb it; Use a pulley; Get an antigravity gun; Cut the flagpole down; etc.

SET 295	**KISS**	1. They increase the intensity of the word. For example "warm*er*" is more warm, and "warm*est*" is the most warm; 2. Volume; 3. India.
	SOS	Rat; Art; Tar.
	ICE	Avoiding the press; Being impeached; Reversing a policy; A gunman is at the bottom of the stairs; He has a hole in the seat of pants; etc.
SET 296	**KISS**	1. That's why they call them tongue twisters; 2. In a desert; but only in one particular desert, the Sonoran Desert in the Mexican state of Sonora, southern Arizona and southeast California; 3. The cacao tree; its seeds are called cocoa beans.
	SOS	Turn the six upside down to make a nine, and the number becomes 931.
	ICE	The moon for cheap cheese; Venus for a romantic getaway; Bottom of ocean for freshest seafood; etc.
SET 297	**KISS**	1. The Guitar; it has six strings; 2. A material's opposition to the flow of electric current; 3. Alcoholic beverages.
	SOS	16 correct; 10 incorrect.
	ICE	Peanut butter with confetti; Sauerkraut; Fish guts; Motor oil; Plastic wrap; Thumbtacks; etc.
SET 298	**KISS**	1. Usher—us, she, he, her; 2. One possible answer: 99+999+9+9+9=1125; 3. Mosque.
	SOS	Scales.
	ICE	The brain, face, paper, clothes, the book *Wrinkle in Time*, etc.
SET 299	**KISS**	1. Mozart, Beethoven, Grieg, Handel, Haydn, Schubert, etc. 2. Core, mantle, crust; 3. Alaska, Washington, Oregon, California, and Hawaii.
	SOS	Orbit; Italy; Lyre; Repeat; Attractive; Venus.
	ICE	If you wake the baby again I'm going to climb up the wall"; "If you startle me again, I'm going to throw up the sauerkraut"; etc.
SET 300	**KISS**	1. The harpsichord; invented in the 16th century; 2. Giraffe and cow; 3. Herbert Hoover.
	SOS	Never; the boat floats on water..
	ICE	Security alarm; Stronger chairs, More porridge; etc.
SET 301	**KISS**	1. They are punctuation marks; 2. Metals are generally denser, more malleable, and conduct electricity and heat better than non-metals; 3. Exxon Valdez.
	SOS	King of diamonds; Jack of hearts; Queen of Spades.
	ICE	Gloves to cool your hands in the hot summer; A novel with a steaming hot plot that needs to be cooled off; Hot chocolate; Window cleaner; etc.
SET 302	**KISS**	1. "Lay"; 2. Alexander Graham Bell; 3. X.
	SOS	$250.
	ICE	Sleepwalking; What elevator button to push; Keeping lumberjacks away; Pesky woodpeckers; etc.

SET 303	KISS	1. The white keys; 2. Smoke and fog; 3. Industrial Revolution.
	SOS	She has a duck/goose/etc. that lays eggs she can eat.
	ICE	Caligon; Texakansas; New Hampshacheusetts; Idatana; etc.
SET 304	KISS	1. Farther-distance; Further-time, quantity or degree.; 2. Penguin; 3. Russia, China, and Canada.
	SOS	27 days.
	ICE	Sequins, flashlights, candles, black eye; moonlight, etc.
SET 305	KISS	1. Did you like this one?; 2. Magma; 3. Theodore Roosevelt and Franklin Roosevelt.
	SOS	1. Whittle; 2. Within; 3. Quit; 4. Shoe it; 5. Witness.
	ICE	Both are small; Both are imaginary; Both can be troublemakers; Goblin has twice as many letters; Goblins get less good press; Tolkien couldn't write without them; etc.
SET 306	KISS	1. Words; 2. 16 x 12 /2 + 3= 99; 3. Harvard.
	SOS	The lawyer is a woman.
	ICE	Chocolate, chocolate, chocolate… etc.
SET 307	KISS	1. I will sit and watch while you set the table.; Sit and watch the sunset.;Set up the folding chair and sit on it.; etc.; 2. Podiatrist; 3. Michigan.
	SOS	Icicle – fire.
	ICE	Can you clean my ring?; I don't pay for soap anymore; Can you eat my fudge?; I don't like the sweets anymore; etc.
SET 308	KISS	1. How did you do?; 2. Annuals; 3. Hippocrates.
	SOS	1. Morse; 2. Darwin; 3. Einstein; 4. Pavlov.
	ICE	Charge people to see it; Ride it shopping; Put it in an imaginary zoo; Introduce it to your agent; etc.
SET 309	KISS	1. Tony Awards; 2. True; 3. Athens.
	SOS	Because her joey has to play inside.
	ICE	Both strong; Keep enemies at bay; Can keep you in one place; etc.
SET 310	KISS	1. "Is" – singular; "are" – plural; 2. 16 packages of gum; 3. The Whig Party.
	SOS	Tears – Sears – Stars – Stare – Stale – Stile – Smile .
	ICE	Emails, marriage, sewing machine, vacuum cleaner, etc.
SET 311	KISS	1. Someone who is left-handed; 2. 93 million miles; 3. The Bible.
	SOS	One or zero.
	ICE	Spoiled food; A temper; A broken heart; etc.

SET 312	**KISS**	1. Desire; 2. Trachea; 3. Portuguese.
	SOS	Between you and me; Good afternoon; Made in Japan.
	ICE	A puddle; Judy Garland or Iz Kamakawiwo 'ole; Gods' paint pallet; Another rainbow; etc.
SET 313	**KISS**	1. 2nd; 3rd;1st; 2. Dandelion; 3. Big Ben.
	SOS	Sue has five cookies, and Roger has seven cookies.
	ICE	Boxes, tubs, chests, etc. are not adequate; the authors wish someone would really come up with a creative solution for this one.
SET 314	**KISS**	1. Bilingual dictionary, Draw pictures, Hire an interpreter, Point, Gestures, etc.; 2. Dolly; 3. Iceland.
	SOS	Clock.
	ICE	Repair a leak; put a hem in a skirt; Make a bracelet; bandage a wound, hold bumper on car; etc.
SET 315	**KISS**	1. Blues, Classical, Country, Jazz, Pop, Rap, Rock and roll, etc.; 2. You would not be able to hear them or talk to them because the lack of air does not allow sound to travel through it; of course if they were in space suits connected by intercoms it might be a different story; 3. Dynasty.
	SOS	Attic: Icicle: Lemonade: Degree: Eerie.
	ICE	Vibrating seats; Add ottomans; Use couches; etc.
SET 316	**KISS**	1. Requirement; 2. Muscles – About 600 of them; 3. Charles Lindbergh.
	SOS	Five people.
	ICE	Glass figurines, egos; butterfly wings, feelings, etc.
SET 317	**KISS**	1. Tips of your shoelaces; 2. Cactus; 3. Washington Monument.
	SOS	Cloe – 12, Jesse – 5, and Mackenzie – 4.
	ICE	F comes before M in the alphabet; Mothers want to know how much the fathers will spend on their gifts; Parent's travel schedule; etc.
SET 318	**KISS**	1. True; 2. Solid, liquid and gas; 3. An early pilot who was the first woman to fly solo across the Atlantic Ocean, and the first person (man or woman) to fly solo from Honolulu, Hawaii to Oakland, California among other records.
	SOS	1) Thomas Alva Edison; 2) Babe Ruth; 3) Betty White.
	ICE	Your bootie, your finger, your head, liquid, salt shaker, rattle, etc.
SET 319	**KISS**	1. Extremely, high; 2. Yes, $400; 3. Asia and Australia.
	SOS	They all have diamonds.
	ICE	Lorene Lenning is really funny; etc.
SET 320	**KISS**	1. Seize the day; 2. The octagon shape of stop signs; 3. Benjamin Franklin – "A penny saved is a penny earned."
	SOS	Pull the bathtub plug.
	ICE	Counting by fives; Spraying bugs; Hot pad holder; etc.

SET 321	KISS	1. Bach; 2. A herbivore, because it eats mostly plants; 3. The Tower of London.
	SOS	Tinkerbell; Bellbottom; barbells or dumbbells.
	ICE	It is an antique shop; Remodeling for a restaurant; They like old tables; The owner is an architect and they are really tables and chairs; etc.
SET 322	KISS	1. Strait; 2. Both are molten rock, but magma refers to the molten rock while it is still underground. Once the molten rock is on the surface, such as after erupting from a volcano, it is considered lava; 3. Oslo.
	SOS	Lettuce, artichoke, etc.
	ICE	Automobiles; Cameras; Flashlights; Hearing aids; Golf carts; etc.
SET 323	KISS	1. Out of one, many, or one from many; 2. 87+65-43-21=88; 3. It is the most holy city of Islam.
	SOS	1,005.
	ICE	Squeaky voice; Uncoordinated; Spit when they talk; Can't remember the order; Serve raw and burned food; etc.
SET 324	KISS	1. Five; 2. Bitter, salty, sour, and sweet; 3. False; it is a free and sovereign state in Mexico.
	SOS	14; using number words, each number is one letter more.
	ICE	The pages are stuck together; Twenty is your favorite number; You hid your money in the book; etc.
SET 325	KISS	1. No place; 2. True; 3. Having the right to vote.
	SOS	Sea.
	ICE	Candy; Evidence; Their face; Money; The truth; Feelings; Gifts; Eggs; etc.
SET 326	KISS	1. Joy of life or joy of living—that's good for your brain!; 2. Krypton; 3. Christianity, Islam, Judaism.
	SOS	How many did you get?
	ICE	For fishing; As a science experiment; To keep his sister away; etc.
SET 327	KISS	1. Examples: Itsy Bitsy Spider, Rudolph the Red Nose Reindeer, How Much is that Doggy in the Window, etc.; 2. It has a gravitational field so strong even light cannot escape; 3. Finland.
	SOS	D-light =delight.
	ICE	Bad omen, Big Oscar, Body odor, etc.
SET 328	KISS	1. Spread out; 2. Above 50%; 3. Samurai.
	SOS	1. Dwayne or Duane, 2. Walter; 3. Phyllis.
	ICE	Keep electronic records; Make sign language the official language; Make paper really expensive; Invest in erasers; etc.

SET 329	KISS	1. Wonder child; 2. The Black Widow spider; 3. Switzerland, where the Red Cross was founded.
	SOS	Template, terminate, or temperate.
	ICE	Have floss attached; Make handle curved to better fit one's mouth; Brush two sides at once; Colored rainbow bristles; Monogram on the handle; etc.
SET 330	KISS	1. Examples: Czech Boys Choir, Mormon Tabernacle Choir, Saint Olaf a Capella Choir; Vienna Boys Choir; etc.; 2. 8,000 hamburger patties; 3. Winston Churchill.
	SOS	Iraq: Aquarius: Usher: Error: Orchestra: Radar.
	ICE	Wrap it in colored bubble wrap; Use glow-in-the-dark paper; Holographic wizard image; etc.
SET 331	KISS	1. Athletic; 2. Move the person to a safer location to avoid getting struck yourself; 3. Hinduism.
	SOS	$42.
	ICE	Credit/debit cards; Money; Grocery list; Driver's license; Insurance cards; Photos; Receipts; etc.
SET 332	KISS	1. Congratulations; 2. Hot; 3. Idaho and Montana.
	SOS	6 horses and 5 clowns.
	ICE	"I'm ahead of you"; "Keep your temper cause no one else wants it"; "Don't follow me, I'm lost"; "I let the dogs out"; etc.
SET 333	KISS	1. Feather; Macaroni; 2. Both; 3. Andrew Carnegie.
	SOS	1. Stan; 2. Oliver; 3. Denise.
	ICE	Form a circle; Circle around; Semi-circle; Circle Drive; Circle of Life; etc.
SET 334	KISS	1. Wrench, written, and wrist; 2. =.03; 3. Mexico City.
	SOS	1. Fair-thee-well 2. Jack-o-lantern 3. Hand-me-down.
	ICE	You could be going in a circle; Hopefully no head-on collisions; Would not have to be concerned about oncoming traffic; Wouldn't need reverse; etc.
SET 335	KISS	1. Pleasantly plump, buxom or full-figured; 2. Jupiter with 60+; 3. The Judicial Branch.
	SOS	Peter is a dog and the doctor is a veterinarian.
	ICE	Comma – Sigh, a comma never feels complete; Question mark – Life is always an adventure for a question mark; etc.
SET 336	KISS	1. Marching band music; he was an American composer and conductor famous for American military and patriotic marches; 2. White horses are better for hot climates. White withstands heat better because it reflects light and heat better than dark colors; 3. Silver.
	SOS	1) Barbra Streisand; 2) William Shakespeare; 3) Irving Berlin.
	ICE	Talking or texting on cell phones; Car horns blaring; Doors slamming; Chewing with mouth open; Gum under desks; etc.

SET 337	**KISS**	1. Bold; 2. Pelican; 3. Arizona, California, New Mexico, Texas.
	SOS	They can all be folded.
	ICE	Eat a lifesaver; Take plane next time; Leave note for loved ones; Curse; Pray; Learn to swim fast; etc.
SET 338	**KISS**	1. Peace, hello/goodbye; 2. One cent; 3. General Douglas Macarthur, upon his arrival in Australia after the Japanese had forced his troops from the Philippines.
	SOS	Sex: Exam: Amuse: Serene: Needle: Levitate.
	ICE	Burn the evidence; Heat; Put your TV in it; Hide something; Give your chimney sweep friend some work; Place for Santa or a wolf to enter; etc.
SET 339	**KISS**	1. A painting or drawing technique in which space and objects depicted on a flat surface seem visually to have depth and distance; 2. Move away from windows and furniture that might fall; drop to the floor and go under a desk or table; if driving stop car; etc.; 3. Peso.
	SOS	Their, fore, errers, and statement says there are four errors—there are only three.
	ICE	"Gotcha!"; "I'm on a blood drive"; "But you let the Red Cross have some"; "Type O, please"; etc.
SET 340	**KISS**	1. Beautify; 2. No, they have white feathers on their heads; 3. Barry Goldwater.
	SOS	The 315th day or November 11th.
	ICE	Since Saturday, silly Sally sold sixty-seven stupendous suede shoes; Simple Simon saw seventy-seven sentimental swans singing slow, sweet songs; etc.
SET 341	**KISS**	1. Goodbye; 2. One gallon; 3. They are all lost cities.
	SOS	John 12/30, Annette 8/4, Sherri 5/7, Joel 6/9.
	ICE	Halt; Pause, Quit; Cease; Whoa; etc.
SET 342	**KISS**	1. **Blue** – indigo, navy, turquoise, etc. / **Red** – crimson, pink, rose, scarlet, etc. / **Yellow** – amber, canary, gold, etc. / **Green** – Jade, cyan, emerald / etc.; 2. The sound of blood surging through the blood vessels in the ear; 3. Russia.
	SOS	Rabbit and turtle.
	ICE	No bullying; Everything is free; Sugar treats only on Wednesdays; Daily royal naps; etc.
SET 343	**KISS**	1. Hypo; 2. Amphibians; 3. Mexicans; San Antonio, Texas.
	SOS	They all have bars.
	ICE	Autumn leaves; Chameleons; Faces; The sky; Rusting metal; Aging bodies; etc.
SET 344	**KISS**	1. Tchaikovsky; 2. Mercury and Venus; 3. Rupees.
	SOS	Mean – Bean – Bead – Bend – Bind – Kind.
	ICE	A Jell-O Giraffe; A worm with allergies; etc.

SET 345	**KISS**	1. Cleopatra, Julius Caesar, Mark Antony, Richard III, Henry IV, etc.; 2. =12; 3. The Stamp Act of 1765, which was so unpopular with the colonists it "sowed the seeds of the American Revolution".
	SOS	Every year there is a Christmas and a New Year.
	ICE	Put your face in ice water; Swallowing a series of sips without interruption, then hyperventilate for a few moments; Just keep the hiccups!; etc.
SET 346	**KISS**	1. Three (k, g, and h); 2. =3/4; 3. Culture.
	SOS	1881.
	ICE	Bring, ringing, ringworm, sharing, swearing, etc.
SET 347	**KISS**	1. *Carousel, Flower Drum Song, King and I. Oklahoma, Sound of Music, South Pacific,* etc.; 2. Dry ice; 3. Israel.
	SOS	1) Chef; 2) Juice factory; 3) Lumberjack; 4) Musician.
	ICE	"How are the authors doing with the activities in this book?"; etc.
SET 348	**KISS**	1. Meeting; 2. 14,700; 3. Amerigo Vespucci, an Italian explorer who played a prominent role in exploring the New World; when sailing near the tip of South America in 1501, he became the first person to realize that North and South America are distinct continents.
	SOS	1) Fishing; 2) Barista; 3) Geologist; 4) Firefighter.
	ICE	Wait until the crowd leaves; Phone their service to locate it using GPS system; Keep looking; Ask the police to find a car matching that description and license plate number in the parking lot; etc.
SET 349	**KISS**	1. Franz; 2. Sternum; 3. Example, Australia, Canada, New Zealand, Singapore, U.S.A.
	SOS	244.
	ICE	Letters, gifts, children, colds, boomerang, the cat that came back; etc.
SET 350	**KISS**	1. Pointed arches, Flying buttresses, Rib vaults, Vaulted ceilings, Rose windows, Towers, Spires and pinnacles, Ornate Style with lots of gargoyles, etc.; 2. False; they swallow it; 3. "All men are created equal".
	SOS	1. Benedict Arnold; 2. August Renoir; 3. Mary Tyler Moore; 4. The Three Stooges.
	ICE	It's a fake to get sympathy; Got caught in barbed wire; Ran through thorny bushes; Brushed against a cactus; Teased the cat; etc.
SET 351	**KISS**	1. Sub; 2. One; 180/180=1; 3. Indentured servants.
	SOS	1. Sleeping Beauty; 2. Yellow Rose of Texas; 3. Les Misérables.
	ICE	Quagmire Leap; Silvertones; Friendly Persuasion; etc.
SET 352	**KISS**	1. Prologue; 2. The kidneys; 3. Great Britain.
	SOS	Sel makes the words "seldom", "select", "seller', and "selves".
	ICE	Toilet paper, aluminum foil, carpet, wheels, dice, etc.

SET 353	KISS	1. Cornet/trumpet; 2. True; 3. A tepee.
	SOS	Block one = 1, 2, 3, 4, 5, and 6; block two =7, 8, 9, 0, 1, and 2.
	ICE	A black outfit with porcupine quills sticking out; Fire on the back and flowers on the front; A slithering snake costume; etc.
SET 354	KISS	1. Hay fever; 2. The islands were formed by volcanoes rising from the bottom of the ocean; 3. A common currency used by a number of European nations that are part of the European Union.
	SOS	Cysts, gypsy, hymns, lymph, lynch, myrrh, myths, nymph, pygmy, rhythm, synch, syncs.
	ICE	Wreath; Bubble; Lost friend; etc.
SET 355	KISS	1. Beethoven; 2. 13 nickels and 7 dimes, 1 nickel and 13 dimes, 25 nickels and 1 dime, etc.; 3. Sandra Day O'Connor.
	SOS	Pep-C = Pepsi.
	ICE	Friends; Chocolate; Love; Endorphins; Success; Humor; etc.
SET 356	KISS	1. A type of verse that usually tells a story and is often put to music and sung; 2. Intensive Care Unit; 3. Arlington National Cemetery.
	SOS	Daisy – Cocker Spaniel; Lucy – German Shepherd; Belle – Miniature Poodle; Rex – St. Bernard.
	ICE	One ornery osprey opened oily orange octagons of oozing offal over outraged ostriches; etc.
SET 357	KISS	1. Bark, bite; 2. White with black stripes; 3. Beijing, China.
	SOS	White, blue, brown, green.
	ICE	Scare them; Push them; Don't put on deodorant; Stare at them; Beg them never to leave you; etc.
SET 358	KISS	1. *Hamlet*; 2. 5200 weeks; 3. Smithsonian Institution.
	SOS	$63.25 – 6 tens, 3 ones, and one quarter.
	ICE	Grapes; People; Flies; Bananas; Trouble; etc.
SET 359	KISS	1. Ballet, Rumba, Modern, Square dance, Cha-cha, Foxtrot, Country line dancing, etc.; 2. The eyes; 3. Iran.
	SOS	They all can be flipped.
	ICE	Work; Think; Play; Stumble; Dazzle; etc.
SET 360	KISS	1. B; R; T; 2. Anywhere in the Southern hemisphere; 3. U.S. Capitol Building.
	SOS	Facetious for one.
	ICE	Shake it up and replace the soft white cloudy thing with bright yellows and oranges or mellow blues and mauves; Polka-dots; Black Tie; etc.

SET 361	KISS	1. The quote "Et tu, Brute?" means "Even you, Brutus?"; 2. 10,080; 3. Republic.
	SOS	Billy the outfielder got four hits. Luis the catcher got one hit. Isabel the shortstop got 5 hits. Mimi the pitcher got two hits. Scott the first baseman got three hits.
	ICE	Giraffes; Yellow polka-dot bikini; Person with measles; Teens with acne; etc.
SET 362	KISS	1. Complementary colors; 2. Oyster; 3. 10 provinces & 3 territories.
	SOS	1. France Dance; 2) Perky Turkey; 3) Damp ramp.
	ICE	Balls; Fish; Colds; Plates falling from the cupboard; etc.
SET 363	KISS	1. I can; 2. Copper; 3. French.
	SOS	The baton of the conductor.
	ICE	Brainstorm; Brain Exercise; Turn on your brain; Brain cells; And of course, "Brain Changers 365"; etc.
SET 364	KISS	1. Mozart; 2. =85; 3. The National Archives in Washington, DC.
	SOS	Butter.
	ICE	The Falling Soufflé Shoppe; Pincher's Shoe Store; Slippery Slope Consulting; etc.
SET 365	KISS	1. Edgar Degas, Mary Cassatt, Paul Cézanne, Claude Monet, etc.; 2. Black, blue, red, white and yellow; they were chosen because at least one of these colors appears on every nation's flag; 3. Paris.
	SOS	1. Flower shower; 2. President's residence 3. Loud cloud; 4) Turtle hurdle.
	ICE	We said we were tired.

About the Authors

Lorene "Renie" Lenning

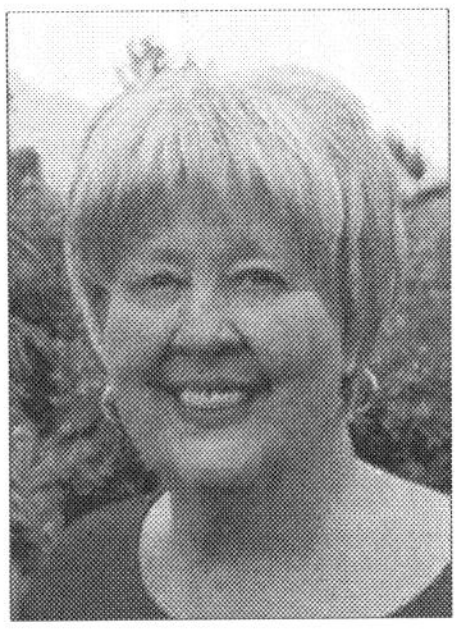

Renie, a retired master teacher of 40 years, has taught in both public and private school settings in Iowa, Colorado, Minnesota, New York, and Oklahoma (also one semester in London, England). In addition, she has taught at the college level at both public and private institutions in New York and Iowa. She has a Masters degree in education and has developed and presented well-received workshops for teachers throughout up-state New York, Iowa, and in Japan. For the last eight years of her career, Renie earned the title of "The Brain Teacher." During that time she worked primarily with gifted and talented students as well as conducting weekly "brain training" visitations to regular classrooms based on the latest brain research. Since her retirement, Renie has developed and taught a weekly "Brain Boosters" class for people in her large (1,700 households) Arizona retirement community. The encouragement of participants in the class asking her to make the activities more widely available was the stimulus for developing *Brain Changers 365*. Mrs. Lenning has authored a previous book, for teachers, titled *More Than Money: An Activities Approach to Economics* (Scott Foresman).

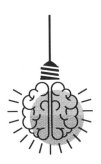

Oscar Lenning

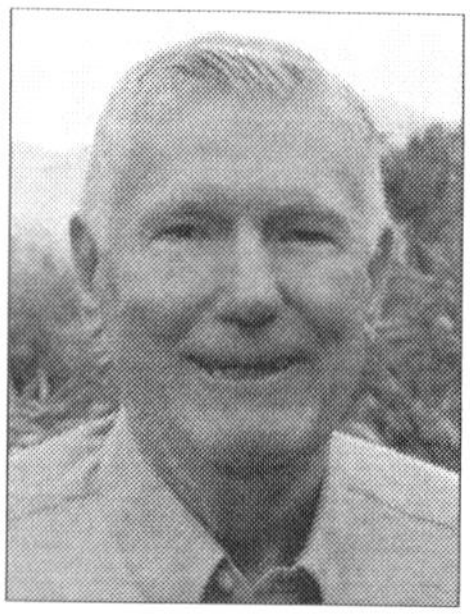

After service as a U. S. Navy Submariner, high school and junior high teacher, and counselor, Oscar became nationally recognized as an educational researcher/scholar and one of the pioneers in the identification and assessment of college and university educational outcomes. He has a Ph.D. in counseling psychology. He thoroughly researched the content of this book to insure that everything throughout was supported by relevant, valid and reliable research findings. After 15 years of research, writing and consulting at the American College Testing Program and at the National Center for Higher Education Management Systems and 20 years as academic VP and dean at colleges in New York, Iowa and Oklahoma, he spent eight years leading development of innovative new programs at three different colleges and universities. Author of 150+ professional publications, including 29 published books/monographs. His 2013 book *Powerful Learning Communities* (Stylus) has relevance for using this current book effectively in group settings. He participates in Renie's "Brain Boosters" class each week.

Alisha Solan

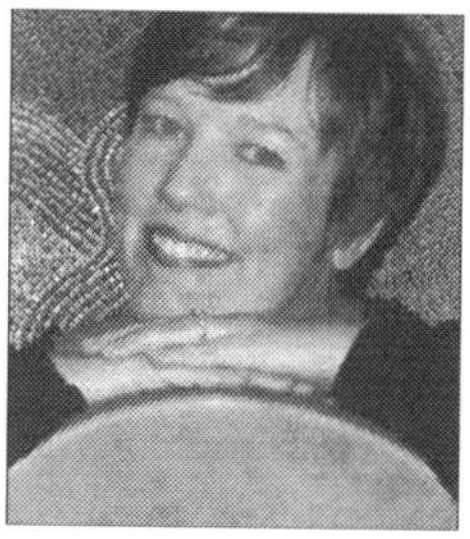

Alisha holds a PhD from the University of Texas at Austin and is currently a Communication professor in San Diego. She brings a strong background in mind-body wellness. Her doctoral dissertation, *Health in Motion* deals with movement and meditation pertaining to good health. She trained as a Nia instructor, leading workshops and holistic group fitness classes. Alisha is co-author of *Powerful Learning Communities*. She also has a chapter in *Ritual and Healing*, which was honored at the Twentieth Annual San Diego Book and Writing Awards in June of 2014.

90285238R00186

Made in the USA
San Bernardino, CA
08 October 2018